# Emergency Transport of the Perinatal Patient

Edited by
**Mhairi G. MacDonald,
M.B.Ch.B., F.R.C.P.(E),
D.C.H.**
*Professor of Child Health and Development,
George Washington University School of
Medicine and Health Sciences;
Vice Chairman for Research and
Postgraduate Education,
Department of Neonatology,
Children's Hospital National Medical
Center, Washington, D.C.*

*Associate Editor*
**Marilea K. Miller, M.D.**
*Associate Professor of Child Health
and Development, George Washington
University School of Medicine
and Health Sciences;
Associate Neonatologist,
Children's Hospital National Medical
Center, Washington, D.C.;
Director of the Nurseries, Holy Cross
Hospital, Silver Spring, Maryland*

Foreword by
James W. Farquhar, M.D., F.R.C.P.(E)
*Professor of Child Life and Health,
University of Edinburgh, Scotland*

Little, Brown and Company
Boston/Toronto

Copyright © 1989 by Mhairi Graham MacDonald and Marilea K. Miller

First Edition

All rights reserved. No part of this book may be reproduced in any form or by any electronic or mechanical means, including information storage and retrieval systems, without permission in writing from the publisher, except by a reviewer who may quote brief passages in a review.

Library of Congress Catalog Card No. 88-82726

ISBN 0-316-54198-2

Printed in the United States of America

EB

The Perinatal Center of
Sarasota Memorial Hospital
917-6259

*Emergency*
*Transport of*
*the Perinatal*
*Patient*

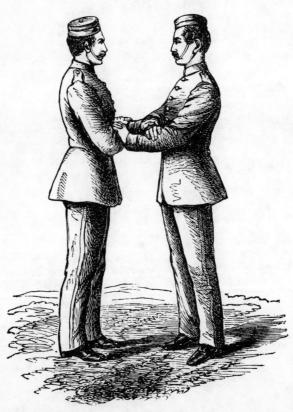

*Position of bearers when forming the four-handed seat with uncrossed arms. (Reproduced from Otis, G. A. A Report to the Surgeon General on the Transport of Sick and Wounded by Pack Animals. War Department, Surgeon General's Office, Circular No. 9, March 1, 1877. Washington, D.C.: Government Printing Office, 1877.)*

***Dedication***

*To Alfred A. Wild, M.B.Ch.B., D.M.R.D., F.R.C.R., without whom this book could never have been conceived, and to the memory of Elspeth Stuart Barnes, M.Sc., A.L.A.A.*

### Special Dedication

*The drive to compile a technical treatise is not exclusively practical. In the case of the editor (M. G. M.) I have suspicion of natal inspiration! As assistant accoucheur and navigator during her first (albeit involuntary) one-way ground transport, it was my untutored task to delay her entry into the world until there was an address to be born at better than the tattered Royal Navy ambulance.*

*On arrival at the nursing home, the ambulance driver/obstetrician was to become god-father as soon as the assistant accoucheur removed his fist from the emerging head. Twenty-seven years later the survivor of this successful naval operation was often seen descending noisily onto a helipad in Baltimore, Maryland, complete with neonate and medical kit.*

*This dedication remembers with gratitude the skill and kindness of Matthew Urie, M.B.Ch.B., of British Columbia, Canada, former Surgeon-Commander, Royal Navy; Monica Evans, R.N., of Swansea, England; and Grace Sutherland, R.N., of Edinburgh, Scotland; all of whom embody the innovativeness, caring, empathy, and drive to provide optimal care to the patient under all circumstances that is the foundation of a successful patient transport system.*

Donald F. MacDonald

# Contents

# *Foreword*

Until recently the fetus was thought to be at best a passenger, at worst a parasite, drowsing in the tropical wet heat of the womb at the receiving end of a simple filter providing, in Professor McCance's words, the essential services of supply and sewage. It seems we have done him an injustice because weightless in his sterile command module, he can monitor a flow of complex signals and make some effective contribution to Mission Control and possibly to his own splashdown.*

The safe launch of the fetus is related to maternal discipline and staff planning. Success on the mission depends on the well-being of craft and crewman as well as on the vigilance of the controlling team. The moment and mode for reentry are critical and the task force must be optimally deployed: ready to react instantly to unpredicted events. The high cost of such a program is justified by success.

Complicated pregnancy may lead to death or, and this outcome may be worse, to a lifetime of severe handicap as well as to parental sorrow and hardship. The community's perinatal mortality responds first to better social and health services, and these depend on economic and political factors. Within such provision, however, advances in reproductive and developmental sciences make possible the best clinical personnel and the improving technology needed to achieve the same order of safety for the uteronaut as can be offered more specifically to voyagers in space.

With advancing technology inevitably comes rising cost. Regionalized care has developed out of the need to contain medical costs and the realization that the pace at which medical knowledge and technical sophistication are developing mandates subspecialization and the concentration of costly equipment in large hospital centers. Regionalized care has led to an increasing need to move high-risk patients between hospitals.

*J. W. Farquhar, Amniotic, urinary and serum hormones in fetal diagnosis. *Can. Med. Assoc. J.* 105:174–176, 1971.

   The editors of *Emergency Transport of the Perinatal Patient* and their talented team offer both the science and the art that can convert a dangerous expedition, which temporarily removes the patient from a controlled therapeutic environment into a safe and sophisticated mobile extension of the perinatal care system.

James W. Farquhar, M.D., F.R.C.P.(E)

# *Preface*

Emergency patient transport has been euphemistically referred to as "swoop and scoop." The sirens and flashing lights may increase the rate of travel and the rate of road accidents; they do not necessarily improve the clinical outcome. Fundamental to an understanding of the need for *Emergency Transport of the Perinatal Patient* is the recognition that the "swoop and scoop" concept of patient transport is not appropriate for the high-risk obstetric or neonatal patient. These patients need to be stabilized as much as possible prior to transport from the referring hospital. Neither the 800-gram fetus delivered in an ambulance while en route to a tertiary level center nor the infant who embarks on an interstate transport in an unpressurized aircraft with an undiagnosed or inadequately treated pneumothorax can, in reality, be said to have benefitted from the availability of a perinatal transport system.

The perinatal transport program cannot exist as a free-standing entity but must be conceptualized and operationally function as an extension of the intensive care unit. The staff and equipment used must be capable of providing highly sophisticated medical care prior to and during transport. However, no matter how efficient the transport system, the patient cannot be optimally cared for unless the personnel at the referring hospital are able to provide adequate patient stabilization prior to the arrival of the transport team. In the case of the neonate, suboptimal care in the first few minutes or hours of life frequently can adversely alter the prognosis, regardless of subsequent therapeutic interventions. A continuum of efficient, effective, cooperative, and educational interaction must thus be achieved between referring and receiving institutions.

History is a silent teacher. Observation and review are the tools of progress. As noted in the first chapter, the field of patient transport owes much to the military experience. In 1869 General Longmore wrote, "The best method of transporting sick and wounded soldiers from one place to another in time of war is one of the most important questions to be studied, as it is one of the most difficult problems to be solved, among the subjects which concern the medical service of armies." One hundred and twenty years later, we recognize that there is no single best method for transporting high-risk mothers and infants. The vehicle and the method must reflect an appreciation of local politics, laws, and geography, as well as the actual distance between facilities and the types of patients to be transported.

Transport of the perinatal patient is an economically costly venture, and in the United States it is not always reimbursed by third-party payers. Thus, the hospital-based medical care coordinators and their administrators must demonstrate a significant degree of individual innovation in locating funds for these programs. These fiscal matters are addressed in Chapter 3, and marketing strategies are discussed in Chapter 5. However, as emphasized in Chapter 13, medical transport should never be misused as a public relations tool. The safety of aeromedical services in the United States, particularly those using helicopters, has come under scrutiny in the past few years because of the unacceptably high accident rates. Unless safety standards are established and enforced, it is probable that insurance carriers will become increasingly reluctant to provide coverage. In the past two years written standards have been developed by both the American Society of Hospital Based Emergency Aeromedical Services (ASHBEAMS) and the National E.M.S. Pilots Association (NEMSPA), but an adequate monitoring system has yet to be devised.

It is well recognized that perinatal patients can be transported with great expertise and favorable outcome by specifically trained nonphysician staff. Perhaps not quite as widely recognized are the responsibilities of the less central members of the transport team, as outlined in Chapter 8, in ensuring that the standards set for patient care and safety during transport are as stringent as those that are adhered to within the referring and receiving hospitals.

The authors have approached their subjects in varying ways, and no attempt has been made to enforce a completely uniform format. There is overlap of subject material between some chapters, but the somewhat different viewpoints presented and the desire to spare the reader from searching for multiple cross-references have persuaded us to permit these minor repetitions.

We hope that we have provided some insights into the basic philosophies underlying optimal medical transport of the perinatal patient as well as a body of knowledge that can be used as a foundation for future evolution and innovation.

M. G. M.
M. K. M.

# Acknowledgments

We acknowledge the invaluable assistance of many individuals in the preparation of this book: for secretarial support, Susan Bender and Nettie Wanda Richardson; for photographic contributions, Richard Reed and David Wooddell; for transport team insights, Arthur Engler, R.N., M.S.N., C.P.N.P., N.N.P., Kathleen Collins, R.N., N.N.P., Sandra Ward, R.N., N.N.P., Barbara Anderson, R.N., N.N.P., and Judith Cannon, R.N.C., N.N.P. We particularly appreciate the aid of Robert Joy, M.D., and Dale Smith, M.D., Division of Military Medicine, the Uniformed Services University of Health Sciences, Bethesda, Maryland who shared their valuable time, expertise, slides, and the university's historical books and manuscripts with us and taught us the intricacies of the library computer system.

Finally, we acknowledge the immense patience and support offered to us by our families—Harold, Rebecca, and James Ginzburg and Michael, Emily, and Sarah Gibson.

M. G. M.
M. K. M.

# Contributing Authors

**Albert L. Bartoletti, M.D.**
*Associate Professor of Pediatrics, Albany Medical College of Union University, Albany, New York*

**Susanne Bennett, L.C.S.W.**
*Psychotherapist, Northern Virginia Psychiatric Group, Fairfax*

**Jean C. Bolan, M.D.**
*Assistant Clinical Professor, Department of Obstetrics and Gynecology, Georgetown University School of Medicine, Washington, D.C.; Director, Division of Perinatology, Washington Hospital Center, Washington, D.C.*

**Carl L. Bose, M.D.**
*Associate Professor of Pediatrics, University of North Carolina School of Medicine; Medical Director, Pediatric Transport Service and Attending Neonatologist, North Carolina Memorial Hospital, Chapel Hill*

**Cheryl Y. Bowen, R.N., M.A.**
*Assistant Director, Maryland Regional Neonatal Program, Maryland Institute for Emergency Medical Services, Baltimore*

**Dennis C. Brimhall**
*Director, University Hospital, University of Colorado Health Sciences Center, Denver*

**Judith A. Cannon, R.N.C., N.N.P.**
*Neonatal Transport Coordinator, Children's Hospital National Medical Center, Washington, D.C.*

**Margaret M. Chou, M.D.**
*Assistant Professor, George Washington University School of Medicine and Health Sciences; Associate Neonatologist, Children's Hospital National Medical Center, Washington, D.C., and Holy Cross Hospital, Silver Spring, Maryland*

**Howard M. Collett**
*Editor and Publisher, Hospital Aviation, St. George, Utah*

**Alasdair K. T. Conn, M.D.**
*Assistant Professor, Department of Surgery, Harvard Medical School; Chief, Emergency Services, Massachusetts General Hospital, Boston*

**Larry G. Dennis, M.D.**
*Assistant Professor, Uniformed Services University of the Health Sciences F. Edward Hébert School of Medicine, Bethesda, Maryland; Chief, Maternal-Fetal Medicine Division, David Grant Medical Center, Travis Air Force Base, Fairfield, California*

**Wendy L. Dorchester, M.P.H.**
*Biostatistician, Memorial Medical Center of Long Beach, Long Beach, California*

**Tom Einhorn**
*Deputy Director, National E.M.S. Pilots Association, Pearland, Texas*

**Anne B. Fletcher, M.D.**
*Professor of Child Health and Development, George Washington University School of Medicine and Health Sciences; Attending Neonatologist and Director, Newborn Intensive Care Unit, Children's Hospital National Medical Center, Washington, D.C.*

**Harold M. Ginzburg, M.D., J.D., M.P.H.**
*Clinical Professor, Department of Psychiatry, Department of Preventive Medicine and Biometrics, Uniformed Services University of the Health Sciences F. Edward Hébert School of Medicine, Bethesda, Maryland; Senior Medical Consultant, Bureau of Health Care Delivery and Assistance, Health Resources and Services Administration, Rockville, Maryland*

**Elisabeth K. Herz, M.D.**
*Associate Professor of Obstetrics and Gynecology and Psychiatry, George Washington University School of Medicine and Health Sciences; Director, Psychosomatic Program, Department of Obstetrics and Gynecology, George Washington University Medical Center, Washington, D.C.*

**Robert P. Howard, M.S.**
*Director, Biomedical Engineering, Children's Hospital National Medical Center, Washington, D.C.*

**Neil K. Kochenour, M.D.**
*Associate Professor, Department of Obstetrics and Gynecology, University of Utah School of Medicine; Chief, Division of Maternal-Fetal Medicine, University of Utah Medical Center, Salt Lake City*

**Mhairi G. MacDonald, M.B.Ch.B., F.R.C.P.(E), D.C.H.**
*Professor of Child Health and Development, George Washington University School of Medicine and Health Sciences; Vice Chairman for Research and Postgraduate Education, Department of Neonatology, Children's Hospital National Medical Center, Washington, D.C.*

**Robert A. Margulies, M.D., M.P.H.**
*Associate Clinical Professor of Preventive Medicine, University of South Carolina School of Medicine, Columbia; Staff, Emergency Medical Services, Naval Hospital, Cherry Point, North Carolina*

## Gerald B. Merenstein, M.D.
*Professor of Pediatrics, University of Colorado Health Sciences Center School of Medicine; Director, Newborn Services, University Hospital, Denver*

## Marilea K. Miller, M.D.
*Associate Professor of Child Health and Development, George Washington University School of Medicine and Health Sciences; Associate Neonatologist, Children's Hospital National Medical Center, Washington, D.C.; Director of the Nurseries, Holy Cross Hospital, Silver Spring, Maryland*

## Houchang D. Modanlou, M.D.
*Associate Professor of Pediatrics, University of California, Irvine; Director, Neonatal-Perinatal Medicine, Miller Children's Hospital Memorial Medical Center, Long Beach, California*

## Nancy M. Nagel, A.C.S.W., L.C.S.W.
*Psychiatric Social Worker, Northern Virginia Psychiatric Group, Fairfax*

## John J. Paris, S.J., Ph.D.
*Professor of Ethics, Holy Cross College, Worcester; Clinical Professor of Community Health, Tufts University School of Medicine, Boston*

## Patricia A. Payne, C.N.M., M.P.H.
*Nurse-Midwife, Durham Women's Clinic; Durham County General Hospital, Durham, North Carolina*

## Gary Pettett, M.D.
*Associate Professor of Pediatrics, Uniformed Services University of the Health Sciences F. Edward Hébert School of Medicine, Bethesda, Maryland; Attending Neonatologist and Director of Fellowship Training, Walter Reed Army Medical Center, Washington, D.C.*

## Nancy E. Rehm, C.N.M., M.S.N.
*Director, Perinatal Department, Utah Valley Regional Medical Center, Provo*

## Herman M. Risemberg, M.D.
*Professor of Pediatrics, Albany Medical College of Union University; Director, Division of Neonatal/Perinatal Medicine, Albany Medical Center Hospital, Albany, New York*

## Oswaldo Rivera
*Assistant Director, Biomedical Engineering, Children's Hospital National Medical Center, Washington, D.C.*

## Don Wright
*Executive Director, National E.M.S. Pilots Association, Pearland, Texas*

**Notice:** The indications and dosages of all drugs in this book have been recommended in the medical literature and conform to the practices of the general medical community. The medications described do not necessarily have specific approval by the Food and Drug Administration for use in the diseases and dosages for which they are recommended. The package insert for each drug should be consulted for use and dosage as approved by the FDA. Because standards for usage change, it is advisable to keep abreast of revised recommendations, particularly those concerning new drugs.

# I

# The History of Patient Transport

# 1 Landmarks in the Development of Patient Transport Systems

Margaret M. Chou
Mhairi G. MacDonald

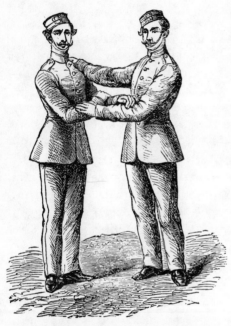

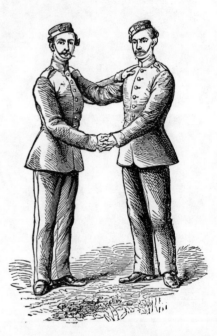

*1A. The bearers with the three-handed seat and back support formed. (Reproduced from Longmore, T. A Treatise on the Transport of Sick and Wounded Troops. London: Her Majesty's Stationery Office, 1869.)*

*1B. Two-handed support by two bearers for carrying a patient in a semirecumbent position. (Reproduced from Longmore, T. A Treatise on the Transport of Sick and Wounded Troops. London: Her Majesty's Stationery Office, 1869.)*

A 45-year-old man collapses, complaining of chest pain. Within minutes he is attended by an emergency medical technician (EMT), given oxygen, and placed on a monitor. He is taken by ambulance to a nearby hospital where he is treated for a myocardial infarction.

A newborn infant, with a large abdominal wall defect, is delivered in a rural hospital 60 miles from the city. Two hours later the infant is flown by helicopter to the metropolitan children's hospital, where he receives emergency surgery to correct his gastroschisis.

In a large metropolitan hospital doctors are unable to oxygenate a 3-day-old infant on maximal ventilatory support. Following consultation, the infant is transferred by jet to a center with facilities for extracorporeal membrane oxygenation (ECMO). A ground ambulance meets the transport team and infant at the airport to complete the transport to the ECMO center.

The examples used above are based on experience in the United States but are illustrative of the level of sophistication of modern patient transport services in many countries in the developed world. Methods for moving the sick and wounded can be traced back to biblical times when the primary methods of transportation were on the shoulders or back of humans or beasts. The inventions of the wheel, cart, automobile, and airplane, and the desire to treat and evacuate the wounded in war, led to the establishment of special organizations (Red Cross) and vehicles (ambulances) designed specifically for the treatment and transportation of the sick and injured. We are indebted to such pioneers as Dominique-Jean Larrey, Jonathan Letterman, Clara Barton, General Thomas Longmore, Captain George Gosman, Lieutenant Albert Rhodes, Martin Couney, Joseph DeLee, and Sydney Segal for their contributions to the history of patient transport. In this chapter we will outline their roles and those of other key individuals in the development of modern-day patient transport systems.

### The Development of Ground Transport*

Before the invention of the wheel (pre-3000 B.C.), the sick and wounded were presumably carried on the shoulders or backs of friends or animals. A hammock suspended between two poles afforded a little more comfort to both patient and porter.

In Western culture, one of the earliest uses of the wheel for patient transport was the Anglo-Saxon wagon hammock (circa 900 A.D.): a hammock suspended between two poles mounted on a four-wheeled platform (Fig. 1-1). The Norman horse litter (circa 1100 A.D.) was an improvement over the Anglo-Saxon wagon hammock, in that a bed was substituted for the

*Sources for this material are listed in the Bibliography.

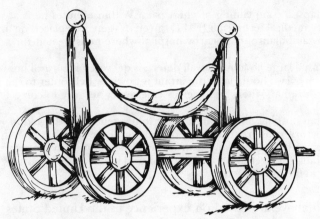

*Fig. 1-1. Anglo-Saxon wagon hammock, circa 900 A.D.
(Drawn by J. Guenther.)*

hammock and the wagon was harnessed to two horses. The patient traded swinging for bouncing.

War casualties were probably the primary stimuli for development of ambulance systems. The English word *ambulance* was derived from the French *l'ambulance,* referring to a military "field hospital" (a mobile unit with associated transport vehicles) that transported, received and treated casualties. This concept may have originated from Ferdinand and Isabella of Spain. During their 1487 campaign against the Moors, they took an unprecedented interest in the welfare of their troops, establishing "ambulances," which were special tents for the wounded.

In the 1790s the French surgeon Dominique-Jean Larrey, appalled at the predicament of the wounded (who were left on the battlefield until they could be moved to the field hospitals at the rear of the army), developed the *ambulance volante* (the flying ambulance). This was a lightweight, two-wheeled, horse-drawn wagon that stayed on the battlefield. The wounded were treated on the battlefield and then transported by the ambulance volante to hospitals. Larrey's ambulance volante was endorsed by Napoleon Bonaparte, who appointed Larrey to direct the ambulance service during his Italian campaign (1797).

It was not until the mid-1800s, however, that the U.S. Army adopted the concept of an organized ambulance service for war casualties. (There was no ambulance system during the War of 1812.) Prior to this, the army improvised using variously designed litters, travais, and cacolets (Fig. 1-2) carried or drawn by animals or men. In their battles against the American Indians, the army frontiersmen recognized that wheeled ambulances were unsuitable for the rough wilderness terrain. Resources were limited: The

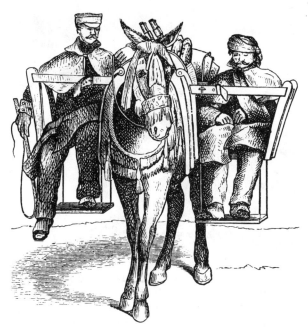

*Fig. 1-2A. British Crimean cacolet ("chair litter") (after Weir). (Reproduced from Otis, G. A.* A Report to the Surgeon General on the Transport of Sick and Wounded by Pack Animals. *War Department, Surgeon General's Office, Circular No. 9, March 1, 1877. Washington, D.C.: Government Printing Office, 1877.)*

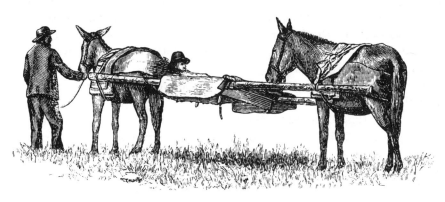

*B. Wounded soldier conveyed on a double mule litter. "The litter with two mules, long in use, I believe to be inferior to the travail. When animals move at an uneven pace, the result is disasterous to the harness and to the patient"—Assistant Surgeon Munn. (Reproduced from Otis, G. A.* A Report to the Surgeon General on the Transport of Sick and Wounded by Pack Animals. *War Department, Surgeon General's Office, Circular No. 9, March 1, 1877. Washington, D.C.: Government Printing Office, 1877.)*

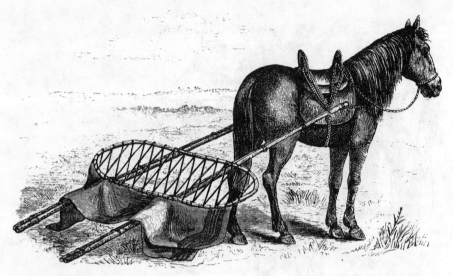

Fig. 1-3. Dakota Indian litter or travais (from a drawing by Dr. J. W. Williams, USA).
(Reproduced from Otis, G. A. A Report to the Surgeon General on the Transport of
Sick and Wounded by Pack Animals. War Department, Surgeon General's Office, Cir-
cular No. 9, March 1, 1877. Washington, D.C.: Government Printing Office, 1877.)

wounded were transported on hastily constructed litters using wooden
poles and canvas or rawhide. The patient could be carried between two
men or two animals. From the American Indians, army personnel learned
how to form a travail by harnessing one end of a litter to an animal (Fig.
1-3). This mode of transportation, requiring only one animal per patient,
was efficient but quite uncomfortable, particularly if the patient had broken
bones. During the Seminole War (1835–1838) the medical director of the
troops of the U.S. Army, Dr. Richard S. Satterlee, organized systematic
transport of the wounded using horse-carried litters. His plan for a uniformly organized system to transport the wounded was, however, rejected
until the Civil War.

It was Jonathan Letterman, medical director of the U.S. Army of the Potomac (1862–1864), who was responsible for the reorganization of the field
medical services during the Civil War. He is credited with developing an
effective plan for the evacuation and treatment of battle casualties. In 1864
the U.S. Congress enacted a law establishing a uniform ambulance service
for all the armies of the United States. The law was based on Letterman's
plan, which included designation and separation of ambulance vehicles, personnel, and equipment from other army transport divisions. The "Rucker
wagon" was designated the official ambulance of the U.S. Army during
the Civil War (Fig. 1-4). After some modifications by a Parisian physician

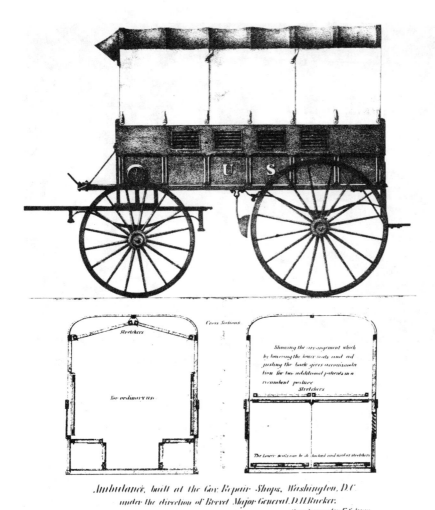

Ambulance, built at the Gov. Repair Shops, Washington, D.C.
under the direction of Brevet Major General D.H.Rucker,
Quartermaster C.S.Army

*Fig. 1-4. The Rucker wagon. (Reproduced from* Reports on the Extent and Nature of the Materials Available for the Preparation of a Medical and Surgical History of the Rebellion. *War Department, Surgeon General's Office, Circular No. 6, November 1, 1865. Philadelphia: J. B. Lippincott, 1866.)*

(springs in the floor, improved ventilation, and seats for attendants), the Rucker wagon was awarded the prize for best ambulance wagon at the 1867 Paris Exposition. Other types of ambulance vehicles used in the Civil War included trains (probably first used for patient transport in Europe in the late 1850s) and steamboats. (Figs. 1-5 and 1-6).

While the Civil War was waged in the United States, a major organization to benefit the wounded was created in Europe. In 1864 The International

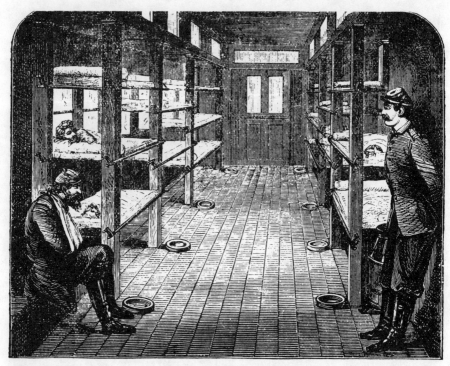

Fig. 1-5. Transport of wounded soldiers by train during the American Civil War. Perspective view of half of the interior of an American hospital car conveying wounded soldiers. (Reproduced from Longmore, C. B. A Treatise on the Transport of Sick and Wounded Troops. London: Her Majesty's Stationery Office, 1869.)

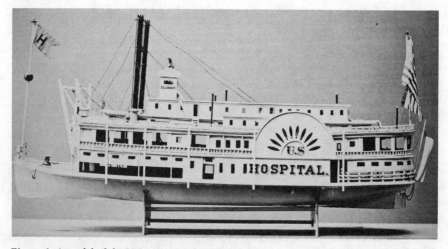

Fig. 1-6. A model of the U.S. Army Hospital Steamer D. A. January. This ship transported hundreds of wounded during the Civil War.

Red Cross Treaty Convention of Geneva (the Geneva convention) was signed by the leaders of France, Switzerland, and a number of other countries, excluding the United States. The purpose of the treaty was to facilitate the creation of permanent societies that were dedicated to providing relief and protection to wounded soldiers. All medical personnel, supplies, vehicles, and sick and wounded were to be recognized as neutral in times of war. A red cross on a white background was adopted as the protective sign that identified the neutrality of those servicing the sick and wounded. The sign (which is the reverse of the Swiss flag) was chosen to compliment the Swiss Henri Dunant, for his support of the treaty. The Geneva convention promoted the concept that there is a need for orderly rescue of wounded from the battlefield.

The Red Cross Society of Britain was formed by members of the Order of St. John represented by John Furley, who had attended the Geneva convention. He, Thomas Longmore, and Colonel Lloyd Lindsey founded the British National Society for Aid to Sick and Wounded in 1870. In 1877 the Order of St. John adopted a proposal made by John Furley to form a volunteer organization for the relief of sick and wounded soldiers in war: the St. John Ambulance Association. The association coined and was the first to use the term *first aid*. It published a manual with a "few plain rules which may enable anyone to act in case of injury or sudden illness, pending the arrival of professional help" [6]. Ten years later the St. John Ambulance Brigade was formed to transport civilian patients.

Although the United States was not among the original signatories of the Geneva convention, a parallel organization called the United States Sanitary Commission (USSC) was already operating under the principles proposed in the Geneva convention. The USSC was under the direction of Dr. Henry Bellows of New York. Following the Civil War, the efforts of Clara Barton resulted in U.S. ratification of the Geneva convention in 1882. The American Red Cross first participated in wartime relief during the Spanish-American War (1898).

The Red Cross in the United States was the first to provide rescue and relief to civilians during peacetime. The number of hospital-based ambulance services in the United States increased concurrently. In 1865 the Cincinnati Commercial Hospital (now Cincinnati General Hospital) introduced the first hospital-run ambulance service, followed a short time later by the New York Bellevue Hospital ambulance service, which transported injured civilians to the hospital after a riot in Elm Park (1869). Most ambulances at this time were horse-drawn, four-wheeled vehicles. Each vehicle was supplied with a first-aid box containing tourniquets, bandages, splints, sponges, and brandy. The ambulances were also equipped with a stretcher, handcuffs, and a straitjacket for transport of the insane. By 1878 the New York City ambulance service was separated into three zones, administered by Bellevue Hospital, New York Hospital, and Roosevelt Hospital, respectively.

The invention of "self-propelled" vehicles at the close of the nineteenth century greatly expedited patient transportation. The first electric ambulance was used in 1899 at the Michael Reese Hospital in Chicago. It was able to reach a maximum speed of 16 miles per hour. A year later the St. Vincent Hospital in New York City acquired the second motor (electric) ambulance. In 1905 Major Palliser designed a bulletproof ambulance automobile for the Red Cross to use on battlefields. It was a three-wheeled van, run by gasoline. Unfortunately, fuel was not easily obtained on battlefields!

The concept of self-propelled ambulances was quickly adopted in Europe. The first British motor ambulance was known as the Straker-Squire van. The French then designed the Boulant mobile surgery vehicle (1912–1918), which was a fully equipped surgical unit on wheels that could travel up to 30 km per hour. These units contained an operating table, scrub sinks, and sterilizers, but their cost made them impractical. However, during World War I buses and taxis in France were modified to resemble the Boulant mobile. Most motor ambulances used by the United States during World War I were modified Model-T Fords (Fig. 1-7).

*Fig. 1-7. An early motor ambulance (1912), manufactured by the Hess and Eisenhardt Company, Rossmoyne (Cincinnati), Ohio. The trademark of "S&S" refers to the original owners of the company, Sayers and Scoville.*

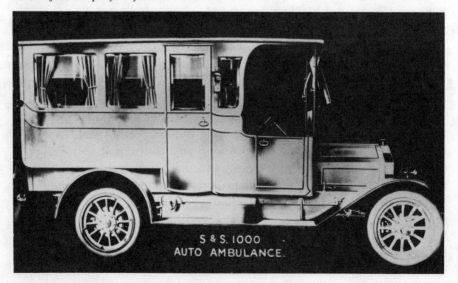

Ground transport improved significantly during World War II. Military ambulance companies were organized to transport casualties, medical personnel, and supplies to triage and treatment stations. The *United States Military Medical Manual* illustrated methods for carrying the wounded manually and on litters. The ambulance used by the United States was a converted Dodge truck called a "Half-tonner." Similar vehicles were used by Great Britain and Germany. The first air-conditioned ambulance in the United States was developed by the Hess and Eisenhardt Company in 1937, and the first ambulance service to carry oxygen as standard equipment was established in 1942.

## The Development of Air Transport*

The concept of air transport for patients dates back to the balloon lift demonstration by the Montgolfier brothers in 1784. Eighty-six years later (in 1870), during the Prussian seige of Paris, 160 Parisians were transported from Paris by balloon. Subsequently, some physicians theorized that patients could benefit from air transport. The invention of the airplane (1903) by the Wright brothers offered an alternative means for patient transport. However, it was almost two decades before the airplane was actually considered practical for this use.

In 1909, Captain George Gosman and Lieutenant Albert Rhodes of the U.S. Army constructed the first aircraft specifically for patient transport. The following year an engine was installed and the aircraft became airborne at Fort Barrancas, Florida. According to their design, the patient was to be carried lying down under one of the aircraft wings (Fig. 1-8). The physician, seated beside the patient, served as the pilot. Unfortunately, the first air ambulance met its demise when it crashed into a tree. The plane was never actually used for patient transport. Lacking funds to build a second aircraft, Gosman and Rhodes were forced to abandon further testing. Nevertheless, the idea that patients could be successfully transported by air was firmly implanted in the mind of Gosman. He approached the U.S. War Department with plans for a larger, more sophisticated plane. However, Gosman and staff from the Office of the Surgeon General, the Association of Military Surgeons, and the Committee on Transportation of the Wounded in War were unsuccessful in their efforts to convince the War Department that the concept of aircraft ambulances should be explored. The War Department, still dubious about the airplane, was unwilling to invest in such a novel and risky idea.

*Sources for this material are listed in the Bibliography.

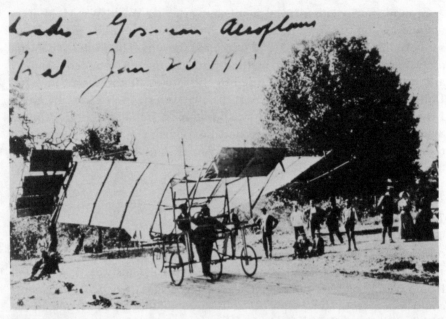

Fig. 1-8. The first ambulance airplane. Constructed by Captain George Gosman, M.C. and Lieutenant Albert Rhodes, C.A.C., officers of the U.S. Army Air Service, using their own funds. The aircraft was constructed and flown in 1910 from Fort Barrancas, Florida. Attaining an altitude of 100 ft, the plane flew 500 yd before crashing. Captain Gosman's efforts to obtain government funding for a second aircraft were fruitless. After one meeting with officials he said, "I clearly see that thousands of hours and ultimately thousands of patients would be saved through the use of airplanes in air evacuation."

The French, on the other hand, were not so reluctant to promote the air ambulance. Mademoiselle Marvingt, a French medical student and aviator, campaigned in the medical community for aeromedical evacuation. In 1912, under pressure from the French Women's Society, aviators, and military experts, the Ministry of War was persuaded to begin experiments in *l'aviation sanitaire*. No patients were actually transported by air, because no appropriate aircraft existed at the time. However, airplanes were used to locate the injured and provide medical supplies. The first actual aircraft evacuation of a patient took place in November 1915 during the retreat of the Serbian army from Albania. Because no other means were available the French were forced to use a French fighter aircraft to evacuate the wounded Serbian Lieutenant Stefanik approximately 80 km. Several months later a dozen wounded were rescued in the same manner.

The successful evacuation of these French soldiers prompted Dr. Chassaing, a French military surgeon, to lobby for money to develop a specific ambulance aircraft. After prolonged effort he was given an old combat plane to convert into an ambulance. His first trial run took place in 1917; Dr. Chassaing volunteered himself as the "patient" to be transported in the hollow fuselage of the plane. His trials were successful, and he was given six more aircraft to convert into air ambulances. One year later he was given 60 additional airplanes for conversion.

Although the War Department was reluctant to endorse the air ambulance, during World War I the U.S. military was subsequently forced to reconsider the use of aircraft for evacuation of the wounded. Fighter pilot practice sessions often took place in deserted and remote areas with poor ground access. Flight surgeons had to be flown to the injured to provide first aid, while awaiting a ground ambulance to transport the patient. By 1918, Captain William Ocker and Major Nelson Drive had convinced the base commander of the Gerstner Field in Los Angeles of the need for an air ambulance. They converted an old JN-4 airplane into the ambulance known as "Jenny" (Fig. 1-9) and successfully completed the first air transport of a patient in the United States. Subsequently, most airfields in the United States converted some aircraft into ambulance planes. There was, however, no standardization or uniformity of design, and the War Department and the surgeon general of the army were still unconvinced that air transport of the sick and wounded was either feasible or safe.

By the late 1920s Jennies had become obsolete and beyond repair. However, proponents of the air ambulance were persistent, and in 1929 the Cox-Kleemmin Aircraft Corporation was commissioned to design two experimental aircraft (XA-1) for patient transportation. These planes were equipped to carry two patients, their attendant, a pilot, and sufficient fuel for 6 hours of flying. Although they received national recognition after assisting in the evacuation of tornado victims in Rock Springs, Texas, economic constraints prevented construction of additional aircraft. Lack of funds also delayed repair of the two existing planes, and by 1930 both XA-1s had been destroyed in accidents and were not replaced.

By the end of World War I, the U.S. War Department had become even less enthusiastic about the development of ambulance aircraft. Medical personnel, however, continued to campaign for the air evacuation of patients. Major C. L. Beaven and Lieutenant Colonel T. E. Darby not only recommended airplanes for patient transport but also proposed use of the autogiro, the predecessor of the helicopter, because it could land and take off without extensive runways. The autogiro was first tested for patient evacuation by the U.S. Navy in Nicaragua. Unfortunately, initial trials were unsuccessful because of lack of power, poor design, and inadequate finances. Without the stimulus of war there was little further development of ambulance aircraft and, at the First International Technical Conference on

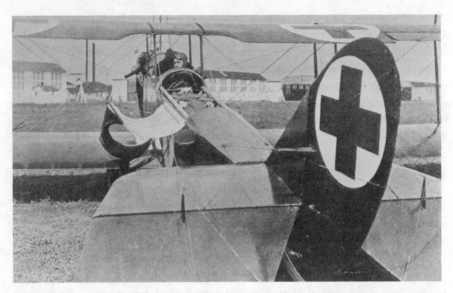

A

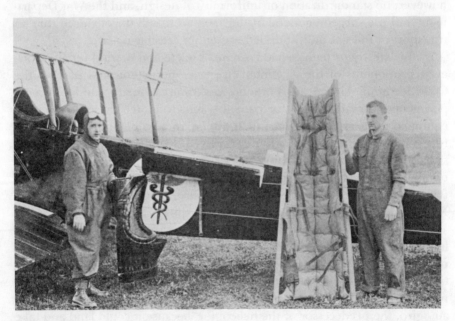

B

1-9A. Ambulance airplane (The "Jenny"), 1918. (Reproduced from Air Service Medical, Washington, D.C.: Government Printing Office, 1919.) B. Ambulance airplane (The "Jenny"), 1918, showing patient litter. (Reproduced from Air Service Medical. Washington, D.C.: Government Printing Office, 1919).

Aerial Relief in 1937 (Budapest), the majority of countries (with the exception of France, Italy, and the Soviet Union) did not have adequately designed aircraft for patient evacuation.

The United States entered World War II with no more advanced air-evacuation equipment than it had had at the beginning of World War I. The majority of those rescued by air were pilots injured during flight training. Converted obsolete aircraft were used. Requests for light planes for use as military air ambulances were rejected by the Department of the Army. Aircraft were, however, approved for use in the observation and control of artillery fire. Although no organized program existed, these planes were sporadically used for the evacuation of patients.

In 1943 British Major General Orde C. Wingate requested and received a squadron of aircraft for evacuation of his troops in Burma. In 1 month (1944) they successfully transported more than 700 wounded from the battlefield. By 1945 more than 19,000 troops, wounded in the Philippine campaign, had been evacuated by air. The large number of air evacuations in the Far East led to the recognition of several disadvantages of the airplane, most notably the need for adequate runways for takeoff and landing. Thus the U.S. Army showed a renewed interest in rotary-wing aircraft. They commissioned the designer of the first operational helicopter, Igor Sikorsky, to produce several helicopters for general military use. This led to the design and production of a helicopter (YR-4) that would transport several patients on litters. In 1943 the first litter-bearing helicopters were tested in Alaska.

The first patient evacuation by helicopter took place in April 1944 in the jungles of Burma. U.S. Technical Sargeant Ed Hladoveaka (Murphy) and three wounded British soldiers were rescued from the Japanese in Burma by U.S. 2nd Lieutenant Carter Harmon of Project 9 and his YR-4 helicopter. No airplane could negotiate and land in the mountainous jungles of Burma, and hiking through jungles full of Japanese soldiers would probably prove unsuccessful. The helicopter rescue took 2 days, four trips, and was complicated by an overheated engine.

During World War II the effectiveness of patient evacuation was further demonstrated in China and the Philippines. Over 100 wounded were safely transported by YR-4 or Sikorsky helicopters. Unfortunately, the conclusion of World War II and debate between the army and air force over responsibility for air evacuation effectively halted development of an organized helicopter ambulance system in the United States. Improved helicopters that were designed specifically for patient transport had been tested and approved at Fort Bragg, North Carolina. However, recommendations for their use were "lost" during disagreements between the army and air force. It was not until the Korean War that the invaluable role of the helicopter in patient evacuation was fully established.

The United States entered the Korean War on June 30, 1950. Initial efforts at air evacuation of wounded were unsuccessful because fixed-wing aircraft were unable to land in the mountains and rice paddies of Korea. Thus the need for helicopter evacuation was thrust on the air force, and rescue of casualties began on August 4, 1950 using H-5 helicopters. By mid-August the effectiveness of the H-5s was obvious. Both the commander of the Far East Air Force and the surgeon general of the army requested and received a number of helicopters for medical evacuations. By the close of the year nearly 1000 wounded had been rescued by helicopter.

As the demand for "Med-Evac" units increased in Korea, a special helicopter unit was created and became attached to the mobile army surgical hospitals (MASH). In 1951 over 5000 casualties were transported by helicopter. The large number of successful evacuations, however, led to unrealistic expectations by the line troops. The limitations of the helicopter units (unarmed, without night-flying capabilities) were recognized by their crews, who issued a bulletin of standard operating procedures for helicopter evacuation. The large number of wounded also led to the establishment of medical regulating agencies to prevent overevacuation and to ensure adequate medical coverage in MASH units. Helicopter ambulance services were reorganized under the direction of the United States Army Surgeon General and Army Medical Department, rather than the line units. In 1953 coordination of helicopter evacuation became the responsibility of the First Helicopter Ambulance Company, which functioned during the last 5 months of the war. This organization became the prototype for contemporary American air ambulance companies. By the conclusion of the Korean War over 30,000 wounded had been "Med-Evaced" by helicopter ambulance, an accomplishment too significant to be ignored.

The lessons learned in the Korean War were well applied in Vietnam. Time and money were invested in improvement of both the helicopter ambulance and air evacuation maneuvers. A plan to manufacture all future aircraft with multiple function capabilities, including patient transport, resulted in design of the "Huey" in 1965 (officially known as the Iroquois), which was later upgraded to a six-litter, four-crew helicopter ambulance. With improved speed and power, the average flight time for an evacuation was only 35 minutes. In addition, formation of a medical radio communications network and a medical regulating facility (MRF) provided in-flight patient triage and forewarned hospitals of the condition and needs of the patient prior to arrival. Almost every wounded man, of the thousands wounded during the Vietnam War, was evacuated by helicopter. Survival statistics neared 100 percent (97.5%) for those reaching medical facilities. The experience gained in wartime helicopter evacuation has subsequently been used to develop civilian emergency rescue programs such as Military Assistance to Safety and Traffic (MAST), in which U.S. military air ambulances provide aid to civilian communities during medical emergencies.

### The Development of Transport Systems for the Sick Neonate

At birth the fetus vacates the safest and most practical means of transportation, the uterus. Ideally, the high-risk fetus is transported in utero to a facility where his or her specialized needs can be met. However, not every high-risk mother can be transported to a tertiary care center for delivery, and some neonates have unanticipated problems that require surgical or other specialized intervention.

Early reports of the transport of premature infants date back to the late 1890s. The Frenchman, Dr. Martin A. Couney, transported premature infants across Europe for exhibition. In 1897, he was invited to display his premature babies in incubators at the Victorian Exposition in Earl's Court, London. Because the London hospitals would not lend British babies for exhibition, but did not object to the use of foreign babies, Couney transported French babies by boat across the English Channel. He placed the infants in wash baskets, keeping them warm with hot water bottles and pillows.

Until the 1890s, most infants in the United States were born at home, in preference to the lying-in hospitals where puerperal infection was rampant and maternal mortality was high. Only the indigent, or those with illegitimate pregnancies, delivered in hospitals. Puerperal fever was largely controlled during the 1880s but delivery in hospitals was common only in urban areas of the United States until the late 1930s (e.g., births in-hospital in Cleveland, Ohio in 1920 = 22%, in 1930 = 55%, and in 1937 = 76%) [15].

In 1899 Dr. Joseph DeLee, obstetrician in-chief at Chicago's Lying-In Hospital, reported the development of the first ambulance incubator to transport premature infants to the hospital [4]: "In connection with the nursery, the society has opened an incubator station for the proper care of weakly and prematurely born infants. We have two of the most modern and improved incubators, and for the transportation of these delicate infants, without exposure, from distant parts of the city and suburbs, we have put in use an ambulance incubator, the first of its kind in this country" [4].

By 1933 Martin Couney, now in the United States with his premature baby exhibitions, had developed a baby ambulance to transport premature babies to his exhibition site. The source of a number of these babies was the Chicago premature station (the first in the United States) founded by Julius H. Hess, who was influenced by studies in Germany and Austria. When Couney left Chicago, his baby ambulance and incubator equipment were donated to Hess and the city of Chicago. In 1935, the Chicago Board of Health instituted a program for comprehensive skilled obstetric and pediatric care. This included a special ambulance with portable incubator, heat, oxygen, and humidity. The transport service was staffed by trained public health nurses and was available 24 hours a day.

A remarkably sophisticated and organized transport service was formed in 1948 under the auspices of the New York City Maternity and Newborn Division of the Department of Health, in conjunction with the New York hospitals [8, 14]. The service was staffed 24 hours a day, 7 days a week, by five rotating transport nurses, four ambulance drivers, a pediatrician, and a transport clerk. Detailed orientation of personnel and precise delineation of responsibilities contributed to the success of the program. For example, the ambulance drivers were responsible for handling equipment, checking and replacing oxygen tanks in the ambulance, and carrying the portable incubator. The role of the transport clerk was to "receive all incoming calls for transport and make out the 'Request for Transfers' card, . . . check with each premature center daily to determine available vacancies . . . check all reports and file all data relating to the transport service. In addition keep an inventory of supplies and equipment . . . and compile . . . the monthly record of babies transported." Not surprisingly, this clerk was assigned solely to the transport service.

The responsibilities of the nurse were to transport the infant (Fig. 1-10), maintain contact with the referring hospital, reassure the family, and record data regarding the transport. In the 2-year period reported, 1209 infants were successfully transported, including 194 infants weighing less than 1000 g! The babies were transported by ambulance in a lightweight aluminum incubator, with windows on both sides to permit access to the

---

*Fig. 1-10A. A transport nurse, 1948. This nurse was a member of a newborn transport service formed by the New York City Maternity and Newborn Division of the Department of Health, in conjunction with the New York hospitals. "Supplies, equipment and transport incubator are kept ready for immediate use at all times." (From Losty, M. A., and Wallace, H. W. A transport service for premature babies, Am. J. Nurs. 50(1): 10–12, 1950. Copyright 1950, American Journal of Nursing. Reproduced with permission.) B. The transport nurse adjusts oxygen flow and checks the temperature of the preheated transport incubator while in transit, 1948. (From Losty, M. A., and Wallace, H. W. A transport service for premature babies. Am. J. Nurs. 50(1): 10–12, 1950. Copyright 1950, American Journal of Nursing. Reproduced with permission.)*

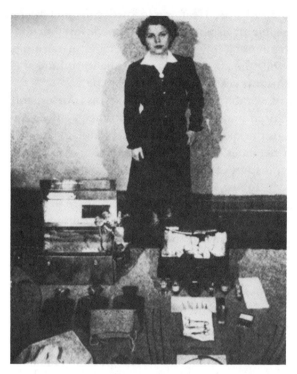

A

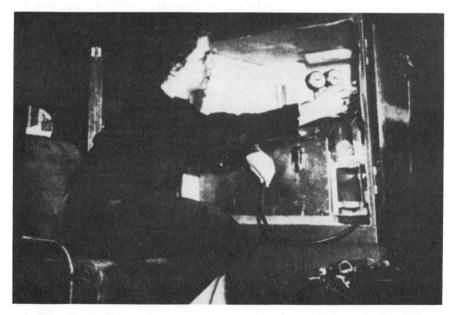

B

infant without opening the incubator. Heat was provided by hot water bottles, and oxygen was available from portable cylinders. Several incubators were set up for immediate use at any time. The average turn around time was just over 2 hours, while the average in-transit time for infants was 27 minutes. The average transport cost per infant was $48.62.

The transport service was favorably received by physicians, nurses, and parents. It was notably advanced and organized for its time, significantly predating the development of the specialized field of neonatology and organized transport teams for neonates.

In France, reports of the transport of premature infants appeared in the medical literature in the early 1960s. In a report by F. Alison the use of heated portable incubators, with portholes for administering care to the infant while in transit, was described, and the need for a centralized transport service to coordinate and triage infant transport among several premature centers was suggested [1]. In a second report, J. Roget described the use of helicopter transport for 78 infants over a 3.5-year period (1960–1964) [10]. Because lengthy ground transport, often lasting 3 to 4 hours, tended to further compromise the condition of sick infants, helicopter transport was initiated in the case of an 1100-g premature infant in a hospital 100 km away from a large metropolitan center. Subsequently the outcomes for 78 infants transported by helicopter were compared to 74 transported by ground. Infants were found to tolerate the shorter air flight as well as, if not better than, the lengthy ambulance ride. The authors reported no complications of flying at altitudes of 50 to 3000 m. This was perhaps the earliest reported series of infants transported by helicopter.

By the mid-1960s Sydney Segal, chairman of the Foetus and Newborn Committee of the Canadian Pediatric Society, had accumulated enough experience from 10 years of neonatal transport at the Vancouver General Hospital to publish guidelines in the *Pediatric Clinics of North America* [11]. Later these guidelines were expanded into a comprehensive manual for infant transport, published by the Canadian Pediatric Society [12]. His guidelines were remarkably similar to those followed today in intensive care nurseries, including an emphasis on the benefits of delivery of the high-risk infant in a referral center and the concept of back transfer for convalescence. Segal also emphasized the need for adequate communication between hospitals, maintenance of infant temperature, airway, and oxygenation, as well as the hazards of trapped air (e.g., pneumothorax) during air transportation.

The Vancouver General Hospital transport inventory included an incubator; battery-operated electric cardiorespiratory monitors; an intravenous pump; medications; oxygen cylinders; and equipment for intubation, suction, assisted ventilation, tracheotomy, and thoracostomy. The transport protocol included details such as copies of the infant's x rays and medical records, a maternal blood specimen, and parental consent for transfer. The options for transport vehicles included commercial or private ambulance, helicopter, fixed-wing aircraft, taxi, train, or snowmobile!

By the late 1960s and early 1970s a number of newborn intensive care referral centers and neonatal transport services were established. Centers reporting specialized transport teams included the University of Utah, Virginia Polytechnic Institute, the University of Iowa, the University of Arizona, Scott Air Force Medical Center (St. Louis), Long Island Jewish Hospital, Hammersmith Hospital (London), and the University of Berlin. Most teams were equipped with portable incubator, heat, oxygen, suction, monitors, and equipment for intubation. The Scott Air Force team was also equipped with microelectrodes for in-transit blood gas determinations. Although portable infant ventilators were available, they were not routinely in use. A 1970 report in *Lancet* described a portable incubator with an attached Vicker's infant ventilator [2]. The device weighed 88 lb, measured $40 \times 14 \times 18$ in. and could fit on the back seat of a car.

Transport vehicles ranged from public or commercial ambulance, helicopter, or fixed-wing aircraft to specialized vans and motor homes. The transport team at Long Island Jewish Hospital converted a nine-passenger Ford Country Squire station wagon into an infant transport vehicle. A variety of vehicles were specially designed as mobile nurseries complete with ventilators, incubators, oxygen, and work space. A mobile baby-care unit of British design is described in a 1968 issue of *Lancet* [9]. The unit was built into a standard ambulance and included "oxygen, suction, resuscitation trolley, a locker for sterile instruments and gowns, a wash basin, special heating and lighting . . . an incubator, a mechanical respirator, and a battery charger." A similar vehicle was designed in 1969 by Dr. George Baker, a pediatrician at the University of Iowa Medical Center, in conjunction with the Iowa State Services for Crippled Children. A large ($6 \times 10 \times 6.5$ ft) van was essentially converted into a nursery on wheels. It was equipped with two incubators, oxygen, monitoring, suction, lighting, air conditioning, medications, intravenous fluids, and a work bench. The initial cost of the van (with modifications) was $12,600, with estimated operating costs of $0.80 to $1.50 per mile. A "flying intensive care nursery" was described in 1970, and one of the first trials of organized aeromedical transport for infants and children in the United States was undertaken by the Children's Hospital in Columbus, Ohio [7, 13].

The deleterious effect of hypothermia on the survival and homeostasis of neonates had been well described. As transport of neonates became more common it was recognized that these patients were placed at significant risk of becoming hypothermic during transport. Various methods for prevention of heat loss in the delivery room had already been devised and were adopted for use during transport. In Europe, the Silver Swaddler, a hooded polyester swaddling suit, laminated on the inside with aluminum, was popular. In the United States a similar heat shield was made of air pockets sealed in plastic (packaginglike material) called the Transparent Baby Bag. Both effectively reduced radiant, convective, and conductive heat loss and were compact. The development of heated transport incubators, as well as heated transport vehicles, has greatly reduced the incidence of hypothermia during transport in all but the very low birth weight (< 1000 g) infant (Fig. 1-11).

## The Transport of High-Risk Obstetrical Patients

The establishment and regionalization of neonatal intensive care in the United States have been recognized as major contributing factors to the reduction of neonatal mortality over the past decade and a half. Simultaneously, observations that the outcome for in-born infants was better than that for transported infants led to the concept of in utero transport of the high-risk fetus. Thus maternal transport programs evolved as a complement to infant transport programs.

In the United States transport of the gravid woman to the hospital for delivery dates back to the 1920s. Transfer of high-risk mothers from community hospitals to regional perinatal centers began in the 1970s. This concept gained further support from the combined recommendations of such prestigious organizations as the American Academy of Pediatrics, the American College of Obstetrics and Gynecology, the American Medical Association, the American Academy of Family Physicians, and the March of Dimes in their 1976 Report of the Committee on Perinatal Health [3]. The rationale behind maternal transport was to provide optimal care for the high-risk mother and fetus before, during, and following delivery. Indications for antenatal referral were maternal, fetal, or both. Transport of the fetus in utero eliminated the additional stress of postnatal transport on an already sick and unstable infant. By the mid- and late 1970s a number of perinatal centers had developed maternal transport programs and had demonstrated reduced neonatal mortality and morbidity for the transported fetus when compared to the transported neonate (see Chap. 14). In addition, overall costs and length of hospitalization were less for the infants referred antenatally. Mother and infant could potentially benefit from spe-

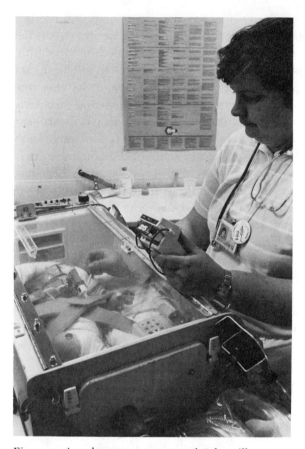

*Fig. 1-11. A modern transport nurse takes the axillary temperature of an infant on arrival at the referral intensive care nursery. Hypothermia remains a significant risk of newborn transport in the 1980s. (Copyright © 1987, David W. Wooddell. Reproduced with permission.)*

cialized perinatal care and avoid separation. The "infant" was transported in a more favorable environment (the uterus) while the mother was transported by ambulance, van, helicopter, or fixed-wing aircraft. The major disadvantage was removal of the patient from her family, community, and physician, as well as the potential for in-transit delivery.

Although some debate still exists as to the cost-benefit ratio of delivery of all high-risk infants in tertiary care centers, most would agree that the very low birth weight infant and those with known surgical emergencies benefit the most from in utero transport.

## Conclusion

The development of effective and organized patient transport systems has been one of the few beneficial results of war. In the last decade the sophistication of neonatal transport has approached the level of an intensive care nursery on wheels. Specially designed transport incubator systems routinely incorporate infant ventilators, transcutaneous oxygen and carbon dioxide monitors, as well as devices for continuous monitoring of heart rate, respirations, and blood pressure. These transport units are remarkably compact and portable, adapting for use in commercial ambulances, helicopter, and fixed-wing aircraft. Transport aircraft now include Lear jets, enabling rapid long-distance transfer of infants to centers specializing in pediatric surgery and ECMO (Fig. 1-12). At the other end of the spectrum, recognition of the positive impact of the maintenance of clinical homeostasis (even over short distances) on the intact survival of small, sick neonates has led to the use of designated transport equipment and personnel to transport infants between hospital departments (e.g., between the intensive care nursery and the operating room).

Future developments will include improvements in the sophistication and portability of the monitoring and support equipment available for transport purposes. As increasing numbers of highly technical therapeutic interven-

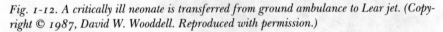

*Fig. 1-12. A critically ill neonate is transferred from ground ambulance to Lear jet. (Copyright © 1987, David W. Wooddell. Reproduced with permission.)*

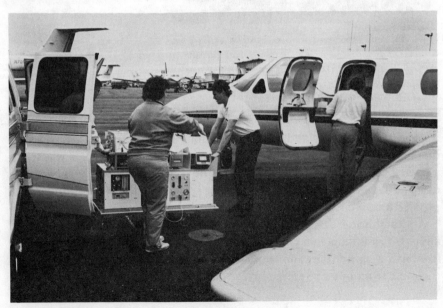

tions (e.g., in-flight ECMO) [5] become more portable, cost-benefit issues will become paramount. The increasing referral of high-risk obstetric and neonatal patients to tertiary care centers inevitably results in a supply and demand imbalance for both Level III and referring hospitals. Of necessity, triage and back transfer of infants no longer in need of intensive care facilities have become routine and optimize use of resources, facilities, and personnel. The existence of organized, efficient, and safe patient transport systems will undoubtedly continue to be integral to our goal to provide the best available care to the largest number of perinatal patients.

## References

1. Alison, F. Le transport des prématurés. *Maternité* 13(12):413–417, 1964.
2. Blake, A. M., et al. Portable ventilator-incubator. *Lancet* II:25, 1970.
3. Committee on Perinatal Health. *Toward Improving the Outcome of Pregnancy: Recommendations for the Regional Development of Maternal and Perinatal Health Services.* White Plains, N.Y.: The National Foundation—March of Dimes, 1976.
4. Cone, T. E. *History of the Care and Feeding of the Premature Infant.* Boston: Little, Brown, 1985. P. 46.
5. Cornish, J. D., et al. In flight use of extracorporeal membrane oxygenation for severe neonatal respiratory failure. *Perfusion* 1:281–287, 1986.
6. Fletcher, I. Aid, first and foremost: A brief outline history of the St. John Ambulance Association and Brigade. *Injury* II:105, 1979.
7. Harris, B. H., Orr, R. E., and Boles, T. Aeromedical transportation for infants and children. *J. Pediatr. Surg.* 10:5, 1971.
8. Losty, M. A., Orlofsky, I., and Wallace, H. A transport service for premature babies. *Am. J. Nurs.* 50:10–12, 1950.
9. Mobile baby care unit. *Lancet* I:1043, 1968.
10. Roget, J., Beaudoing, A., and Gilbert, Y. Le transport héliporté des prématurés. *Maternité* 13(12):418–423, 1964.
11. Segal, S. Transfer of a premature or other high-risk newborn infant to a referral hospital. *Pediat. Clin. North Am.* 13:1195–1205, 1966.
12. Segal, S. (ed.). *Manual for the Transport of High-risk Newborn Infants.* Sherbrooke, Quebec: Canadian Pediatric Society, 1972.
13. Shepard, K. S. Air transportation of high-risk infants utilizing a flying intensive care nursery. *J. Pediatr.* 77:148, 1970.
14. Wallace, H. M., Losty, M. A., and Baumgartner, L. Report of two years experience in the transportation of premature infants in New York City. *Pediatrics* 22:439–447, 1952.
15. Wertz, R. W., Wertz, D. *Lying-In: A History of Childbirth in America.* New York: Free Press, 1977.

## Bibliography

Anderson, C. L., et al. An analysis of maternal transport within a suburban metropolitan region. *Am. J. Obstet. Gynecol.* 140(5):499–504, 1981.
Arp, L. J., et al. An emergency air-ground transport system for the newborn with respiratory distress syndrome. *J. Indiana State Med. Assoc.* 62(6):547–549, 1969.
Baker, G. L. Design and operation of a van for the transport of sick infants. *Am. J. Dis. Child* 118:743, 1969.

Barkley, K. T.: *The Ambulance: The story of Emergency Transportation of Sick and Wounded through the Centuries.* Hicksville, N.J.: Exposition Press, 1978.

Barnes, J. K., Otis, G. A., and Huntington, D. L. *The Medical and Surgical History of the War of the Rebellion, Part 3, Surgical History* (1st ed.). Washington, D.C.: Government Printing Office, 1883.

Baum, J. D., and Scopes, J. W. The Silver Swaddler. *Lancet* 1: 672, 1968.

Besch, N. J., et al. The transparent baby bag. *N. Engl. J. Med.* 243(3):121, 1946.

Blake, A. M., Pollitzer, M. J., and Reynolds, E. O. R. Referral of mothers and infants for intensive care. *Br. Med. J.* 2:414–416, 1979.

Boehm, F. H., and Haire, M. F. One-way maternal transport: An evolving concept. *Am. J. Obstet. Gynecol.* 134(4):484–492, 1979.

Brady, E. R. The thread of a concept. *Marine Corps Gazette* 55:35, 1971.

Chance, G. W., O'Brien, M. J., and Swyer, P. R. Transportation of sick neonates, 1972: An unsatisfactory aspect of medical care. *Can. Med. Assoc. J.* 109:847–851, 1973.

Cone, T. E., Jr. *History of the Care and Feeding of the Premature Infant.* Boston: Little, Brown, 1985.

Cunningham, M. D., and Smith, F. Stabilization and transport of severely ill infants. *Pediatr. Clin. North Am.* 20(2):359–366, 1973.

Description of Perot and Company's improved medical wagon (1862). J. Morris Perot and Company, Wholesale Druggists, Philadelphia, Pa., 1876.

Dorland, P., and Nanney, J. *Army Aeromedical Evacuation in Vietnam.* Washington, D.C.: Center of Military History, U.S. Army, 1982.

Elliott, J. P., O'Keefe, D. F., and Freeman, R. K. Helicopter transportation of patients with obstetric emergencies in an urban area. *Am. J. Obstet. Gynecol.* 143(2): 157–162, 1982.

Evans, T. W. *History and Description of an Ambulance Wagon.* Paris: E. Brière, 1868.

Frank, H. D., Ballowitz, L., and Schachinger, H. Ambulance with intensive care facilities for the transport of infants at risk. *J. Perinat. Med.* 1:125–132, 1973.

Giles, H. R., et al. The Arizona high-risk maternal transport system: An initial view. *Am. J. Obstet. Gynecol.* 128(4):400–407, 1977.

Harris, B. A., et al. In utero versus neonatal transportation of high-risk perinates: A comparison. *Obstet. Gynecol.* 57(4):496–499, 1981.

Harris, T. R., Isaman, J., and Giles, H. R. Improved neonatal survival through maternal transport. *Obstet. Gynecol.* 52(3):294–300, 1978.

Kanto, W. P., Jr., et al. Impact of a maternal transport program on a newborn service. *South. Med. J.* 76(7):834–845, 1983.

Lam, D. M. From Balloon to Black Hawk: Part I—The Origins. *U.S. Army Aviation Digest* 27, June 1981. P. 41.

Lam, D. M. From Balloon to Black Hawk: Part II—World War II. *U.S. Army Aviation Digest* 27, July 1981. P. 44.

Lam, D. M. From Balloon to Black Hawk: Part III—Korea. *U.S. Army Aviation Digest* 27, August 1981.

Lam, D. M. From Balloon to Black Hawk: Part IV—Vietnam. *U.S. Army Aviation Digest* 27, September 1981.

Letterman, J. *Medical Recollections of the Army of the Potomac.* New York: Appleton, 1866.

Longmore, T. C. B. *A Treatise on the Transport of Sick and Wounded Troops.* London: Her Majesty's Stationery Office, 1869.

Merenstein, G. B. An analysis of air transport results in the sick newborn. *Am. J. Obstet. Gynecol.* 128(5):520–525, 1977.

Miller, T. C., Densberger, M., and Krogman, J. Maternal transport and the perinatal denominator. *Am. J. Obstet. Gynecol.* 147(1):19–24, 1983.

Modanlou, H. D., et al. Perinatal transport to a regional perinatal center in a metropolitan area: Maternal versus neonatal transport. *Am. J. Obstet. Gynecol.* 138(8): 1157–1164, 1980.

Modanlou, H. D., et al. Antenatal versus neonatal transport to a regional perinatal center: A comparison between matched pairs. *Obstet. Gynecol.* 53(6): 725–729, 1979.

Neonatal ICU reaches out via air lift. *Hosp. Pract.* 115–117, 1972.

Otis, G. A. *A Report to the Surgeon General on the Transport of the Sick and Wounded by Pack Animals.* Washington, D.C.: Government Printing Office, 1877.

Pettett, M. G., et al. An analysis of air transport results in the sick newborn infant: Part I: The transport team. *Pediatrics* 55(6):774–782, 1975.

Redard, P. *Transport Par Chemins de Fer Des Blessés et Malades Militaires.* Paris, 1889.

Snook, R. Transport of the injured patient: Past, present, and future. *Br. J. Anaesth.* 49:651, 1977.

Sorima, M. L. Maternal transport: Behind the drama. *Am. J. Obstet. Gynecol.* 134(8): 904–910, 1979.

Special van gives babies head start on survival. *J.A.M.A.* 209(12):1826, 1969.

Storrs, C. N., and Taylor, M. R. H. Transport of sick newborn babies. *Br. Med. J.* 3:328–331, 1970.

## Chapter Appendix I: History of Medical Transport— Time Line

Margaret Chou
Mhairi G. MacDonald

### A Historical Chronology of Medical Transport*

Biblical references—transport of patient on litter, on shoulders, or on beasts

Throughout history—litters drawn by horse or other animal

| | |
|---|---|
| 1487— | Queen Isabella of Spain—ambulances or "field hospitals" |
| 1784— | Montgolfier brothers—balloon lift |
| — | Jean Francis Picot theorized patients could benefit from and tolerate flight |
| 1792— | "Ambulances volantes"—French carts for carrying wounded from battlefield |
| 1862— | Jonathan Letterman reorganizes field medical services |
| 1864— | Geneva convention |
| 1865— | Cincinnati Commercial Hospital introduces first hospital-based ambulance service in United States |

*Major American wars, nineteenth century to the present: Civil War—1861–1865, World War I—1914–1920, World War II—1939–1945, Korean War—1950–1953, and Vietnam War—1961–1975.

1869—        First civilian ambulance service at Bellevue Hospital, New York

1870—        Balloon evacuation of 160 during Bismarck's siege of Paris

1877—        Founding of St. John Ambulance Association—transport of sick in mining and pottery districts in England

1882—        Ambulances for noninfectious patients—run by London Horse Ambulance Service—too costly to be hired. Most injured transported by hand litters or wheeled litters

—            Geneva convention ratified by U.S. Senate

1887—        St. John Ambulance Brigade founded—trained personnel in first aid and nursing

1894—        Auckland St. John Ambulance—horsedrawn—very bumpy

1897—        Martin Couney transports infants for exhibition in France

1899—        First "self-propelled" electric ambulances (Chicago)

—            Joseph DeLee develops ambulance incubator for transport of infants to Chicago Lying-In Hospital

1900–1932—   "Micawber's Navy"—river ambulance service, United States

1903—        Wright brothers

1904—        London medical profession urges unified system of ambulance services—turned down by Parliament because of cost

1907—        City of London forms own ambulance service—including an electric ambulance

1909—        400 wheeled litters in London

—            Captain Gosman (Florida) designs aircraft specifically to carry patients—called Gosman-Rhodes aircraft

1910—        Gosman-Rhodes aircraft airborn without engine; towed along by ground vehicle. Engine added—crashed—inadequate funds. Gosman goes to Washington, D.C. to present concept to War Department—turned down

—            French propose air transport of patients from battlefield—"l'aviation sanitaire" (balloon-lifted platform pulled by horsemen)

1912—        Surgeon general makes recommendation to War Department (unsuccessfully) for reevaluation of aircraft for patient evacuation

—            French design air ambulance for testing

1913—        French military medical officer and English captain urge development of air ambulances—published in *Journal of the Royal Army Medical Corps*

1915—        Retreat of Serbian army from Albania—forced to use French fighter aircraft for evacuation of wounded

—            November—first air ambulance evacuation of wounded from Mitrovitra to Prizrend, then Vallona

—            Formation of ambulance service in London under fire brigade, with motor ambulance donated

| 1917— | French physician, Dr. Chassaing, converts old aircraft to air ambulance (patients carried in hollow fuselage—volunteers himself as first patient from Villacoublay)—then evacuates casualties from Aisne front |
| 1918— | Evacuation of Flanders |
| — | Dr. Chassaing receives 60 aircraft to convert to air ambulances |
| — | World War I—United States forced to train pilots in remote areas—crash response aircraft carry physicians to wounded pilots to stabilize patients |
| — | U.S. military aircraft converted to air ambulance under supervision of Major Driver and Captain Ocker—the "Jenny" |
| — | All U.S. airfields ordered to convert a service aircraft to an air ambulance |
| 1918–1925— | U.S. revisions of aircraft for patient transport gains acceptance from medical community—believed too risky by military |
| 1922— | Establishment of Hortense Schoen Joseph Premature Station in connection with Michael Reese Hospital in Chicago |
| 1927— | Air evacuation of victims of tornado in Texas—gains national coverage and recognition |
| 1928— | Plane evacuation of wounded in Nicaragua |
| 1931— | Major Beaven recommends testing autogiro for air evacuation |
| 1932— | Navy tests autogiro—unsuccessful |
| 1933— | Martin Couney develops baby ambulance for transporting infants on exhibition |
| 1935— | Chicago Board of Health—infant ambulance and transport service |
| 1936— | Pennsylvania—field test of autogiro—believed to be too expensive and machinery inadequate (not enough power) |
| 1937— | First International Technical Conference on Aerial Relief. Aircraft of most countries inadequate for patient transport |
| 1939–1940— | Soviet Union uses air evacuation in Finland |
| 1939— | Redesign of helicopter |
| — | London Auxiliary Ambulance service formed to deal with air raid casualties—volunteer staff. After war used to transport patients to hospital and midwives to laboring mothers |
| 1940— | Plans for airplane ambulance shuttle squadron—convert obsolete aircraft into ambulance aircraft to rescue training pilots after crashes |
| 1942— | First ambulance to carry oxygen as standard equipment in United States |
| 1943— | Two aircraft converted to ambulance aircraft and used in Pacific |
| 1944— | First helicopter evacuation in jungles of Burma |

1947–1951—   Arguments over responsibility for air evacuation—U.S. Army versus Air Force

1948—        New York City Department of Health 24-hour infant transport service

—            U.K. National Health Service requires local authorities to provide free ambulance service to community

1949—        Fort Bragg, N.C.—army evaluates helicopter as medical evacuation vehicle—concludes practical and desirable

1950—        U.K. city of Bath Ambulance Service (vans)

1950–1953—   Korean War—more than 20,000 evacuations by helicopter

—            U.S. fixed-wing aircraft not able to function in Korean terrain (rice paddies and mountains)—sent helicopters. Surgeon general requests helicopters for medical evacuation. Landing pads constructed

1951—        Creation of mobile army surgical hospital (MASH). Evacuate more than 5000 casualties by helicopter

—            Standard operating procedures for helicopter evacuation written to educate troops on capabilities and limitations of helicopters (i.e., night flying, unarmed, etc.)

1953—        Centralization of helicopter units—First Helicopter Ambulance Company organized—prototype for modern air ambulance companies

1955—        Design contest sponsored by army for helicopter ambulance

—            Practice exercises for forward aeromedical evacuations

1962—        First helicopter ambulance unit sent to Vietnam

1964—        Montreal Children's Hospital transport service

—            French report use of helicopter for infant transport

1965—        U.S. military medical radio network to coordinate flights established (medical regulation office [MRO])

1966—        Sydney Segal publishes guidelines for infant transport in *Pediatric Clinics of North America*

1967—        Formation of Maryland helicopter evacuation plan by University of Maryland

1967–1972—   Report of Scottish Air Ambulance transports from islands to mainland

1968—        Design of ambulance for patient comfort—effects of motion on patients studied

—            Helipad built on roof of University of Maryland Hospital

1969—        Maryland helicopter evacuation plan put into practice—"Maryland Air Med-Evac"—Maryland state police and University of Maryland used for traffic accident victims, interhospital transfers, transfer of premature babies, medical supplies, and organs

| | |
|---|---|
| — | Sick baby van developed by University of Iowa Health Center and Iowa State Services for Crippled Children |
| — | Rome—Needs of airline company in transporting neonates outlined. Case report of transport Milan to London |
| 1970s— | Establishment of multiple newborn intensive care referral centers and transport services |
| 1970— | Military Assistance to Safety and Traffic (MAST)—U.S. military air ambulance units aid in civilian medical emergencies |
| — | U.S. Air Force jet designated for transfer of infants—carries oxygen, monitors, respirator, blood gas analyzer, IV pump |
| — | Portable ventilator-incubator for infant transport described in *Lancet* |
| 1971— | Report of infant transport team in San Diego using commercial ambulance, fixed wing, or helicopter |
| — | Long Island Jewish Hillside Medical Center uses Ford Country Squire stationwagon as transport vehicle, with a Bird respirator and transport incubator |
| 1972— | Canadian Pediatric Society publishes manual of transport of high-risk newborns |
| — | Denver air transport review |
| — | Ambulance recognition factor—flashing lights and audible warning device |
| 1977— | U.S. Department of Transportation and the Federal Aviation Administration publish proposed regulations governing "the transportation in small aircraft operated for compensation or hire of persons who may need assistance in meeting their medical needs while in flight" in the *Federal Register*. |
| 1986— | Report of inflight extracorporeal membrane oxygenation (ECMO) |
| — | American Society of Hospital-Based Emergency Air Medical Services (ASHBEAMS) drafts standards for aeromedical services |
| 1987— | (United States) National Emergency Medical Service Pilot's Association (NEMSPA) holds first safety conference |

# II

*Administrative Aspects of a Medical Transport Program*

# 2

# An Overview of the Organization and Administration of a Perinatal Transport Service

Carl L. Bose

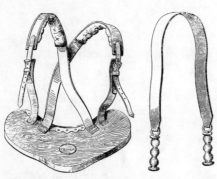

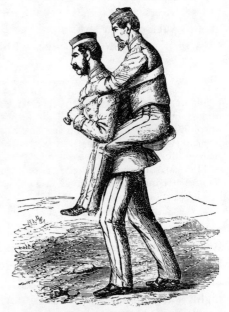

2A. Left. Fisher's apparatus for carrying a wounded man en cheval *on a bearer's back.* A class 1 sick transport conveyance (conveyance borne by men). (Reproduced from Longmore, T. A Treatise on the Transport of Sick and Wounded Troops. *London: Her Majesty's Stationery Office, 1869.)*
Right. Supporting belt used with the apparatus. A class 1 sick transport conveyance (conveyance borne by men). (Reproduced from Longmore, T. A Treatise on the Transport of Sick and Wounded Troops. *London: Her Majesty's Stationery Office, 1869.)*

2B. Mode of using the Fisher apparatus. A class 1 sick transport conveyance (conveyance borne by men). (Reproduced from Longmore, T. A Treatise on the Transport of Sick and Wounded Troops. *London: Her Majesty's Stationery Office, 1869.)*

## The Role of Transport in Regionalized Perinatal Care

Intensive care first became available for critically ill neonates in the late 1950s and early 1960s at selected centers in the United States. These centers proliferated during the latter half of the 1960s as the scope of neonatal care expanded. The coincidental decline in neonatal mortality appeared to justify this rapid growth of neonatal intensive care units (Fig. 2-1). In addition, since this decline in neonatal mortality resulted primarily from the improved care of premature infants, neonatal intensive care became increasingly linked to complicated obstetrical care. This relationship stimulated the evolution of perinatal centers caring for both high-risk mothers and infants.

The value of such centers was soon recognized by many professional groups, including organizations such as the American Medical Association (AMA). In 1971, the AMA adopted the following policy statement [11]:

Application of recent advances in scientific knowledge and skills in the intensive care management of high risk pregnant women and high risk newborn infants will result in reduction of present maternal and infant mortality. A major contribution to such a program is the development of a centralized community (or regional) hospital-based newborn intensive care unit. Concentration of high risk infant care programs in a hospital specially staffed and equipped to provide optimal care is a proven life-saving mechanism for infants at risk.
The AMA urges that in every community (or if more appropriate, geographical region) attention be directed to the development and operation of such centralized special care facilities. . . .

Unfortunately, the growth of perinatal care services did not proceed in a systematic fashion. With a few exceptions, this early growth was not carefully planned. Knowledge was inadequate at some centers. Technology was misapplied in others. Because of tremendous costs and the demand for highly skilled and trained personnel, perinatal intensive care could be made available in selected centers only. The result was maldistribution of resources, with the lack of availability of intensive care in some areas and costly duplication in others.

This problem was soon recognized, and efforts were made to establish some order to the further evolution of perinatal health care delivery systems. The National Foundation–March of Dimes convened a study group to collect available data on the advantages of regional systems of perinatal care. Their report, *Toward Improving the Outcome of Pregnancy*, formally described the concept now known as regionalized perinatal care:

Regionalization implies the development, within a geographic area, of a coordinated, cooperative system of maternal and perinatal health care in which, by mutual agreements between hospitals and physicians and based upon population

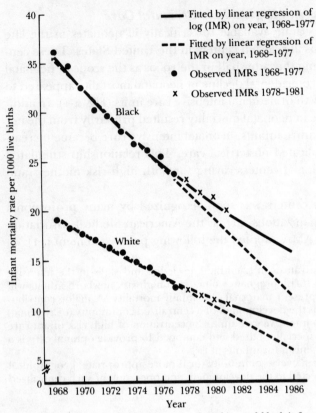

*Fig. 2-1. Comparison of mortality rates for white and black infants in the United States, 1968–1981, including both observed rates and rates fitted to linear and log-linear models. (From Kleinman, J. C. Am. J. Public Health 76:682, 1986.)*

needs, the degree of complexity of maternal and perinatal care each hospital is capable of providing is identified so as to accomplish the following objectives: quality care to all pregnant women and newborns, maximal utilization of highly trained perinatal personnel and intensive care facilities, and assurances of reasonable cost effectiveness [10].

This report objectively defined three levels of perinatal care and the appropriate contributions that hospitals delivering each level of care should make to perinatal care within a geographical region (Chapter Appendix I and Table 2-1). Level I hospitals were defined as those hospitals providing primary care for uncomplicated neonatal and maternal patients. Level II hospitals provided primary care but also provided care for patients with moderately severe complications of pregnancy and neonates with some illnesses of moderate severity. Level III centers provided all the resources

Table 2-1. Levels of program development (I, II, III).

| Levels of basic perinatal network | Activity | Locations | Usual physician leadership |
|---|---|---|---|
| I | Usual focus of patient entry into system<br>Risk assessment<br>Uncomplicated perinatal care<br>Stabilization of unexpected problems<br>Data collection<br>Sponsor of local education | Community hospital or co-located at level II or level III facility | Primary care physician or specialist |
| II | Level I activities, plus:<br>Diagnosis and treatment of selected high-risk pregnancies and neonatal problems<br>Patient transport<br>Education efforts for part of network | Large community hospitals with many support services or co-located at level III facility | Specialist or subspecialist |
| III | Usually level I and level II activities,* plus:<br>Diagnosis and treatment of most perinatal problems<br>Research and outcome surveillance<br>Regional education<br>Regional administration | Large medical centers with comprehensive academic programs | Subspecialist |

*Some level III facilities, such as level III neonatal units in children's hospitals, may not provide level I and level II services. Regional Resource Centers provide specialized knowledge and skills in academic medical centers (level III) at a subspecialty (academic) level.

Reproduced with permission from American Academy of Pediatrics Committee on Fetus and Newborn and American College of Obstetricians and Gynecologists Committee on Obstetrics: Maternal and Fetal Medicine. *Guidelines for Perinatal Care.* Evanston, Ill.: American Academy of Pediatrics and American College of Obstetricians and Gynecologists, 1983.

available in Level I and II centers, in addition to caring for patients with severe complications of pregnancy and critically ill neonates. A regional system should include hospitals delivering different levels of care. The March of Dimes Study Group recommended formal relationships between these hospitals such that each patient would be cared for in a facility best able to provide the requisite care.

Numerous reports, some in the early 1970s, documented improved outcome among premature or critically ill infants provided with neonatal intensive care [1, 5, 18, 27]. Further, the benefits of this care appeared to outweigh the risks of transport [22, 24, 25]. However, neonatal transport was not without inherent risks and several more recent studies have indicated further overall improvement in the outcome for neonates as a result of maternal-fetal transport, when compared to delivery in a community hospital followed by neonatal transport. Merenstein et al. reported a significantly lower-than-predicted mortality among infants delivered following maternal transport compared to infants cared for in their perinatal center following neonatal transport [21]. Harris et al. demonstrated that the greatest benefit of maternal-fetal transport was derived by the very low birth weight infant [14]. Other investigators have demonstrated a lower incidence of respiratory distress syndrome and other morbidity and shorter hospitalization of neonates as a result of maternal-fetal transport [13]. Although none of these studies report controlled trials, the hypothesis that maternal-fetal transport is preferable to neonatal transport has been widely accepted.

Therefore, it has been recommended that community hospitals without in-house neonatal intensive care services should assess each mother to determine her medical needs and the likelihood of her delivering an infant with a degree of illness beyond the capabilities of that hospital. Maternal patients identified as being high risk should then be transferred to institutions delivering more complex care. Similarly, neonatal patients delivered in Level I or II hospitals whose medical needs exceed the capabilities of the hospital of birth should be transferred to a center capable of providing more intensive care.

Enthusiasm for these well-defined systems of regionalized perinatal health care was so great that, by the late 1970s, the federal government and the majority of states had adopted legislation either encouraging or mandating the development of regionalized perinatal care. Therefore, by the end of 1970s, the transport of perinatal patients from community hospitals to perinatal centers was an integral part of the delivery of perinatal health care throughout the country.

A significant disadvantage of the widespread practice of referral of high-risk obstetrical patients to regional centers is the inherent likelihood of transferring some patients who, in retrospect, do not benefit from perinatal intensive care. Assessment of the mother and fetus is often an unreliable predictor of problems in the neonate. Harvey and Bowes reported that, in 1977, 44 percent of maternal referrals to the University of Colorado Medical Center did not require the resources of their perinatal center [15]. There were reasons other than medical necessity for the referral of many of these patients. Some inappropriate referrals could have been avoided by a tighter screening method. However, of the appropriately referred patients, only 36 percent delivered infants who required neonatal intensive care. Therefore, overuse of perinatal center resources appears to be an unavoidable consequence of regionalized care. The financial impact of this problem is compounded by the increased cost of care in most regional centers compared to community hospitals. Maternal transport may also result in disruption of the nuclear family and removal of the mother from her psychological support system.

The bulk of evidence appears to favor maternal transport *if* patients are carefully selected. Therefore, a major emphasis of regionalized care should be the identification of mothers with complications of pregnancy, particularly those complications that are likely to result in preterm delivery. In *Toward Improving the Outcome of Pregnancy*, suggested criteria for the identification and transfer of maternal patients between Level I, II, and III hospitals are listed [10]. Unfortunately, the recommended criteria cannot be uniformly applied to all perinatal regions. Many regions have unique geographical features and illogical political boundaries. Most regions have certain hospitals that cannot be clearly categorized as Level I, II, or III. Therefore, it is essential that, within each region, the limits of complexity of maternal and neonatal care provided in each hospital be defined. This is best done by the medical and nursing staffs of the individual hospitals. Consultation by the perinatal staff at the regional center may be helpful to the community hospital staff. However, it is unwise and usually unsuccessful for the perinatal center staff to offer consultation when it has not been solicited or to attempt to mandate patient care preferences in community hospitals. Since the limiting factor in the care of a maternal patient is often the ability to care for the infant, criteria for the transfer of maternal patients from community hospitals to perinatal centers must be developed as a collaborative effort between the obstetrical and pediatric care providers.

Transfer criteria should be appended with detailed information about the regional perinatal center or other centers available to assist with more complex care. The regional center should provide each community hospital with a description of its services and the location of an alternate center if a particular service is unavailable. Also, a precise plan should be developed with each community hospital that details the methods by which patients should be transferred to the perinatal center.

Even the most aggressive programs of prenatal risk assessment do not obviate the need for neonatal transport. Illness in the neonate may not be apparent until after delivery (e.g., congenital heart disease) or may occur as a result of a problem late in the intrapartum period (e.g., meconium aspiration). Even in areas where regionalized perinatal care programs are well established, a significant percentage of very low birth weight infants are delivered in Level I or II hospitals. For example, after the inception of regionalized perinatal care in North Carolina in the mid-1970s, the percentage of very low birth weight infants ($<1500$ g) delivered in Level I and II hospitals steadily declined but reached a plateau at about 30 percent around 1980 (Fig. 2-2). No further decline has been observed. The reason for the continued birth of very low birth weight infants in hospitals unprepared to manage their degree of illness is unclear. It may result from the conscious choice of some obstetrical care providers not to transfer maternal patients or from an inherent inability to identify a mother likely to deliver prematurely early enough to facilitate transfer. This latter possibility seems more likely since the percentage of infants with birth weights less than 1000 g born in Level I and II hospitals in North Carolina is nearly identical to the percentage with birth weights less than 1500 g born in those hospitals

*Fig. 2-2. Comparison of the percentage of live births of infants with birth weights less than 1500 g born in Level I, II, and III hospitals in North Carolina in the years 1968 to 1984. (Personal communications, Richard Nugent, M.D., Department of Human Resources, North Carolina.)*

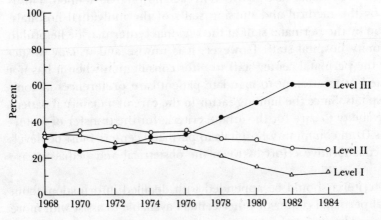

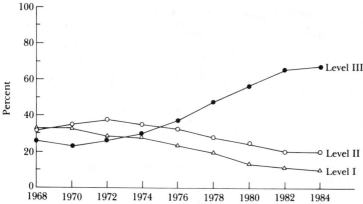

*Fig. 2-3. Comparison of the percentage of live births of infants with birth weights less than 1000 g born in Level I, II, and III hospitals in North Carolina in the years 1968 to 1984. (Personal communications, Richard Nugent, M.D., Department of Human Resources, North Carolina.)*

(Fig. 2-3). It seems highly unlikely that obstetrical care providers would choose to deliver infants with birth weights less than 1000 g in community hospitals. It is probable that a significant percentage of women in preterm labor appear at community hospitals too late in the intrapartum period to permit transport. In either case, it seems clear that a significant number of both preterm infants and critically ill term infants will be born in Level I and II hospitals who will then require transport to a perinatal intensive care center. Therefore, as with high-risk maternal patients, community hospitals should develop criteria for the transport of neonatal patients to a regional perinatal center.

In many parts of the country, locating an appropriate site for care of a perinatal patient is attended by many practical problems. Some of these are geographical, some are financial. In other regions, a severe shortage of beds (particularly neonatal intensive care unit beds) exists or subspecialty services may be unavailable. These regions may benefit from more formal systems of communication to facilitate the transfer of perinatal patients. In some areas, sophisticated communication networks linking neighboring perinatal centers have been developed to assist in the referral of patients. For example, since 1980, North Carolina has operated a network that provides each perinatal center with up-to-date information about the services and beds available in all other centers in the state [4]. This information is constantly displayed on a terminal in each perinatal center (Fig. 2-4). The staff at each center is responsible for updating information regarding their center when appropriate. Updated information is disseminated at frequent

NEONATAL TELECOMMUNICATIONS NETWORK

| HOSPITAL-CITY | BEDS OB-PED | | NOTES | PHYSICIAN OB-PED | TELEPHONE OB-PED |
|---|---|---|---|---|---|
| MISSION-ASHEVILLE | Y | Y | A | CALL CHARGE R.N. | 704-255-6232/6233 |
| CHAR MEM-CHARLOTTE | N | N | 3 | OB RES/SMITH | 704-331-2121/3000 |
| BAPTIST-WINSTON-SAL | Y | Y | | THOMAS/ICN ADM RES | 919-773-3210/7482 |
| CONE-GREENSBORO | N | N | | OB RES/PEDS ADM RES | 919-378-4188/4190 |
| NCMH-CHAPEL HILL | Y | Y | 12 | JONES/HARRIS | 919-966-4131/3481 |
| DUKE-DURHAM | N | N | 3 | OB RES/WILSON | 919-684-3461/5551 |
| WAKE-RALEIGH | N | N | | OB RES/JOHNSON | 919-755-8466/8467 |
| N HAN MEM-WILMINGT | M | M | ABE | OB RES/CHARGE RN | 919-343-7394/7391 |
| PITT CTY-GREENVILLE | N | N | 14 | ROBERTS/CHARGE RN | 919-757-4553/4665 |

NOTES

| A.NO CARDIAC PATIENTS | 1.NEONATAL TRANSPORT AVAILABLE |
|---|---|
| B.NO PEDIATRIC SURGERY PATIENTS | 2.MATERNAL TRANSPORT AVAILABLE |
| C.NO PRETERM-OTHERS OK(PEDIATRIC) | 3.BEDS AVAIL FOR CARDIAC & PED SURGERY |
| D.NO IMMINENT PRETERM (MATERNAL) | 4.BEDS AVAIL FOR PED SURGERY |
| E.NO VENTILATORS AVAILABLE | X.NOT CONTACTED LAST POLL |

**REFERRING UNIT MUST CALL ACCEPTING UNIT BEFORE INITIATING TRANSPORT**

*Fig. 2-4. Sample of information displayed on the screen of the terminal in each perinatal center participating in the North Carolina neonatal/perinatal telecommunication network. Information is provided regarding both bed availability and specialty services. (From Bostick, J. S., et al. Pediatrics 71:274, 1983. Reproduced by permission of Pediatrics.)*

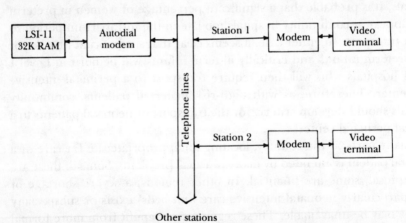

Other stations

*Fig. 2-5. System configuration for the North Carolina neonatal/perinatal telecommunication network. The central computer (LSI-II) links video terminals via telephone lines in each perinatal center in the state. (From Bostick, J. S., et al. Pediatrics 71:273, 1983. Reproduced by permission of Pediatrics.)*

intervals via telecommunications by a centrally located computer (Fig. 2-5). If the perinatal center to which a patient is first referred is unable to accommodate the patient, information is immediately available about alternate locations for the necessary service. Such communication networks are most efficacious in regions where several perinatal centers are in reasonably close proximity to one another and are only of benefit if the demand for beds frequently exceeds the supply within a given region.

## One-way Versus Two-way Transport

Neonatal transport has evolved in a manner similar to that of other aspects of regionalized care. At first, transport was almost exclusively the responsibility of the referring hospital and consisted primarily of conveying the sick patient, with little care provided en route. The hazards of this approach were soon appreciated [7] and the advantages of the provision of intensive care during transport were documented. At least two controlled studies have demonstrated that neonatal mortality and morbidity can be reduced among infants referred to tertiary centers if the infants are attended during transport by skilled and properly equipped professionals [6, 16]. The decision regarding who provides the equipment and the skilled professionals is largely dependent on a variety of practical constraints.

Responsibility for providing these resources may be left to the referring hospital (termed "one-way transport"). Conversely, the regional perinatal center may send out a team (termed "two-way transport"). The disadvantages of one-way transport relate primarily to the comparatively small number of transports conducted by any given referral hospital. With a small number of transports it is difficult to justify the expense of equipment dedicated exclusively to patient transport. Physicians are usually not available to participate in transport, and nonphysician personnel generally do not have sufficient experience in managing critically ill infants to provide skilled care en route. Finally, suitable emergency vehicles may not be available to provide transportation. If local emergency medical services (EMS) vehicles are used, gaps in the continuity of local emergency services may occur.

The availability of two-way transport circumvents most of these problems. The transport service from a single perinatal intensive care center can provide service to many communities and, therefore, appreciate the benefits of the economy of scale. The purchase of expensive equipment becomes cost-effective. Teams of skilled attendants, sometimes dedicated exclusively to patient transport activities, become practical. These individuals are usually recruited from within the perinatal center and have a broad experience in neonatal intensive care. They can be trained to perform transport activities and can expect to perform enough transports to maintain their skills. Most tertiary centers can also justify the expense of a vehicle (or vehicles) dedicated exclusively to two-way patient transport.

The major disadvantage of two-way transport is the time delay in moving the patient from the community hospital to the tertiary center. This delay may be compounded at the inevitable points in time when multiple requests for transport coincide. The impact of this disadvantage of the time delay in beginning the transfer of the patient can be minimized by requesting that referring personnel call for assistance as soon as the need for transport is evident. They can also minimize impact by using the time between the request for transport and the arrival of the transport team to stabilize the patient to the extent of their capabilities and resources. Outreach education programs should focus on this particular aspect of neonatal care. In addition, the tertiary center should consider the use of rapid transportation (e.g., helicopters or fixed-wing aircraft) if a significant number of referral hospitals are at great distances from the tertiary center.

For the majority of regionalized perinatal care programs, the advantages of two-way neonatal transport far outweigh the disadvantages. The choice between one-way and two-way transport of maternal patients is not as clear-cut. The sole purpose of many maternal transports is to facilitate the immediate care of the neonate in an appropriate intensive care environment. Often the mother has no significant health problem other than a complication of pregnancy likely to result in preterm delivery (e.g., preterm labor, chorioamnionitis, rupture of membranes). In these situations, the only objective is to transport the mother to the tertiary center prior to delivery and this can often be best accomplished by a system of one-way transport. Even in situations where the mother is moderately ill (e.g., preeclampsia, congestive heart failure), one-way transport may be indicated because local hospitals usually have personnel available for transport who are reasonably competent in the management of adults with medical emergencies. In addition, special medical equipment, other than that available in most ambulances, is usually not necessary.

In the past, systems of two-way maternal transport have typically evolved only in those areas where great distances exist between the tertiary center and referring hospitals and where air transportation was available at the tertiary center. With the recent proliferation of hospital-based helicopter programs, more perinatal centers are offering two-way maternal transport by air. Use of the aeromedical helicopter for the transport of high-risk maternal patients has been demonstrated to be efficacious even in an urban area and may become more widespread in the future [12].

In the remainder of this chapter, the organization and administration of two-way perinatal transport programs will be discussed. For the purposes of this discussion, it will be assumed that the staff of the regional perinatal center has made the decision that two-way transport is efficacious and has taken the responsibility for operating such a program.

### Administration of a Perinatal Transport Program

The success of any transport program is dependent on the integration of many components that can be divided into two general categories: nonmedical and medical.

The nonmedical components include transportation, communications/dispatch, billing/accounting, and marketing.

The medical components include transport teams, equipment, and outreach education.

Figure 2-6 depicts the organization of a typical regional, hospital-based transport program. This scheme is based on the assumption that neonatal and maternal transport systems are part of a multipurpose program that is capable of transporting patients with a variety of illnesses. Although two-way transport began as the exclusive province of the neonatology service, at many medical centers maternal and neonatal transports are performed by specialty teams from programs serving a variety of critically ill patients. Such multipurpose programs generally have a specialty team to transport neonatal patients and one or more other teams to transport other types of patients. A separate team for neonates can usually be justified, based on the number of transports and the uniqueness of these patients. The decision to

*Fig. 2-6. An example of the organizational structure of the administration of a transport service that includes specialty teams for neonatal, maternal, and other critical care medicine patients.*

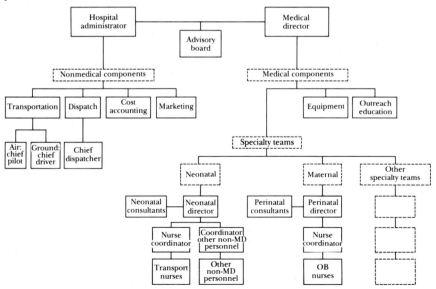

develop other specialty teams (e.g., maternal) will depend on the number of these patients and the availability of personnel with special training in their care.

Direction of the nonmedical components of the program is usually the responsibility of a member of the administrative staff at the sponsor hospital. Direction of the medical components is best assumed by an individual involved in some aspect of critical care medicine and an individual with expertise in program administration. This scheme proposes distinct divisions of responsibility that may be neither practical nor advantageous in many medical centers. The expertise and availability of the individuals will usually determine precise assignment of duties. A discussion of each of the key administrative positions and their relationships to various components of the program follows.

ROLE OF THE HOSPITAL ADMINISTRATOR
The nonmedical components of a transport program are characterized by those aspects of the program that are not directly related to patient care. Because of the constraints on physicians' time and their frequent lack of expertise in administration, these components of the program are usually best managed by a hospital administrator. Many decisions regarding the operation of the program require an analysis of costs and benefits. While the medical representatives of the program are better prepared to assess the benefits, a hospital administrator is usually better prepared to assess the financial impact. Therefore, the administrator must receive advice from medical personnel and develop and operate the nonmedical components of the program within the limits of the financial resources of the institution.

The administrator will develop contracts with parties responsible for providing rapid, safe, readily available transportation. This individual will develop a communication network that integrates all components of the program. Someone on the hospital administrative staff will usually develop the strategies for marketing the program. Finally, the administrator must ensure the financial solvency of the program or at least understand the monetary losses and justify these on the basis of the contribution of the program to the institution. It is essential that the administrator be fully cognizant of the legal and safety aspects of providing patient transport (see Chaps. 8 and 13).

ROLE OF THE MEDICAL DIRECTOR
The magnitude of the role of the medical director will depend primarily on the complexity of the program. In the very simplest model, a program may provide only two-way neonatal transport. In this situation, the medical di-

rector is usually a neonatologist on the hospital staff. However, many programs now provide transport for a broad spectrum of patients, using two or more specialty teams. In these situations, the medical director should first and foremost be an individual with proved administrative ability. This individual should also be able to appreciate the needs of all medical specialties served by the program. Such an individual is logically a member of the staff of one of the critical care medicine services.

The primary role of the medical director is to ensure quality patient care. This individual must establish training programs for transport personnel. This area of responsibility is particularly important for those programs that primarily use nonphysician transport teams. The medical director must ensure that the training program will prepare personnel to provide for the needs of the patients. This training must also satisfy regulatory agencies that govern the limits of care that may be provided by nonphysician personnel (e.g., nursing boards). The director should develop some method of determining that an individual trainee has successfully completed the training program and reached an adequate level of proficiency.

The medical director should also develop some strategy for reviewing the quality of care provided during transport. Ideally, a thorough review of each transport should be conducted using the paper record and interviews with the attendants. This is clearly not practical for programs transporting a large volume of patients. An alternative may be to review in detail only transports of the most critically ill patients or transports during which the transport team had questions regarding appropriate care. It is also prudent to review in detail any case in which a medical-legal question might arise. Oral case presentations at team meetings provide an additional means by which the medical director can assess the quality of care provided by an individual team member and assess their understanding of the principles of care.

The assurance of quality care should be the ultimate responsibility of the medical director. However, in programs with several specialty teams, this responsibility should be delegated to a physician director of each team. Other aspects of the review of the performance of transport personnel may be delegated to nonphysician personnel. For example, the professional conduct of a neonatal transport nurse, if it does not impact directly on patient care, might be best reviewed by a nurse supervisor (e.g., nurse coordinator of the transport team).

The medical director is also responsible for ensuring that the transport team is properly equipped. The director should seek assistance in selecting equipment from those who will actually use the equipment and from biomedical engineers. The director must also consider financial constraints.

However, since the cost of equipment is usually relatively small in comparison to the operating costs of most programs, and because safe transport is highly dependent on adequate equipment, few compromises should be made in the selection of equipment.

ROLE OF THE ADVISORY BOARD

Transport programs are best viewed as an extension of the inpatient services to which they transport patients. As such, the program should be the servant of the inpatient critical care unit. Therefore, it is absolutely essential that a variety of personnel representing the affected inpatient units be involved in program administration in an advisory capacity. It is clearly impractical for a large number of individuals to participate directly in the day-to-day management of a transport service. However, representative input must be solicited on issues of broad impact.

The advisory board should include representatives from all inpatient services to which patients are transported. For multipurpose programs, this board might include the following representatives:

Directors of intensive care units
Director of perinatal medicine
Director of the emergency room
Representatives of other hospitals to which patients might be transported
Nursing administrator
Respiratory therapy administrator
Hospital communications director
Outreach education director
Director of public relations

The advisory group for programs that provide only neonatal transport can be less formal and more limited in size but should, nonetheless, appreciate the need for the cooperative effort of a variety of hospital-based services.

SPECIALTY TEAMS

The training and expertise of transport personnel determine the character of a transport program and define the complexity of care that can be provided during transports. Because of the wide variety of diseases encountered in the critically ill patients referred to most medical centers, many transport programs have developed two or more specialty teams. One team is usually a neonatal transport team. In recent years, neonatal teams have more frequently been composed of nonphysician personnel, which include some combination of nurse clinicians, nurse practitioners, specialty trained neonatal intensive care unit nurses, and respiratory therapists.

Two individuals are pivotal in the management of a neonatal transport team: the physician director and the nurse coordinator. The physician director is particularly important when transport is conducted exclusively by nonphysician personnel. The director is responsible for education, development of patient care protocols, and quality assurance. The nurse coordinator should assume responsibility for scheduling personnel, ordering supplies and equipment, and record keeping. The nurse coordinator should also supervise a system of peer review and, along with the physician director, should participate in the selection and training of other nursing personnel. Programs that use other types of nonphysician personnel (e.g., respiratory therapists) should also consider appointing an individual to coordinate the activities of these team members. Nonnursing personnel must have a supervisor appreciative of their unique contribution and background who can assist in their selection, training, and the review of their performance.

The composition of the team designated to transport maternal patients will often determine the complexity of illness of the maternal patients transported, as well as the supervision required by a member of the perinatal medical staff. In programs that depend on personnel with general training to transport all adult patients, members of the transport team are generally not expected to provide specialized diagnostic skill for perinatal medical problems and usually provide limited therapeutic intervention. In these programs, patient transport is typically by air; the service is used primarily as a rapid conveyance. In such a program, assistance from a member of the perinatal staff should be solicited for patient care review and personnel training, but physician directorship is best performed by an intensivist with a broader background. However, in programs with a sufficient number of maternal transports to justify a maternal transport team, a physician director with special training in perinatology and an obstetrical nurse coordinator are essential.

Specialty teams, composed of personnel skilled in the evaluation of maternal patients in the intrapartum period permit the two-way transport of a broader range of patients. In these programs, the perinatal consultant supervising a transport is no longer totally dependent on information provided by the referring physician. Further evaluation of the patient in the community hospital can be provided by the transport team. This results in the more precise identification of the risks and benefits of transport for each patient. A specialty team designated to transport maternal patients might include labor and delivery nurses, nurse midwives, intensive care nurses, obstetrical residents, and postdoctoral fellows in perinatology. This team should develop an administrative structure similar to a typical neonatal transport program.

THE PERINATAL/NEONATAL CONSULTANT

Success of a transport program is absolutely dependent on a responsive communication system. Referring personnel must have a single point of access to the program. Most programs provide a toll-free telephone number that connects referring personnel to a dispatch center or an operator capable of triaging calls. An alternative is for calls to be received directly in the perinatal center. A single phone call should provide the referring physician with all necessary services. This may begin with consultation regarding care of a patient or assistance in making the decision to transport the patient. The individual providing this consultation should logically have greater expertise and training than the referring physician. For this reason, a neonatologist, perinatologist, or postdoctoral fellow should provide this service for community physicians referring neonatal and maternal patients.

To properly advise a referring physician, the consultant must have an accurate knowledge of the resources of the community hospital and of the expertise of the referring physician. Once the decision has been made to transfer the patient, the decision to perform a one-way or a two-way transport must be made. In some programs, the appropriate mode of transportation must also be selected. This decision is particularly important in programs using helicopters because the cost of helicopter transportation, and its inherent risk, must be weighed against the potential benefit to the patient. The consultant or medical control officer must be knowledgeable in all these issues.

If two-way transport is indicated, the responsibility for the further communications required to initiate the transport rests entirely with personnel at the perinatal center. The sole responsibility of the referring physician should be to further evaluate and stabilize the patient to the limits of the capabilities of the referring hospital and staff. The consultant should minimize the impact of any delays in arrival of the transport team by providing extensive advice about further stabilization.

In many perinatal centers, adequate space, equipment, and staffing exists to accommodate nearly all referrals. At these centers, the consulting perinatologist or neonatologist need only make the decision that transport is necessary and activate the system. However, in a significant number of perinatal regions there is a critical shortage of neonatal intensive care unit beds. In these regions, the consultant must first make the decision that transport is indicated and then decide whether, at that point in time, the perinatal center can accommodate the patient. The consultant should always have this information. If beds are unavailable, the responsibility to locate an available bed should rest with personnel at the perinatal center.

During the transport, it is absolutely essential that a physician be identified to provide consultation to the transport team. This is particularly important for nonphysician-attended transport. In most states, nurse practice acts demand that a physician have direct communication with nursing personnel providing extended nursing care. This is almost always the case when nurses are performing invasive procedures. This medical control officer for each transport is logically the same perinatal or neonatal consultant who has provided consultation to the referring physician. This person will already have a reasonably precise understanding of the problems of the patient and the care provided by the referring personnel. He or she will have begun to advise the referring physician about further care, and therefore, should logically continue this advisory role with the transport team.

OTHER KEY INDIVIDUALS
*Chief Pilot or Chief Ambulance Driver*
The transportation vendor should provide a representative to contend with the transportation problems that will invariably arise. A designated individual with whom these problems can be dealt with directly is absolutely mandatory.

*Chief Dispatcher*
Communication problems are also fairly common in most transport programs. Because of the critical contribution of communications to the success of the transport program, an individual responsible for responding to these problems is essential.

## Transportation
SELECTION OF A VEHICLE
A variety of vehicles may be used for two-way transport of neonatal and perinatal patients. They include EMS ambulances, specially retrofitted vans, helicopters, and fixed-wing aircraft. The choice of a vehicle depends on the unique needs and features of each program, the resources of the sponsor institution, and the expected subsidies from patient reimbursements and government agencies.

When selecting a mode of transportation, one must consider the advantages and disadvantages of each in relation to the needs of the program.

Ambulances are available at most medical centers and are relatively inexpensive to operate. Vehicle maintenance and drivers' salaries are less costly than the costs of aircraft operation. Ambulances are almost always properly equipped to transport maternal patients but may not be ideally suited to accommodate neonates. Some centers circumvent this problem by using vehicles designed for and dedicated to neonatal transport. The disadvantage of ground transportation may be the excessive time required to travel between hospitals. This disadvantage is greatest when the distance between hospitals is great; when terrain, weather conditions, or traffic congestion slow travel; or when the resources of the referring hospital are extremely limited. Travel times in excess of 1 or 2 hours severely compromise the value of neonatal transport and make two-way maternal transport by ground almost totally ineffective.

The nonavailability of air transportation generally limits the scope of a transport program. For example, few maternal patients and almost no trauma patients will benefit from two-way ground transport. However, ground transport of neonatal patients may be quite satisfactory for regions that are relatively small. If the primary need of sponsor institutions in these regions is to transport neonates, then a program dependent on ground transportation may be a wise choice. Unfortunately marketing factors may also influence decisions regarding the choice of transportation. If institutions within a region compete for patients, the center with more rapid transportation and shorter response time will preferentially receive referrals. This is often true even when air transport offers little or no real benefit to the patient.

Hospital-based helicopters offer the most rapid door-to-door service. Under usual circumstances they travel about 3 times as fast as ground vehicles, and most hospitals now have some type of landing facility. Nearly all hospital-based helicopters are dedicated exclusively to air ambulance service and are, therefore, specially retrofitted to accommodate a variety of critically ill patients. However, noise and vibration levels in helicopters make auscultative assessment and manipulation of the patient difficult. An ambulance can be stopped at the roadside, if necessary, to permit a procedure to be performed or for the patient to be better evaluated. The patient compartment usually provides adequate space for two attendants to have access to the patient. Interruption of a helicopter flight is rarely practical, and the patient compartment in many aeromedical helicopters is too small to provide good access to the patient by more than one attendant. These disadvantages can be overcome by better preparation of the patient prior to transport and extensive electronic monitoring during transport.

There are both intuitive and proved benefits of helicopter transportation.

The most hazardous period in the care of a perinatal patient is often during the transport between institutions. Delivery of an infant en route is usually a catastrophe. Deterioration of a neonate may be equally life-threatening. With proper evaluation and preparation of the patient, neither of these situations is more likely to occur in a helicopter than in a ground vehicle. Because of the contracted time in transit in a helicopter, therefore, this form of transportation appears to offer theoretical advantages. Unfortunately this hypothesis has not been subjected to critical analysis.

An additional advantage of speed in the transport of maternal patients is the ability to transfer patients who, because of impending delivery, would not be eligible for ground transport. This advantage was demonstrated by Elliott et al in their report of 100 maternal patients transported by helicopter to a regional perinatal center in Southern California [12]. These patients were all transported from hospitals within 90 miles of the regional center. Seventy-five were attended during transport by an obstetrician from the regional center. They estimated that 25 patients would not have been transported, had helicopter transportation not been available, because of an imminent obstetrical emergency or impending delivery. Seven additional patients required stabilization prior to transport that was beyond the capability of the community hospital staff. The regional center was able to provide this care by rapidly transporting the perinatal staff to the patient. No patients delivered en route; all were delivered aseptically at the regional center. These findings are closely related to the problems of urban transportation and may not be applicable to all settings. However, the principles demonstrated in their study permit one to evaluate the potential benefits of helicopter transport for maternal patients in other regional perinatal programs.

A major disadvantage of helicopter transportation is the extremely high operational cost, which may be prohibitive for many medical centers. A helicopter prepared for medical use can cost more than $1.2 million, and operational expenses usually exceed $25,000 per month. The resulting cost for each transport, including personnel and equipment, often exceeds $2000, even in programs with a very high volume of transports. Costs of this magnitude can rarely be recovered by direct patient reimbursement. Although there are often long-term financial benefits to the sponsor institution, subsidization of the helicopter transport program may be a significant problem, thus, only institutions with substantial operating budgets can afford to sponsor such programs.

Another disadvantage of transport by helicopter is the inherent risk of this mode of transportation. Between 1980 and 1986, 66 serious aeromedical helicopter accidents occurred; 21 of these resulted in fatalities [9].

The accident rate during this period was 19.2 accidents (6.1 fatal accidents) per 100,000 patient transports. These rates are approximately 3 times the rates experienced by other commercial helicopter operations. Although the likelihood of mishap during any individual flight is extremely small, at the time of each request, the risks of the transport must be weighed against the potential benefit to the patient. Helicopters should not be used as a vehicle to transport patients with all varieties and acuities of illness, but rather should be reserved for those patients for whom the speed of transport is likely to affect outcome. Therefore, the selection of a helicopter for aeromedical transport should only be contemplated by medical centers who anticipate transporting a significant number of the most critically ill patients.

Ground ambulances, in contrast to helicopters, are typically already available to most medical centers, either through a private vendor or as a service of the institution. To dedicate a ground ambulance to perinatal transport may require little additional expense. Even the purchase of a dedicated vehicle is usually not a prohibitive expense. The usual cost per transport in a ground-based program is in the $300 to $600 range. These costs can often be recovered through reimbursements or, if unrecovered, will have less impact on the operational budget of the sponsor institution than the cost of air transportation.

Fixed-wing aircraft have limited application in perinatal transport. Since their speed is 5 to 6 times that of ground vehicles and about twice that of helicopters, their greatest utility is when hospitals are long distances apart. Fixed-wing aircraft usually offer time advantages only when hospitals are separated by more than 120 miles. The difficulty in coordinating ground transportation at each end of the flight and the necessity to disrupt care during the transfer between vehicles also create logistical problems. Currently, fixed-wing aircraft are in widespread use only in the western part of the United States, where distances between hospitals sometimes exceed 300 miles. At these distances, fixed-wing aircraft offer the only reasonable means of transporting perinatal patients.

Many successful transport programs have integrated two or more modes of transportation. These programs have the unique capability of matching the needs of individual patients with the most efficacious mode of transportation. Even programs that rely primarily on a single form of transportation should consider alternate forms or sources of transportation for those times when their primary vehicle is unavailable. Dependence on a single vehicle results in the complete interruption of the program when the vehicle is unavailable because duplicate requests for transport are received or when the vehicle is out of service for repair or because of weather conditions. The latter situation is a particular problem for programs dependent on aircraft. Backup transportation may be provided through contractual arrangement with the primary vendor. For example, most hospital-based helicopter vendors will, as part of their contractual arrangement with the sponsor hospital, provide a backup helicopter during periods when the primary helicopter is out of service for repairs. Collaborative arrangements for backup service may also be developed with neighboring helicopter programs, if distances are not prohibitive. It is advisable for all hospital-based helicopter programs to prearrange for the availability of ground transportation when inclement weather prevents air travel.

VEHICLE OWNERSHIP
Issues related to hospital ownership of transport vehicles are very different for ground vehicles versus aircraft. Many municipal hospitals have owned and operated EMS ground vehicles for years. For these institutions, adding a vehicle for perinatal transport is generally less costly than procuring this service from an outside vendor. Even institutions that have never sponsored any type of patient transport system can generally afford the start-up costs of a ground transportation system. In addition, the operation of ground vehicles is not as complex as the operation of aircraft and is within the limits of expertise of many hospital administrators. An alternative to hospital ownership is to contract with a local ambulance service to provide a vehicle and drivers dedicated to perinatal transport. The sponsoring institution will then benefit from the economies of scale appreciated by the ambulance service. This arrangement is sometimes more cost-effective for institutions without existing transportation systems.

Hospital ownership of aircraft is a much more complicated proposition. The potential advantages of ownership are almost exclusively financial. Proprietary, for-profit medical centers may gain a tax advantage from ownership. However, since nearly all medical centers that sponsor perinatal transport are nonprofit or state institutions, this advantage is usually lost. The few institutions that can afford to purchase the vehicle outright can appreciate substantial savings by avoiding costly finance charges. The major risk of ownership in these situations is the possibility that, after a period of time, the hospital may wish to change to a different vehicle.

Although hospital *ownership* of aircraft may be desirable in some situations, *operation* of the vehicle by a hospital is very seldom a wise choice. Few hospitals employ personnel who have any experience in the operation of aircraft, and those hospitals that attempt to provide this service may encounter several difficulties. The hospital staff is burdened with the responsibility of hiring mechanics and pilots and evaluating their performance, a responsibility that they are usually ill equipped to perform. Most hospital-based programs have only one vehicle [8], and, thus, cannot provide a backup vehicle during periods when the primary vehicle is out of service. A vendor who supplies vehicles for several hospitals will usually provide this vital service. The financial risk involved in maintaining helicopters is significant. Because of the relatively large number of close tolerance parts in a helicopter, the potential for premature and unexpected parts failure is great. This can result in unexpected and prolonged periods of vehicle downtime for hospital operators who have limited parts inventories. Out-of-service time can cause a significant loss of revenue and tarnish the image of the medical center. In addition, the cost of the purchase of parts beyond the warranty period can be substantial. Further, financial incentive for ownership is diminished because of the significantly higher insurance premiums charged to inexperienced operators without a proved safety record. Most hospitals sponsoring aeromedical helicopter programs have agreed that the disadvantages of operating helicopters outweigh the advantages. Fewer than 10 percent of these programs own and operate their own vehicles [8].

Although a variety of contractual arrangements exist between aircraft vendors and medical centers, the most common is a "turnkey" lease. Under this type of lease arrangement, the hospital typically is responsible for providing the medical personnel and equipment. The aircraft operator (vendor or company) provides an aircraft chosen by the hospital and retrofitted to the specifications of the medical staff. The operator also hires pilots and mechanics and is entirely responsible for the safe operation of the vehicle. The contract generally requires the hospital to pay a fixed amount per month to cover the operator's fixed costs. The hospital also pays an amount for variable costs, depending on use of the service per month. This type of lease arrangement decreases costs somewhat during periods of low volume but also creates financial incentives for high use because the fixed operational costs can be apportioned to more transports. Lease arrangements also minimize start-up costs and permit hospitals to discontinue the service if it proves to be unsuccessful. The hospital also has the option of changing vehicles at the end of the lease period without penalty.

Even with strict attention to the potential economies in program management, patient transport systems are extremely expensive to operate. However, unlike most other intensive care services, transport services are highly portable and may be shared by several medical centers. Consortium arrangements have been constructed in many parts of the country. These arrangements vary considerably. Vehicles provided by a single vendor may be shared by several institutions, each of which provide their own transport personnel and equipment. Each institution participates in the contract with the vendor. This concept can be extended by using specialty teams from designated participating institutions to deliver patients to any institution within the consortium. For example, a consortium including a children's hospital, a general hospital, and an academic medical center might develop a neonatal/pediatric transport team at the children's hospital and an adult/maternal transport team at the academic medical center. These teams might use a common vehicle to transport patients to the most appropriate available bed. The expense of such a program might be shared, based on the relative use of the service by each institution. Another model for shared transport services is exemplified by the program administered by the Maryland Institute for Emergency Medical Services. This is a government-funded program, with vehicles and teams distributed throughout Maryland. These vehicles and teams are available to transport patients to the closest appropriate medical center.

Consortium arrangements are most efficacious when the user medical centers are in close proximity to one another and are only possible if significant "political" barriers can be overcome. Participating institutions always sacrifice some identity in such programs, and hence some public relations benefits, but may appreciate substantial financial benefits. Inherent in any successful consortium arrangement is a highly sophisticated communication system that includes the capability to triage calls equitably so that easy access to the system is available to all participants.

### Relations between the Perinatal Centers and Community Hospitals

A transport program often dramatically affects the relationship between a perinatal center and its catchment area hospitals and may be a major determinant of referral patterns. However, many other factors affect the quality of this relationship. These may include the following:

Geographical proximity of the institutions to the center
Nature of regionalization of perinatal care
Facilities, personnel, and services available at the perinatal center
Location of training of personnel at the community hospital
Admission policy of the perinatal center
Educational opportunities for community hospital personnel provided by the perinatal center

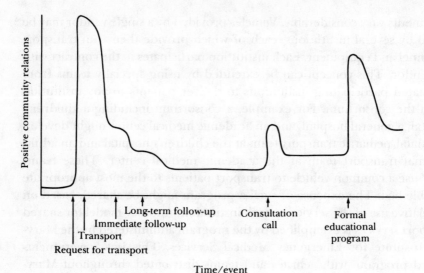

Fig. 2-7. Graphic representation of the potential impact of a transport program on relations with referring hospitals. Events or points in time that may affect relations are listed below the horizontal axis.

The relative contribution of each factor is highly dependent on the unique features of each institution and the environment in which they deliver perinatal care.

In general, events or points in time when direct contact between personnel at the community hospital and the perinatal center occur have the greatest impact on the relationship between institutions. A transport program and its related activities include many such events. Therefore, transport programs have the potential to dramatically improve relations between institutions or may cause irreparable damage. The following section examines the manner in which transport program activities may affect the relationship between a perinatal center and community hospitals. Figure 2-7 depicts graphically the potential positive influence these activities may have on this relationship.

The moment that a perinatal center advertises the existence of a transport program, even before the transport of a patient, the relationship between the center and the hospitals it serves may begin to change. The assumption is often made by community health care professionals that, because the perinatal center has offered this new service, other new services must be available within the institution. Similarly, since patient transport often involves very sophisticated technology, many may assume that the services within the perinatal center are equally sophisticated. This perception is usually correct and is advantageous to the perinatal center. However, announcing the existence of a transport program is not without certain liabilities. The perinatal center must provide the service that it has advertised. Unfulfilled promises are worse than promises never made. In addition, the perinatal center must be prepared for the invariable influx of additional new patients and, possibly, some negative reaction from competing perinatal centers in the region.

Each request for transfer or consultation represents an opportunity for success or failure. For this event to be a success, the referring personnel must have easy access to the required resources of the perinatal center. If consultation is sought, an appropriate and knowledgeable consultant must be readily available. If transport is necessary, the transport team and vehicle should respond within a reasonable period of time. Since there are times when either the team or the vehicle will be unavailable, personnel at the perinatal center must be prepared to offer alternatives. Finally, the necessary inpatient services must be available. Since many perinatal centers have chronic bed shortages or may lack certain subspecialty services, plans for alternative sites for perinatal care must be well established.

The event that has perhaps the greatest impact on the relationship between institutions is the transport of a patient. The image of the perinatal center will be bolstered if response to a transport request is prompt; it may be tarnished if there are avoidable delays. Rapidity of response often seems critical from a public relations standpoint, even when the patient's medical needs do not necessitate speed. Although perinatal center personnel usually consider response time to be the time between the decision to transport a patient and departure from the perinatal center, referring personnel consider this interval to be the time from the request for transport to the arrival of the team. All reasonable efforts should be made to constrict this latter time interval. Perhaps of greatest importance is that the community hospital be *accurately* informed about the estimated time of arrival of the transport team.

It is imperative that the team dispatched to transport a patient has the requisite training and skills to adequately care for that patient. This generally means that the care provided by the team will either be a continuum of the ongoing care in the referral hospital or an improvement on that care. In the past, many have felt that physician attendance during transport was mandatory. Recent experience has demonstrated that this is neither practical nor necessary, particularly for neonatal patients [26]. In most parts of the country, community health care providers now also believe in this principle. They have become confident in nonphysician transport through repeated exposure to skilled transport professionals. However, this confidence can easily be eroded through a very limited number of experiences when the referring personnel perceive that the expertise of the transport team does not meet the needs of the patient.

Everyone involved in the conduct of a transport must appreciate the psychological milieu surrounding this event. The transport is often emotionally charged because of the acute and critical illness of the patient. Emotions may be somewhat fragile because of the invariable feelings of inadequacy on the part of the personnel in the community hospital. Referring personnel may be very sensitive to criticism. The consultant receiving the request for transport and the members of the transport team should be very attentive to the manner in which they communicate with referring personnel. This should begin with appreciation for the contribution that the community hospital personnel have made to the care of the patient. For example, the transport team should seek information from referring hospital personnel regarding the needs of the patient and ask for their assistance in preparing the patient for transport. The team should explain the need for performing all procedures. Referring personnel may have elected not to perform certain procedures (e.g., endotracheal intubation) because of a lack of appreciation of the transport environment. An explanation of the unique features of this environment will usually convince referring personnel that a particular procedure is necessary and also eliminate any feeling on their part that it was a procedure that they should have known to perform. Disagreements between transport personnel and referring physicians will invariably arise, generally concerning the necessity of further stabilization and observation prior to transport. Transport personnel, particularly nonphysician personnel, should avoid confrontation in these situations. Direct communication between the consultant and the referring physician is generally the best way to resolve such disagreements.

Communication between the perinatal center and the community hospital should not cease at the end of a transport. A major source of frustration for many conscientious community practitioners is the referral of patients about which they receive no follow-up information. Providing this information may be a valuable educational tool and is another opportunity to recognize the importance of the primary care provider in regionalized care. Failure of the perinatal center to provide follow-up is one of the most common complaints made by community hospital personnel.

There are at least two critical periods of time during which information should be provided, immediately after the transport and prior to anticipated discharge or back transport. Communication after the delivery of an obstetric patient is also essential. Direct phone communication, although time consuming, is usually most beneficial. It affords an opportunity for a more extensive explanation of the patient's problems and for an exchange of questions and answers. Plans for further communication can also be discussed. Prior to discharge, the referring physician will need to have a complete understanding of the problems encountered during the hospitalization to provide appropriate follow-up care. A phone call at this time is usually appreciated by the community physician. However, since detailed information generally needs to be transmitted, it is wise to follow this conversation with a letter or discharge summary.

It is also imperative that community hospital personnel be notified of the death of a patient. This notification should rarely be delayed for any significant period of time. Immediate phone communication should occur with caretakers of a mother whose infant has died following neonatal transport. Failure to fulfill this obligation may result in embarrassment for the referring physician and anger toward the perinatal center.

Any system of communication should recognize the contribution of all perinatal health care professionals. For example, nurses in community hospitals often play an integral role in the care of perinatal patients and have a keen interest in their outcome. Communication with these professionals is logically the responsibility of the appropriate nonphysician members of the transport teams. Many transport programs have developed schemes for communicating with community hospital nonphysician personnel that parallel the efforts made by physicians at the perinatal center.

### Relationship between Outreach Education and Transport Program

An integral component of regionalized perinatal care is an educational program designed to maintain the competency of health care professionals at a level commensurate with the demands of patient care. The responsibility for the development of these programs often rests with the regional perinatal center. This responsibility was proposed by the professional organizations of pediatrics and obstetrics and is detailed in the publication *Guidelines for Perinatal Care:* "Each regional perinatal care center is responsible for organizing an education program tailored to the identified needs of the perinatal health professionals employed in community institutions in its area" [2].

Many perinatal centers have chosen to integrate the activities of transport programs and outreach education programs. This is often a logical choice. Transport activities represent one of the few points in time when perinatal center staff interact directly with personnel in community hospitals. In addition, the transport of a patient requires a thorough retrospective review by members of the staff at the perinatal center that includes the care provided for the patient by the community hospital. These interactions provide an opportunity to develop the close relationships necessary for successful outreach education and permit direct observation of the resources and needs of the community hospital.

Many transport programs systematically review transport records to identify the needs of individual community hospitals. For example, indicators of the degree of stability (e.g., body temperature, arterial pressure, pH, blood sugar, and blood oxygenation) of referred infants on arrival of the transport team at a community hospital might be tabulated over a period of time. Recurrent hypothermia might indicate the need for education about this aspect of care. The frequent need for further stabilization by the transport team, particularly for the performance of invasive procedures, might indicate the need for instruction about appropriate intervention in preparation for transport. Although this type of surveillance is only representative of the care provided to a small segment of the entire patient population of a community hospital, it may accurately reflect deficiencies in care provided to patients not requiring transport as well. In this manner, education programs can be tailored to identified deficiencies.

The formal review of the care of all patients transported between a community hospital and a perinatal center (transport conference) has also been used as a forum for outreach education [23]. The Dartmouth-Hitchcock Medical Center in conjunction with the Vermont College of Medicine has used this educational format in communities in the two states served by these centers. The details of the preparation for these conferences and the format of the conference are outlined in Tables 2-2 and 2-3. Active participation is required by members of the medical staffs of both the perinatal center and the community hospital. Records from the transport program provide the database for selection of patients. The identification of high-risk perinatal patients and their preparation for transport are a major focus of discussion. From their experience, the perinatal/neonatal staff at Dartmouth and Vermont have concluded that outreach programs that involve a critique of the care of transported patients are an effective means of peer education.

Regardless of the format of educational programs, transport personnel are often a vital educational resource. Although usually not educators by training, transport personnel are often among the most knowledgeable and skilled members of the perinatal center staff. They generally have a close relationship with the staffs of the community hospitals. Because they make repeated visits to community hospitals at times when deficiencies in

Table 2-2. *Sample protocol and timetable for a transport conference**

| Protocol | Responsible personnel | Time prior to conference |
|---|---|---|
| Set up<br>Written confirmation<br>Explanation of format<br>Request for suggested cases for discussion | Nurse coordinator | 1 month |
| Selection of patients for discussion | Nurse coordinator<br>Community hospital nursery nurses and pediatricians<br>Regional perinatal program physician | 3–4 weeks |
| Mail conference materials<br>Case summaries, one per local physician<br>Case summaries, two per unit for nursing staff | Nurse coordinator | 2 weeks |
| Review clinical details of<br>Transport<br>Hospital stay<br>Disposition<br>Follow-up clinic | Regional perinatal program physicians (neonatologist, obstetrician)<br>Regional perinatal program nurse coordinator | 1 week |
| Review clinical details of care at referral hospital | Community hospital pediatrician and obstetrician | 1 week |

*Adapted from Little, G. A., and Webb, R. P. In B. S. Raff (ed.), *Perinatal Outreach Education: Methods, Evaluation, and Financing*. White Plains, N.Y.: March of Dimes, 1981. P. 41.

care are most likely to be apparent, they are ideally suited to identify the educational needs of the hospital. This is particularly true of deficiencies that are not easily identified through retrospective review of the care of transported patients (e.g., the improper use of equipment). They are also in a good position to recognize local limitations regarding available equipment and services, which may ultimately limit the beneficial impact of peer education. Finally, the interaction between the transport team and the community hospital staff at the time of a transport offers a unique opportunity for educational exchange that cannot be duplicated in another setting.

Many outreach education programs do not have a formal relationship with the perinatal transport program at their sponsoring institution. Although these programs may be highly successful, they probably do not achieve their maximum impact if they fail to use the resources of the transport service.

*Table 2-3. Format for a transport conference*

| Activity | Participants |
| --- | --- |
| CONFERENCE | |
| Review of birthweight gestational age grid and problem list, including all patients transported to center | Regional perinatal program (RPP) physicians<br>Community hospital staff |
| Presentation of clinical history through time of transport | Community hospital physician |
| Presentation of clinical history from transport to disposition from intensive care nursery | Regional perinatal program physicians |
| Discussion of clinical details at community hospital and center | Community hospital staff<br>Regional perinatal program staff |
| Didactic presentation on specific topic (optional) | Regional perinatal program staff |
| Completion of conference evaluation forms | Community hospital staff |
| FOLLOW-UP (2–4 WEEKS LATER) | |
| Information requests answered and requests for education input from RPP program processed | Nurse coordinator |
| Continuing education certificates processed | Nurse coordinator |

Source: G. A. Little, and R. P. Webb. In Raff, B. S. (ed.), *Perinatal Outreach Education; Methods, Evaluation, and Financing.* March of Dimes, 1981. P. 41.

## Neonatal Back Transport

The evolution of regionalized perinatal care has resulted in a dramatic increase in the number of infants cared for in perinatal centers; much of this increase has been in low birth weight infants. In addition, the survival of these infants has increased dramatically. The net result has been an exponential growth in the demand for neonatal intensive care beds. In many regions of the country, the addition of resources has not kept pace with the demand. An effective means of managing this problem has been to transfer convalescing infants to Level I and II centers after the resolution of their acute illness and prior to their discharge home. This is a concept commonly referred to as "back transport."

The benefits of back transport in relation to the improved efficiency of bed use at the perinatal center have been extensively studied for the perinatal region associated with the University of Utah Hospital (UUH) [17]. During 1980, 172 infants, or 65 percent of eligible infants, were back transported to Level I and II community hospitals. Infants returned to Level II hospitals were smaller and required more complex care than those returned to Level I hospitals. Back transport deferred 3892 days of hospitalization from the UUH to community hospitals. This equated to eliminating the need for at least 10 beds at full occupancy at the UUH. Although these results cannot necessarily be extrapolated to all perinatal regions, it is apparent that back transport is a means of preserving the often scarce resources of the perinatal center for those patients in greatest need.

Other potential advantages of back transport include the more efficient use of nursery beds in community hospitals, improved relations between the perinatal center and community hospitals, and greater opportunity for parental visitation with facilitation of parent-infant attachment. Back transport affords an opportunity for the continuing care physician to become familiar with the infant prior to discharge home. In addition, the cost of convalescent care in community hospitals is usually less than in the perinatal center. Thus, back transport can result in substantial cost savings even when the expense of transport is subtracted from the cost of convalescent care [3].

There do not appear to be significant disadvantages to a well-organized and properly supervised system of back transport. Although the safety of returning relatively healthy infants to community hospitals has been reported [19, 20, 28], the outcome of back-transported infants with complex illnesses has not been examined. However, it seems likely that, if prudent decisions are made regarding the location of continued care for individual infants, back transport can be both safe and efficacious.

Because of the unique features of each perinatal care region and the varying capabilities of community hospitals, it is unreasonable to create narrowly defined categories of infants eligible for back transport. However, general guidelines may be helpful. Infants should have recovered from the acute phase of their major disease process. The evolution of a new significant problem should be unlikely. Infants should have reached the point in convalescence when major complications (e.g., bronchopulmonary dysplasia, patent ductus arteriosus, intraventricular hemorrhage) will have been recognized. Some community hospitals are capable of managing these latter complications. In these situations, stability of the problem should be ensured and a treatment plan well established. From these general principles, it may be useful to create specific criteria for back transport. These might include the following:

No requirement for mechanical ventilation
Removal of endotracheal tube
Removal of central catheters
Requirement for less than 40 percent oxygen
Initiation of enteral feedings
No requirement for hyperalimentation

Stable body weight or gaining weight
Absent or occasional mild apneic episodes

To make appropriate decisions about individual infants, one needs an accurate knowledge of the resources of the community hospital. Communication with the local pediatric caretaker is invaluable. It may also be useful to catalogue the resources of each community hospital. This practice has been useful in perinatal care regions that are very large, with hospitals of diverse capability.

Unlike the transport of acutely ill neonates, back transport can be safely conducted by most community hospitals. However, various practical constraints often determine the assignment of this responsibility. Community hospitals usually rely on local EMS ambulances for transportation. Removing this vital resource from the local community can be hazardous to its service area. If backup service is not available, transport may have to be performed by the perinatal center. In spite of the relative well-being of most back-transported infants, attention to certain aspects of care during transport is necessary. The community hospital must provide equipment sufficient to transport the infant in a neutral thermal environment and a caretaker who can manage minor emergencies. By using the transport service of the perinatal center, one can eliminate nearly all the hazards of the transport, but it may interfere significantly with the primary responsibility of the service to transport acutely ill patients.

### References

1. Alden, E. R., et al. Morbidity and mortality of infants weighing less than 1000 grams in an intensive care nursery. *Pediatrics* 50:40, 1972.
2. American Academy of Pediatrics Committee on Fetus and Newborn and American College of Obstetricians and Gynecologists Committee on Obstetrics: Maternal and Fetal Medicine. *Guidelines for Perinatal Care.* Evanston, Ill.: American Academy of Pediatrics and American College of Obstetricians and Gynecologists, 1983. P. 45.
3. Bose, C. L., LaPine, T. R., and Jung, A. L. Neonatal back-transport. Cost effectiveness. *Med. Care* 23:14, 1985.
4. Bostick, J. S., Hsiao, H. S., and Lawson, E. E. A minicomputer-based perinatal/neonatal telecommunications network. *Pediatrics* 71:272, 1983.
5. Carrier, C., et al. Effect of neonatal intensive care on mortality rates in the province of Quebec (abstract). *Pediatr. Res.* 6:408, 1972.
6. Chance, G. W., et al. Neonatal transport: a controlled study of skilled assistance. *J. Pediatr.* 93:662, 1978.
7. Chance, G. W., O'Brien, M. J., and Sawyer, P. R. Transportation of sick neonates, 1972: An unsatisfactory aspect of medical care. *Can. Med. Assoc. J.* 109:847, 1973.
8. Collett, H. M. (ed.). Hospital-based helicopter programs. *Hosp. Aviat.* 5:25, 1986.

9. Collett, H. M. Aeromedical accident trends. *Hosp. Aviat.* 6:6, 1987.
10. Committee on Perinatal Health. *Toward Improving the Outcome of Pregnancy.* White Plains, N.Y.: National Foundation—March of Dimes, 1976. P. 2.
11. Committee on Perinatal Health. *Toward Improving the Outcome of Pregnancy.* White Plains, N.Y.: National Foundation—March of Dimes, 1976. P. 36.
12. Elliott, J. P., O'Keefe, D. F., and Freeman, R. K. Helicopter transportation of patients with obstetric emergencies in an urban area. *Am. J. Obstet. Gynecol.* 143:157, 1982.
13. Harris, B. A., et al. In utero versus neonatal transportation of high-risk perinates: A comparison. *Obstet. Gynecol.* 57:496, 1981.
14. Harris, T. R., Isaman, J., and Giles, H. R. Improved neonatal survival through maternal transport. *Obstet. Gynecol.* 52:294, 1978.
15. Harvey, K., and Bowes, W. A. Maternal-fetal transport. Reflections on experience at University of Colorado Medical Center. *Perinat. Neonat.* 5:53, 1981.
16. Hood, J. L., et al. Effectiveness of the neonatal transport team. *Crit. Care Med.* 11:419, 1983.
17. Jung, A. L., and Bose, C. L. Back transport of neonates: Improved efficiency of tertiary nursery bed utilization. *Pediatrics* 71:918, 1983.
18. Kitchen, W. H., and Campbell, D. G. Controlled trial of intensive care for very low birth weight infants. *Pediatrics* 48:411, 1971.
19. Leake, R. D., Loew, A. D., and Oh, W. Retransfer of convalescent infants from newborn intensive care to community intermediate care nurseries. *Clin. Pediatr.* 15:293, 1976.
20. Lynch, T. M. Back Transport of Infants From Neonatal Intensive Care Units for Convalescent Care: Is It Safe? Dissertation, University of Utah, 1984.
21. Merenstein, G. B., et al. An analysis of air transport results in the sick newborn. II. Antenatal and neonatal referrals. *Am. J. Obstet. Gynecol.* 128:520, 1977.
22. Pettett, G., Merenstein, G. B., and Battaglia, F. G. An analysis of air transport results in the sick newborn infant. *Pediatrics* 55:774, 1975.
23. Philips, A. G. S., Little, G. A., and Lucey, J. F. The transport conference as a teaching strategy. *Perinat. Neonat.* 8:63, 1984.
24. Ramamurthy, R. S., et al. Transport of high-risk neonates. Part I: clinical and metabolic observations. *I.M.J.* 150:518, 1976.
25. Roy, R. N. D. Neonatal transport. *Med. J. Aust.* 2:862, 1977.
26. Thompson, T. R. Neonatal transport nurses: An analysis of their role in the transport of newborn infants. *Pediatrics* 65:887, 1980.
27. Vapaavouri, E. K., and Raiha, N. C. R. Intensive care of small premature infants. I. Clinical findings and results of treatment. *Acta. Paediatr. Scand.* 59:353, 1970.
28. Zarif, M. A., Rest, J., and Vidyasagar, D. Early retransfer: A method of optimal bed utilization of NICU beds. *Crit. Care Med.* 7:327, 1979.

## Chapter Appendix I: Perinatal Care Programs

| | Level I | Level II | Level III |
|---|---|---|---|
| GENERAL<br>Function | Risk assessment<br>Management of uncomplicated perinatal care<br>Stabilization of unexpected problems<br>Initiation of maternal and neonatal transports<br>Patient and community education<br>Data collection and evaluation | Level I plus:<br>Diagnosis and treatment of selected high-risk pregnancies and neonatal problems<br>Initiation and acceptance of maternal-fetal and neonatal transports<br>Education of allied health personnel<br>Residency education (affiliation) | Levels I and II plus:<br>Diagnosis and treatment of all perinatal problems<br>Acceptance and direction of maternal-fetal and neonatal transports<br>Research and outcome surveillance<br>Graduate and postgraduate education<br>System management |
| Types of patients | Uncomplicated, emergency, and remedial problems such as lack of progress, immediate resuscitation of asphyxiated neonates, uterine atony, nursery care of large premature neonates (>2000 g) without risk factors, physiologic jaundice | Level I plus:<br>Selected problems such as preeclampsia, premature labor at 32 weeks and later, mild-to-moderate respiratory distress syndrome, suspected neonatal sepsis, hypoglycemia, neonates of diabetic mothers, postasphyxia without life-threatening sequelae | Levels I and II plus:<br>Premature rupture of membranes at 24–26 weeks, severe maternal medical complications, pregnancy with concurrent cancer, complicated antenatal genetic problems, prematurity at 26–32 weeks (500–1250 g), severe respiratory distress syndrome, sepsis, severe postasphyxia, symptomatic congenital cardiac and other systems disease, neonates with special needs such as hyperalimentation, prolonged mechanical ventilation |

|  | Level I | Level II | Level III |
|---|---|---|---|
| Location and number of births, neonatal beds | Located within Level II or III hospital or in sparsely populated or isolated areas; at least 1 birth/day unless in isolated area | Medium and large communities, may be part of Level III facility, several births/day, 3–4 neonatal beds/1000 births served | Medium and large communities, usually in academic centers, several births/day, 1 intensive care neonatal bed/1000 births served in addition to Level II |
| **SPACE** Sq ft/bed | Delivery/resuscitation (120) Admission/observation (40) Newborn nursery (20) Postpartum unit (100) | Level I plus: Intermediate nursery (50) Continuous/convalescent nursery (30) | Level I and II plus: Intensive neonatal (80–100) |
| **PERSONNEL** Chief of service | One physician responsible for perinatal care (or codirectors from obstetrics and pediatrics) | Joint planning: Obstetrics: Board-certified obstetrician with certification, special interest, experience, or training in maternal-fetal medicine; Pediatrics: Board-certified pediatrician with certification, special interest, experience or training in neonatology | Codirectors: Obstetrics: Full-time board-certified obstetrician with special competence in maternal-fetal medicine; Pediatrics: Full-time board-certified pediatrician with special competence in neonatal medicine |
| Other physicians | Physician (or certified nurse-midwife) at all deliveries, Anesthesia services, Physician care for neonates | Level I plus: Board-certified director of anesthesia services Medical, surgical, radiology, pathology consultation | Levels I and II plus: Anesthesiologists with special training or experience in perinatal and pediatric anesthesia Obstetric and pediatric subspecialists |

*Chapter Appendix I: (continued)*

| | Level I | Level II | Level III |
|---|---|---|---|
| Supervisory nurse | RN in charge of perinatal facilities | Obstetrics: RN with education and experience in normal and high-risk pregnancy only responsible<br>Pediatrics: RN with education and experience in treatment of sick neonates only responsible | Supervisor of perinatal services with advanced skills<br>Separate head nurses for maternal-fetal and neonatal services |
| Staff nurse–patient ratio | Normal labor (1:2)<br>Delivery in second stage (1:1)<br>Oxytocin inductions (1:2)<br>Cesarean delivery (2:1)<br>Normal nursery (1:6–8) | Level I plus:<br>Complicated labor/delivery (1:1)<br>Intermediate nursery (1:3–4) | Levels I and II plus:<br>Intensive neonatal care (1:1–2)<br>Critical care of unstable neonate (2:1) |
| Other personnel | LPN, assistants under direction of head nurse | Level I plus:<br>Social service, biomedical, respiratory therapy, laboratory as needed | Level I plus:<br>Designated and often full-time social service, respiratory therapy, biomedical engineering, laboratory technician<br>Nurse-clinician and specialists<br>Nurse program and education coordinators |
| OBSTETRIC UNITS<br>Admission/observation | Close to labor and delivery, comfortable, room to ambulate | Level I plus:<br>Beds, space for diagnostic procedures, possible emergency delivery | Levels I and II plus:<br>Other bed designated for observation |

| | | | |
|---|---|---|---|
| Family waiting | | Level I | Level I |
| Labor | Nearby/adjacent<br>Single: 140 sq ft multiple, 80 sq ft/patient<br>Beds adjustable and moveable to delivery, may be used as birthing bed<br>Full utilities, including auxilliary electrical, oxygen, suction<br>Communication system<br>Full routine patient care and CPR equipment<br>Secure medication area<br>Monitoring capabilities | Level I | Level I |
| Birthing (labor/delivery/recovery) | Combined equipment for labor and delivery, may be concealed<br>Adequate space, equipment for ambulation, support person | Level I | Level I |
| Delivery (vaginal and operative) | Contiguous to labor; at least 2 available, with 1 equipped for cesarean delivery<br>Operating room in design<br>Equipment/supplies necessary for normal delivery and management of complications, including surgical intervention | Level I (actual number of delivery rooms depends on total births) plus:<br>Intensive care room in labor/delivery area for patients with significant complication | Levels I and II plus:<br>Intensive care area |

*Chapter Appendix I: (continued)*

| | Level I | Level II | Level III |
|---|---|---|---|
| Antepartum and postpartum area | Contiguous with nursery<br>Large enough to accommodate mother, baby, visitors<br>Maximum 2 mothers/room<br>100 sq ft/patient in multiple patient rooms<br>Communication system<br>Hospital standard utilities | Level I | Level I |
| **NURSERY**<br>Resuscitation | 100 footcandles illumination<br>Overhead radiant heat<br>Heating pad<br>Wall clock<br>Resuscitation and stabilization equipment<br>Designated area (40 sq ft) or room (120 sq ft)<br>Full utilities, including suction, oxygen, compressed air, electrical outlets | Level I | Level I |
| Admission/ observation | Near or adjacent to delivery/cesarean birth room, may be part of maternal recovery area<br>40 sq ft/neonate<br>Equipment as in resuscitation area | May be located in newborn or continuing care area | Level II |

| | | | |
|---|---|---|---|
| Newborn nursery | Close to postpartum area<br>Beds and equipment to exceed obstetric beds by 20–30%<br>20 sq ft/neonate<br>Resuscitation equipment 1 electrical outlet/2 beds<br>1 $O_2$, air suction/5–6 beds | Level I | Level I |
| Continuing care | Usually not located in Level 1 | Near intermediate nursery<br>30 sq ft/neonate<br>Resuscitation equipment<br>4 electrical outlets, 1 $O_2$, 1 air, 1 suction/neonate | Level II |
| Intermediate care | Not present | Near delivery and intensive care nurseries<br>Full life support and monitoring in addition to resuscitation equipment<br>50 sq ft/neonate<br>8 electrical, 2 $O_2$, 2 compressed air, 2 suction outlets/neonate | Level II |
| Intensive care | Not present | Present in some hospitals | Near delivery/cesarean birth rooms<br>80–100 sq ft/neonate<br>12 electrical, 2 $O_2$, 2 compressed air, 2 suction outlets/neonate<br>Full life support, monitoring, and resuscitation equipment |
| ANCILLARY SUPPORT<br>Operating room | Technicians on call 24 h/day, available within 15–30 min | Technicians immediately available for emergency situations | Level II, may be in delivery room area |

# Chapter Appendix I: (continued)

| | Level I | Level II | Level III |
|---|---|---|---|
| **Laboratory (microtechnique for neonates)** | | | |
| Within 15 min | Hematocrit | Blood gases, blood type and Rh | Level II |
| Within 1 h | Glucose, BUN, creatinine, blood gases, routine urinalysis | Level I plus: Electrolytes, coagulation studies, blood available from type and screen program | Levels I and II plus: Special blood and amniotic fluid tests |
| With 1–6 hr | CBC, platelet appearance on smear, blood chemistries, blood type and cross matched, Coombs' test, bacterial smear | Level I plus: Coagulation studies, magnesium, urine, electrolytes, and chemistries | Levels I and II |
| Within 24–48 hr | Bacterial cultures and antibiotic sensitivity | Level I plus: Liver function test, Metabolic screening | Levels I and II |
| Within hospital or facilities available | Viral cultures | Level I | Level I plus: Laboratory facilities available |
| **Radiography and ultrasound** | Technicians on call 24 hr/day, available in 30 min; Technicians experienced in performing abdominal, pelvic, and OB ultrasound examinations; Professional interpretation available on 24-hr basis | Experienced radiology technicians immediately available in hospital (ultrasound on call); Professional interpretation immediately available; Portable x-ray equipment; Ultrasound equipment may be in labor and delivery or nursery areas | Level II plus: Computerized axial tomography |

| | Level I | Level II | Level III |
|---|---|---|---|
| | Portable x-ray and ultrasound equipment available to labor and delivery rooms and to nurseries | Sophisticated equipment for emergency gastrointestinal, genitourinary or CNS studies available 24 hr/day | Level II plus: Resource center for network; Direct line communication to labor and delivery area and nurseries |
| Blood bank | Technicians on call 24 hr/day, available in 30 min, performing routine blood banking procedures | Experienced technicians immediately available in hospital for blood banking procedures and identification of irregular antibodies; Blood component therapy readily available | |
| Examination and treatment room | Pelvic examination; Culture of cervix and uterus | Level I plus: Amniocentesis; Equipment for removal of suture for cerclage | Levels I and II plus: Services within unit |
| Auxiliary areas | Parent education; Conference room; Locker room (may be remote); Physician on-call room nearby | Level I plus: Breast-feeding area within unit; Parent waiting room for intensive care | Levels I and II plus: All areas within unit; Conference/lecture room as necessary for professional/regional education commitments |
| | Laboratory within unit for hematocrit, centrifuge for dip stick for urine, albumin, glucose, microscope | Level I plus: Refrigerator to hold cultures, materials; Gram's stain material | Levels I and II |

Reproduced with permission from American Academy of Pediatrics Committee on Fetus and Newborn and American College of Obstetricians and Gynecologists Committee on Obstetrics: Maternal and Fetal Medicine *Guidelines for Perinatal Care.* Evanston, Ill.: American Academy of Pediatrics and American College of Obstetricians and Gynecologists, 1983.

# 3

# Financing a Perinatal Transport Program in the United States

Herman M. Risemberg

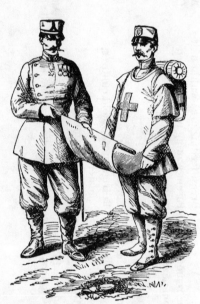

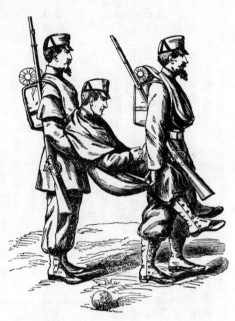

3A. *Manner of wearing the "mandil de socorro." The staff is inserted in its hem. A class 1 sick transport conveyance (conveyance borne by men). (Reproduced from Longmore, T.* A Treatise on the Transport of Sick and Wounded Troops. *London: Her Majesty's Stationery Office, 1869.)*

3B. *Manner of using the "mandil de socorro." A class 1 sick transport conveyance (conveyance borne by men). (Reproduced from Longmore, T.* A Treatise on the Transport of Sick and Wounded Troops. *London: Her Majesty's Stationery Office, 1869.)*

In the late 1960s, dramatic progress in the art and science of perinatal medicine and the development of neonatal intensive care units motivated leaders in obstetrics and neonatology to devise and use new methods to improve perinatal care.

In 1972 a national task force on perinatal health was formed, assisted by the National Foundation of the March of Dimes. A plan entitled *Toward Improving the Outcome of Pregnancy* was completed by the Perinatal Task Force in 1976. Thereafter the organization of perinatal centers began and included the active interhospital transport of mothers and infants. During this period there was an underlying philosophical belief that the expenses generated by the perinatal centers should be absorbed by the university hospitals, and that the financial cost-benefits of the perinatal programs would eventually make them self-supporting.

Subsequent cost-benefit analysis has shown that regionalization of neonatal care does indeed have a positive economic outcome [5, 9]. Nevertheless, a number of investigators in the field have expressed a need for further evaluation, using rigorous scientific methods to determine the cost-benefit impact of such programs on perinatal morbidity and mortality [7, 8].

The financing of perinatal programs remains an important challenge to their survival. The challenge will persist beyond the 1980s unless proper strategies are devised.

Thomas Parris points out key trends that have appeared [6]:

1. Rapidly increasing government intervention
2. Increasing regulatory measures, some of which are conflicting
3. Requirements for integrated health planning
4. Reimbursement constraints
5. Demand for cost-effectiveness
6. Higher bed occupancy, ensuring a census with at least 85 percent bed use

In the United States, there is a mandate placed on physicians and administrators to secure the availability of perinatal services. At the same time the system of prospective payment to hospitals, based on diagnosis-related groupings (DRGs), is likely to expand. Concurrently, insurance benefits and state health programs providing for maternal and child health will probably be reduced, thus increasing the economic burden on hospitals and creating uncertainty about their financial stability. In the final analysis, the total responsibility for securing financial support for perinatal services is placed on the perinatal centers.

Although it is impossible to separate maternal-infant transport costs from the overall costs of a perinatal program, it is important to map strategies that will enable the transport component of the program to obtain financial support from sources other than per diem hospital revenues.

This chapter will concentrate on financial planning for a neonatal transport service. However, the same logic and budget planning can be used for maternal transport programs.

## The Budget Process

The development of a transport budget is of paramount importance, not only to identify expenses but also to have a programmatic source of information to locate revenues. The size of the final budget will primarily depend on the size of the catchment area, whether or not there is sharing of transport resources among perinatal centers (e.g., large metropolitan areas), and the type of transport personnel and vehicles used.

During the budgeting process it is important to identify and recognize the individual components of overall cost including

1. Payments to physicians, salaries and overtime payments for nursing staff, and insurance costs, if applicable. Transport personnel may be expected to receive their regular salary plus an on-call premium, because of the 24-hour nature of the transport service.
2. Equipment costs, including maintenance and replacement.
3. Communications costs, including correspondence and telephone expenses.
4. Costs for training of personnel at the perinatal center and continuing education at local hospitals.
5. Vehicle and carrier personnel (e.g., ambulance drivers) expenses, if applicable. In addition, security staff may be needed to assist the transport team in preparing the ambulance or helicopter for departure or arrival.
6. Costs for return transport [4].
7. Hidden costs (unexpected expenses).

ACCOUNTING FOR COST

To be able to control costs it is important to establish a cost center for accountability. The hospital should consider setting up a separate account from others pertaining to the neonatology or pediatrics department and should, if possible, separately track costs for labor, transportation, capital equipment, and transport supplies. By establishing a separate cost center for transport the hospital administration is able to readily determine what the transportation costs are and, therefore, what should be charged to the patient for this service. Hidden costs are also more easily defined.

## *Types of Perinatal Transport Programs*

There are four main categories of perinatal transport programs in the United States. Examples of each of these will be used to illustrate the different means by which these programs obtain financial support. General methods for planning and mapping of strategies to obtain program revenues will then be reviewed.

### PERINATAL REGIONAL PROGRAMS SERVING LARGE DEMOGRAPHICAL REGIONS

The most common type of perinatal program found in the United States is probably that serving large geographical regions. There are five such service systems in upstate New York (see Fig. 3-1).

Albany Medical Center Hospital (AMCH) provides tertiary level peri-

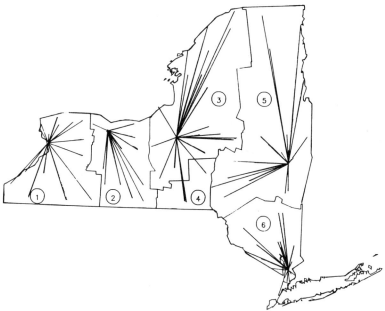

*Fig. 3-1. Regional Perinatal Networks, Upstate New York. 1 : HSA1 — Western New York (Children's, Buffalo). 2 : HSA2 — Finger Lakes Region (Strong Memorial, Rochester). 3 : HSA3 — Central New York (Central NY Perinatal Center, Syracuse). 4 : HSA4 — New York — Pennsylvania (same as HSA3). 5 : HSA5 — Northeastern New York (Albany Medical Center, Albany). 6 : HSA6 — Mid-Hudson Region (Westchester County Medical Center, Valhalla). (From New York State Health Department, Bureau of Biostatistics, February, 1986.)*

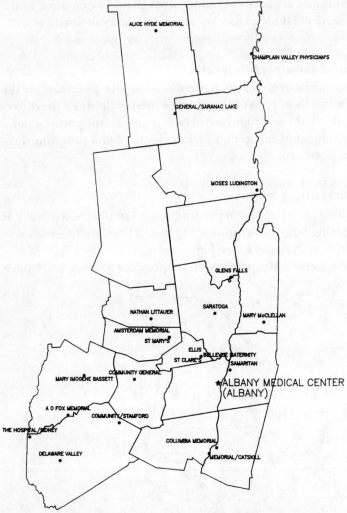

*Fig. 3-2. Northeastern New York–HSA5, Perinatal Network.*

natal care to the population of northeastern New York (NENY), a large region of upstate New York, southern Vermont, and areas of western Massachusetts. There are a total of 24,000 deliveries per year, of which 2400
babies are born at AMCH (Fig. 3-2). Between 800 and 850 infants are admitted per year to the neonatal intensive care unit at AMCH; of these, 40
percent are transported as neonates, 35 percent as maternal transports,
and 25 percent are delivered in-house from the Albany catchment area.

   Ten percent of the neonatal transports are accomplished using helicopters provided by the state police or by the National Guard. Medical care

during transport is provided by a transport team that consists of a physician, a nurse, and a respiratory therapist. Rarely, one-way transports are performed by the community hospital (see Chap. 2).

In 1979 the AMCH Administration established an estimated cost of $900 per neonate transported, with $400 representing manpower costs and an average of $500 representing the cost of the ambulance service. In 1987 the cost was estimated to be between $1000 and $1500 per transport. AMCH and the ambulance company each pay half of any unreimbursed transport cost. Agreements were made with Blue Cross health insurance carriers to obtain compensation for vehicle costs. The original plan incorporated transport costs into the per diem hospital charges.

In 1980, the state of New York declared a freeze on medical costs; at that time AMCH was transporting approximately 350 infants per year. By 1984, the number of transports had increased to approximately 570 per year. Since 1980, the AMCH program has incurred $525,800 of unrecouped expenses attributable to neonatal transport. These expenses include costs for transport personnel and $150,000 net loss for unpaid vehicle costs.

In 1984 alone, the hospital lost $126,000, of which $19,200 was the "bad debt" write off for ambulance services. A 3-month sample of transports in 1986 is shown in Table 3-1, and it should be noted that 43 percent of transports involved either third-party payers that had not developed specific agreements with the medical center or families who did not have health benefits and provided direct payment.

During 1985 a program was developed at AMCH to increase the number of infants transferred back to the hospital of delivery or to the hospital closest to the patient's home. By 1986, more than 55 percent of out-born neonates were returned to the originating hospital for a period of care prior to discharge home. During the last 6 months in 1986 188 babies with weights

Table 3-1. Albany Medical Center Hospital (AMCH):
reimbursement sources for neonatal transports by ambulance in 1986

| Month | Blue Cross | Blue Shield | Medicaid | Personal pay* | Total patients |
|---|---|---|---|---|---|
| January | 9 | | 1 | 9 | 19 |
| February | 12 | | 1 | 13 | 26 |
| March | 14 | 2 | 2 | 9 | 27 |
| TOTALS | 35 | 2 | 4 | 31 | 72 |
| Percentage of total transports | 49% | 2% | 6% | 43% | 100% |

*Third-party payers that do not have an agreement with AMCH or "self-pay" by the family.

below 1500 g were admitted to AMCH, 81 of whom were returned to the referring hospital.

When an infant is returned to the hospital where the mother originally sought perinatal care or where the baby was born, significant benefits accrue:

1. Family-infant interaction is facilitated.
2. Patient care characteristics of the community hospital receive a stimulus to improve.
3. The cost of medical care decreases.
4. Bed availability at the tertiary center increases.

The per diem rate for the neonatal intensive care unit at AMCH is $475 and that for the average community hospital is $275. Following back transfer, the average length of stay at the community hospital is 12.5 days. This represents an average savings of more than $250,000 per patient per diem for bed charges alone.

STATEWIDE REGIONAL PERINATAL PROGRAMS
Because of the demographics of certain states, a single regional perinatal center may provide statewide services [6]. Since these perinatal centers receive referrals from a large territorial area, it is particularly necessary to provide for air transportation as well as ground transportation. The transport programs run by the University of New Mexico School of Medicine and the Maryland Regional Neonatal Program (MRNP) are examples.

The New Mexico program is responsible for the supervision of 28,000 births per year with approximately 550 admissions per year to the neonatal intensive care unit. The program is directly subsidized by the state, with a budget that includes the salaries for neonatal and perinatal staff equivalent to 21 full-time equivalents (FTEs) as well as transport allocations to compensate carriers when there is no third-party coverage. Outreach education and a toll-free WATS line are also financed. The transportation allocations may be used to transport either mothers with high-risk pregnancies or sick neonates.

The MRNP is organized somewhat differently. This service transports approximately 600 premature and sick neonates per year to seven regional intensive care nurseries located in the city of Baltimore. Two-thirds of the MRNP transports are by ambulance and one-third are by specially equipped Maryland State Police helicopters. Eight specifically trained neonatal transport nurses are essential to the program. They are divided into two teams;

one based at the University of Maryland and the other at Johns Hopkins Hospital.

The Maryland Institute of Emergency Medical Services (MIEMS) administers the MRNP grant funds and provides the communication and transportation components. It is estimated that the average cost of transporting an infant is approximately $1000. This does not include communication and other administrative costs. On an annual basis, the overall cost is approximately $600,000, part of which is paid for by a state grant. The itemized budget includes salaries for the transport nurses, secretarial staff, a nurse, ambulance drivers, and partial support for neonatologists, in addition to costs of equipment and supplies, vehicle operation, and van and transport unit depreciation and maintenance.

The remaining expenses are borne by the departments of pediatrics and the nursing administrative services of the two institutions. In the future, billing will occur for the professional component (doctors, nurses, and respiratory therapists) to reimburse the MIEMS and the participating institutions.

## REGIONAL PROGRAMS THAT SHARE A STATE SYSTEM OF EMERGENCY MEDICAL SERVICES

Illinois has 12 regional perinatal centers, 8 of which are located in Chicago [3]. The Illinois Department of Public Health has a regionalized perinatal care program that is subsidized by permanent block grants from the state. Regulations that define the scope of these regional networks establish that the regional centers shall

1. Maintain a communication system 24 hours per day.
2. Provide consultation and advice regarding support services.
3. Provide for transfer of high-risk intrapartum and newborn patients.
4. Provide or arrange emergency transportation, and determine whether ground or air transport will be used.
5. Determine the composition of the transport team.

Each perinatal center may contract with a private ambulance service or use the Division of Emergency Medical Services (DEMS), or both. The DEMS is used primarily for air transport. Thirty percent of all patients transported by DEMS are high-risk neonates. The DEMS is supported by four helicopters from the Department of Transportation (which are based at strategic locations throughout the state), two fire department helicopters in Chicago, and a helicopter owned by the University of Chicago. Each institution is responsible for its own transport team.

The Department of Public Health allocates funds, in the form of grants,

to the regional programs. This is done through a network of regional perinatal management groups or by direct reimbursement to the regional centers. The DEMS is in the process of transferring coordinating functions to
the regional trauma centers.

REGIONAL PROGRAMS IN LARGE METROPOLITAN AREAS
THAT DO NOT SHARE TRANSPORT SYSTEMS
New York City (NYC) has several regional perinatal programs that do not
share a transport system. Through the NYC Health and Hospital Corporation the city supports a unified high-risk infant transport system that is
located at Bellevue Hospital—a New York University Medical Center–
affiliated hospital. From the budget standpoint this program is deemed
a separate entity. The program coordinates the transport of any infant
at high risk in the city of New York to any of the seven regional perinatal
centers. The program budget supports personnel (including two neonatologists, one neonatal fellow, five nurses, five technicians, one part-time
clerk/typist, and an administrator), equipment, and maintenance. In spite
of this, parallel transport systems have been developed by other tertiary
care centers in the city.

The Albert Einstein College and affiliated hospitals use private ambulances. The ambulance companies bill separately for each transport. The
medical center bills for physician services and absorbs the expenses of the
patients who are unable to pay for the transport or who do not have an
insurance carrier.

The New York Hospital has also developed a parallel high-risk infant
transport system [2]. The hospital accepts patients from 20 hospitals within
and outside the limits of New York City. Because of dissatisfaction with
their original system, which used private ambulances, often without proper
equipment, the hospital now owns a high-risk infant transport ambulance
that was designed and built to their specifications. The neonatal transport
team consists of 10 specially trained medical technicians, nurses, and physicians. The total capital expenditures were $93,000, and the yearly operat-
ing expenses amount to $293,500. The costs attributable to the neonatal
transports are not directly reimbursed but are included as part of the hospital per diem charges. Older infants and obstetric patients who are transported are charged a flat fee of $350.

The Rainbow Babies and Children's Hospital in Cleveland has developed
a similar pediatric emergency transportation program. They have two vehicles with pediatric modules. They are staffed by 12 paramedic drivers,
pediatric residents, and specially trained nurses. The original cost of the
vehicles in 1981 was $75,000. Their annual transport budget is $192,138.

Initially, they had a grant from the Cleveland Foundation, but they have since negotiated reimbursement agreements with the Ohio Health Department and Blue Cross/Blue Shield Insurance carriers.

INTERTERTIARY NEONATAL TRANSPORT
In the past 5 years several new technologies, such as extracorporeal membrane oxygenation (ECMO) and high-frequency jet ventilation (HFJV), have become available. These techniques are currently available at a relatively small number of centers in the United States, leading to an increased number of long-distance transports of critically ill neonates between centers [1]. Among the problems associated with intertertiary transport, the economic issues are significant. The cost of the transport is usually very high, particularly if long-distance air transport is required. Most third-party insurers in the United States will reimburse the bulk of the expenditure, as long as they are convinced that the care rendered at the receiving hospital cannot be provided at the referring institution. However, very few third-party payers currently reimburse the cost of the return transport. In the case of patients who are not covered by health insurance the financial loss incurred by the receiving hospital can be significant. It is fairly common for a convalescing baby to be kept at a great distance from the family because there are no funds for back transfer. Additional, hidden costs include those for such items as long-distance phone calls and inability to accept acutely ill local patients because of decreased bed availability.

## The Accessibility of Program Revenues
In the United States, it is estimated that the cost of a patient transport varies from 1000 to $1500, depending on the distance and type of vehicle used. Long-range air transport costs may be up to 4 to 5 times this amount (see Chap. Appendix 3-1 for sample invoice).

Traditionally, medical centers have been willing to absorb financial losses emanating from transport services. Initially, the prestigious position of being a referral center played an important role in producing this attitude toward economic losses. It was believed that, since transport costs were only a small fraction of the total expenses of perinatal care, the losses could be absorbed by the institution. However, subsequent to the intense economical restraints imposed on the referral institutions, administrators have transferred the responsibility for obtaining revenues to the department chairmen of neonatology/pediatrics and obstetrics.

The most conventional access to funds has been the incorporation of the transport costs into the per diem hospital charges. This source seldom covers equipment replacement costs, continuing education, or professional expenses. In some states, a freeze on the per diem revenues will increase the budget deficit for transport.

There are several programs that have successfully negotiated agreements with local health departments, Blue Cross/Blue Shield, or other third-party payers. It is important that professional fees are included when such agreements are secured. Private foundation grants have been obtained by a number of programs, but they are usually intended to facilitate the development of the transport system and have a limited life span. Block grants are probably the best and most permanent source of financial support for the transport system, especially if associated with state agencies such as the Department of Transportation, the Fire Department, state or city police, and the Department of Conservation.

MAPPING STRATEGIES
Two premises should be agreed on before establishing a funding strategy:

1. It is the ultimate joint responsibility of the hospital administrators, department chairmen of neonatology/pediatrics and obstetrics and gynecology, and the directors of the perinatal programs to provide leadership in financing their programs.
2. Attempts should be made to finance the perinatal program as a whole, rather than to individually fund the components.

Mapping a strategy starts with establishing a cost center for accountability and developing a comprehensive budget. This budget should acknowledge all existing revenues, including what is derived from the per diem of each involved medical institution. Transport costs should be carefully itemized and formal agreements should be signed with third-party payers. These agreements should cover transport expenses as well as professional fees. Once these steps are formalized, the expected annual net losses can be calculated. They should not exceed 30 percent of the total cost of the program.

To offset the losses, the hospitals benefiting from the regional program might be requested to allocate funds to help defray the expenses for their patients who are ineligible for third-party reimbursement of transport costs. It is feasible to calculate the number of transports coming from each institution and report a proportional sum, not to exceed 5 percent of total net loss. Another 5 percent may be obtained from the counties where the hospitals are located. The approach to the county commissioners should be similar to the approach to the administration at the community hospitals, and the formula to arrive at a proper amount is the same.

When regional programs involve the provision of care in large metropolitan areas, the plan recommended to city government officials might be similar to that supported by New York City. However, competing regional centers must agree to share the benefits and costs. Duplication of services only adds to the expense. In some instances, regional programs extend beyond the immediate city limits, and it may be necessary to provide different transport services for patients originating outside the metropolitan area.

It is possible to finance up to 80 percent of a transport program from available local resources. However, for total reimbursement it is necessary to obtain government subsidies through block grants. The government will provide the opportunities but perinatal organizations must provide the leadership. In most states in the United States the state governor's office will originate proposals either directly or via the Bureau of Reproductive Health, the Division of Maternal and Child Health, or the Office of Management of the Health Department. Because of the complexity of the issues involved, it is preferable to obtain support from an individual appointed by the governor who reports directly to the executive office. That individual will call on members of different departments (e.g., health, budget, transportation, and education) and provide a coordinated approach.

In many states, block grant advisory committees and perinatal advisory councils may provide avenues to obtain support. There is a reluctance on the part of government agencies to sponsor new programs; however, requests for up to 20 percent support for net losses will usually gain a sympathetic ear from the executive branch. The governor will propose monetary allocations. The legislature will then revise and ultimately allocate the necessary monies. Legislators tend to consider favorably programs that go beyond parochial geographical areas or that include suburban and rural areas proportionately, especially if many age groups will be served.

### Use of Perinatal Advocates

There are a number of state and national perinatal organizations that, although created for different purposes, have essentially developed to represent the interests of the mother, fetus, and neonate. Such organizations can serve as the voice of perinatal communities. They may be the vehicle for widely organized advocacy and for support of perinatal programs.

However, it must be realized that, because we live in a political world, advocacy is becoming a political science. These lobbyist organizations must be professionally organized and should develop support in the local community. Staffing should include full-time personnel with expertise in the areas of executive direction, field coordination, legislative coordination, and medical care. Through such perinatal organizations a planning initiative should be developed to support the financing of perinatal programs as a whole or to finance the transport system. Some of the steps involved are outlined below.

1. Develop the proposed initiative
   A. Select the title of the proposal.
   B. Formulate a budget.
   C. Develop funding projections.
   D. Prepare the supporting documents.
2. Plan the campaign strategy
   A. Make political assessments, including the identification of groups and individuals to target.
   B. Demonstrate the potential number of beneficiaries in the state.
   C. Plan the public relations program.
   D. Obtain broad-based and bipartisan statewide support.
3. Focus on the governor
   A. Identify a gubernatorial staff member to introduce the proposals.
   B. Meet with gubernatorial staff, budget director, health staff members, and influential advisors.
   C. Obtain organizational endorsements and letters to the governor.
   D. Secure endorsements from prominent individuals.
4. Revisit the governor's staff
   Lobby key advisors to the governor and obtain commitments.
5. Focus on the legislature
   A. Meet with legislative leaders and staff.
   B. Lobby in districts.
   C. Obtain petitions and letters reflecting statewide support.

In the past health professionals have been somewhat reluctant to organize themselves to petition for their patients. The time is now ripe to get together and request help from other organizations with the same goals and to make an impact on the development of policies to improve the outcome of pregnancy.

### Future Trends
In the United States a complex system is usually required to obtain revenues to support perinatal transport programs. This system may encompass

any or all of the following: the inclusion of transport expenses in the per diem hospital charges, agreements with third-party payers, contributions from community and metropolitan hospitals, and fiscal support from counties, states, and cities. The opportunity for innovation also exists.

A DRG system will be fully implemented for neonatal patients in the near future. It may be possible, for example, to incorporate certain incentives in the form of credits that will not only help defray the costs of transport but also stimulate hospitals to upgrade their services. For example, whenever there is an intrauterine fetal transport, the cost of returning the infant back to the community hospital could be reimbursed. When neonates are transported from a community hospital for intensive care the return transport costs could be totally reimbursed if the subsequent care is concluded within the average length of hospitalization determined by the DRG system. As previously stated, the total cost of patient care can be reduced by transferring infants back to their original hospitals. Incentives to do so may provide both necessary funding and serve to strengthen the relationship between the regional center and the community hospital. In the case of intertertiary transports, it would seem reasonable that the referring and receiving hospitals share the expense of unreimbursed two-way transport in some equitable manner.

## References

1. Donn, S. M. Intertertiary neonatal transport. *Perinatol.-Neonatol.* 11:35–50, 1987.
2. Greene, W. T. Organization of neonatal transport services in support of a regional referral center. *Clin. Perinatol.* 7:187, 1980.
3. Illinois Department of Public Health. *Rules for Regionalized Perinatal Care.* Illinois Perinatal Care Program.
4. Jung, A. L., and Bose, C. L. Back transport of neonates: Improved efficiency of tertiary nursery bed utilization. *Pediatrics* 71:918, 1983.
5. McCarthy, J. T., et al. Who pays the bill for neonatal intensive care? *J. Pediatr.* 95:755, 1979.
6. Parris, T. G., Jr. *Maternal and Child Health. Part II: Organizing for Advocacy. Perinatal Press* Aug. 1982. Pp. 95–100.
7. Sinclair, J. C., et al. Evaluation of neonatal-intensive care programs. *N. Engl. J. Med.* 305:489, 1981.
8. Spitz, A. M., et al. The impact of publicly funded perinatal care programs on neonatal outcome, Georgia, 1976–1978. *Am. J. Obstet. Gynecol.* 147:296, 1983.
9. Walker, D. J. B., Vohr, B. R., and Oh, W. Economic analysis of regionalized neonatal care for very low-birth-weight infants in the state of Rhode Island. *Pediatrics* 76:69, 1985.

## Chapter Appendix I: University of Utah Hospital Patient Transport Charges

Patient name _____

Patient account number _____

Date of patient transport _____

Trip from _____ to _____

*Transport Team*

NBICU ☐   Adult ☐   Obstetrics ☐   Transplant ☐

*Patient Transport for*

University hospital ☐

Primary children's medical center ☐

YAH ☐

Other receiving hospital ☐ _____

*Type of Transportation*

Helicopter ☐   Fixed wing ☐        Ground (ambulance) ☐

222 ☐   Cheyenne ☐ MU=2 ☐

206 ☐   Lear 25 ☐   Lear 35 ☐

University hospital supplies/equipment   $_____

University hospital transport personnel   No. on team _____

Trip hours _____

Helicopter mileage charges   $_____

Helicopter call-out fee   $_____

Fixed wing charges   $_____

Helicopter shuttle to airport   $_____

Total charges: No. of hours × No. on team   $_____

Equipment charges   $_____

Total transport charges   $_____

# 4

# The Communications
# Network for
# Perinatal Transport

Alasdair K. T. Conn
Cheryl Y. Bowen

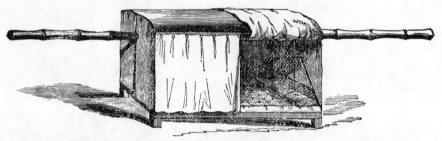

*4A. Bengal dhooley and bamboo pole with half of the side curtain thrown over the top to show the interior with mattress and pillow. A class 1 sick transport conveyance (conveyance borne by men). "It is not possible to place a patient within it, nor can surgical attention be given to him, especially in the instances of injuries to the upper or lower parts of the body, without great inconvenience to all concerned." (Reproduced from Longmore, T.* A Treatise on the Transport of Sick and Wounded Troops. *London: Her Majesty's Stationery Office, 1869.)*

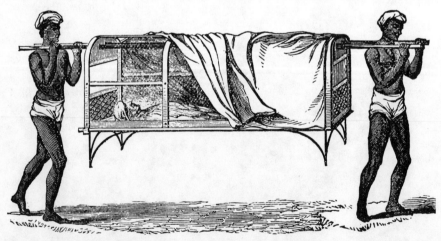

*4B. Dr. Francis' improved dhooley. A class 1 sick transport conveyance (conveyance borne by men). (Reproduced from Longmore, T.* A Treatise on the Transport of Sick and Wounded Troops. *London: Her Majesty's Stationery Office, 1869.)*

In 1966 the Highway Safety Act was passed by the Congress of the United States. As part of this legislation (Standard II) every state was mandated to establish and operate emergency medical services (EMS). To operate a functioning EMS system there are several essential components that must be in place and smoothly integrated; the communications link is essential (Table 4-1). After passage of the Highway Safety Act, networks of transmitters and base stations were established to allow both medical direction and telemetry to pass between mobile ambulances and paramedic vehicles and participating hospitals.

Although some aspects of the communications network required for a perinatal transport system are unique, knowledge of the general requirements for an EMS communications system are essential.

## EMS Communications
GENERAL CONSIDERATIONS
At the local level of the EMS communication, responsibilities cover the following areas [5]:

### The Patient Notification Call
This call allows the patient or patient representative access to the system and is the point of first contact. Calls are screened to ensure that they are appropriate and are then relayed to the dispatcher for vehicle response. Most areas of the United States are using a 911 access number. Some are using "enhanced 911," meaning that the caller's phone number and location can be identified within seconds by computer; the computer can also determine the nearest ambulance available to go to the location (see box). Perinatal patients do not usually enter the system in this way. However, a similar dispatch/coordinating center can be established to receive calls and maintain updated information on the bed status at hospitals in the regional perinatal referral network.

### Ambulance Dispatch
Ambulances are dispatched either by radio or by dedicated land telephone line. Types of vehicles include:

First responder vehicles (fire or police)
Basic life support ambulances
Advanced life support vehicles
Helicopters and fixed-wing aircraft in some systems—appropriate for transports requiring greater than 30 minutes travelling time one way.

*Table 4-1. Elements of an emergency medical services system*

Advisory councils
Public information/education
Dispatch centers
Ambulance services
Provider training programs
Instructor training programs
Categorized hospital emergency facilities
Communication
Documentation
Disaster plans

---

**Computer-aided dispatch**
Computer-aided dispatch is currently used by several urban EMS systems in the United States.

The initial step to upgrading to a full system is to initiate an "enhanced" emergency telephone number, often designated as an E-911. In this system a computer will automatically determine the address and location of the calling party from the calling number. Thus, as the specifics of the request are being obtained by the dispatcher, the address from which the call is being made comes up on the computer screen. More sophisticated systems include the following capabilities: As the emergency call is answered a time appears on the screen and the ambulance in closest proximity to the caller's district is identified. Depending on the nature of the emergency, e.g., a cardiac case, a few pertinent questions for the dispatcher to ask will also appear on the screen. The answers (yes or no) to these questions will then allow the computer to determine a priority for the call. The computer has thus determined the location of the emergency, the ambulance that should respond, the priority of the call, and is keeping track of response times. If the designated ambulance is already in use, the computer will then determine the next closest ambulance. With this system in place paperwork is reduced and analysis of response times, priority of calls, and use of equipment is greatly simplified. However, the capital cost of such equipment means that it is only cost-effective when used in a consolidated system.

---

The response can be tailored to the call. In an optimally tiered response the patient may expect arrival of a basic life support ambulance in 2 to 4 minutes and a paramedic response in 4 to 8 minutes.

In most regions of the United States dedicated vehicles and specially trained transport teams are used for neonatal transport. Maternal transport may also be carried out by a special vehicle and team or by the local advanced life support ambulance. The first responder and basic life support vehicles are rarely used except in case of home delivery.

*Intercommunication Between Responding Emergency Units*
This includes communication with other EMSs in case of disaster or multiple requests and communication with the civil defense and military systems.

*Communications Between the Transport Ambulance*
*and Consulting Hospital Personnel*
Communications between the ambulance and the tertiary care center can be critical for the perinatal patient.

ROLE OF THE FEDERAL COMMUNICATIONS COMMISSION
The Federal Communications Commission (FCC) has the authority, as contained in the Communications Act of 1934, to regulate radio transmissions and issue licenses for radio stations and transmitters [3]. The FCC limits both the power of transmitters and also the wavelengths that are used. This is to ensure, for example, that commercial air traffic, local taxi services, and EMS communications are on completely different wavelengths and that EMS communication in one region does not overlap or interfere with neighboring communication systems. To this end the FCC regulates band width and transmission power and can monitor frequencies to promote compliance. Emergency medical communications use both very high frequency (VHF) and ultra-high frequency (UHF) bands that cover frequencies of 30 to 175 MHz (VHF) and 300 to 3000 MHz (UHF), respectively. The VHF is divided into low band (30–50 MHz), which has a range of up to 2000 miles but is subject to interference, and high band (150–175 MHz). The UHF band has better penetration of buildings but has shorter range.

The FCC has assigned certain frequencies on the VHF and UHF bands for EMS access channels and medical consultation. The exact frequencies in any region are delineated within the state communications plan and may be ascertained by contacting the state office of emergency medical services.

In many cases the transport vehicles are provided by a commercial operator. The ambulance is then not dispatched on an EMS frequency (unless prior arrangement has been made) but on a commercial wavelength from the carrier's own dispatch center. The ambulance should have access to the EMS communications system for entry notification. Preprogrammable radios are now available that can store several thousand frequencies that can be changed at the touch of a button (Fig. 4-1).

ACCESS TO THE COMMUNICATIONS NETWORK
In most cases the perinatal patient is referred from a primary care hospital, and the referring physician requires immediate access to consultative services at the tertiary care center and to the transport team. To provide these

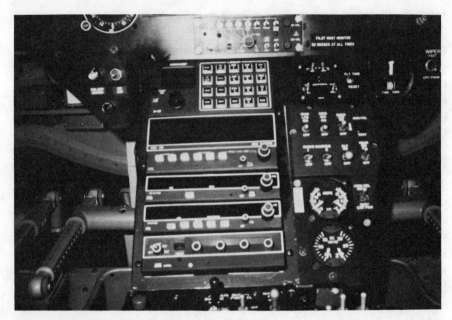

*Fig. 4-1. A Wulfsburg radio. These radios can be preprogrammed and enable the transport nurse to contact medical control for specific orders. They are widely used on helicopters that transport critically ill patients.*

services an access number must be available. Most commonly this is a toll-free number (hot line), which must be open 24 hours a day for the planned geographical area. These lines take from 1 month to 6 weeks to install.

Although mnemonics are not essential, it is helpful if the number is easy to remember. This number should be publicized in brochures and via outreach programs, and its use encouraged. If possible, the hot line should be supervised at all times by trained personnel. Inquiries should be answered promptly and professionally and every call should be documented (see Chap. Appendices I–IV for examples of transfer record forms). Immediate access to an attending physician is crucial. The line should have an automatic call forwarding feature so that the caller will not receive a busy signal. Conference call capability is a desirable feature. For quality control purposes, the record of calls should be reviewed on a regular basis.

### Lines of Referral for Perinatal Transport
ROLES AND RESPONSIBILITIES
*Dispatch Center*
The dispatch/coordinating center is often the first point of contact for perinatal referrals. In regions with multiple participating tertiary care centers,

a single dispatch center should receive and direct all incoming calls. Calls should be referred according to preset guidelines. There may be a simple rotation for receiving referral calls or a more complex set of guidelines including patient condition, geographical proximity to family and referring hospital, referring physician preference, bed availability, and family preference.

Delays in transport of both maternal and neonatal patients can often be attributed to difficulties in locating beds within the neonatal centers. The dispatch center can facilitate arrangements for neonatal transport and significantly reduce delays. Data reported by Vogt suggest that improvements in perinatal mortality may be related to improved efficiency in locating neonatal intensive care beds via the use of a dispatch center [6]. Bostick et al. have described the use of a communications network to provide information on available beds to all tertiary care centers in the region (Fig. 4-2) [2] In this system, the referring physician calls the regional neonatal center of choice and, if that center is unable to accept the infant, their personnel are able to immediately locate a bed in one of the other centers.

Ideally, this first call should be the only call that the referring physician has to initiate. The dispatch center should have the capability of telepatching calls to any of the participating perinatal centers. In the event that beds

*Fig. 4-2. Bed availability. This computer is on-line with nine hospitals. (Copyright © 1987, David W. Wooddell. Reproduced with permission.)*

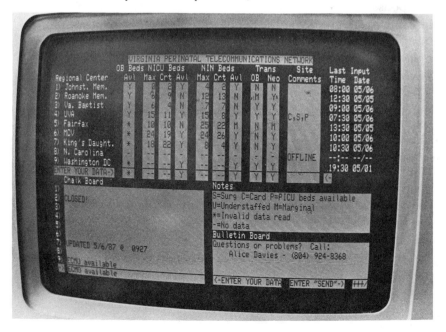

are fully occupied the dispatch center should then contact neighboring regions. It should be emphasized that dispatching a perinatal transport team is not a decision that should be given to an EMS dispatcher; this is a complex medical judgment and should be made by the transport team or transport coordinator in conjunction with the perinatal consultant.

When air ambulances must connect with ground ambulances, it is desirable for a single dispatch center to coordinate the movements of all involved vehicles.

### Transport Coordinator

The roles of the transport coordinator (see also Chap. 15), perinatal consultant, and transport team often overlap and vary in different regional systems. Frequent communication between these members of the referral system is necessary for the system to operate smoothly. Routine scheduled meetings, attended by the entire transport staff, can provide an opportunity to address any problems that occur and to keep all personnel well informed.

The communication responsibilities of the transport coordinator include the following:

Orientation and training of the transport team regarding the elements and function of the communication system.
Ensuring that all requests for transport receive an appropriate and timely response.
Ensuring that all records pertaining to transport are complete and filed.
Ensuring appropriate backup equipment and personnel if multiple requests are made simultaneously.
Developing protocols for dispatch and communications.

### Perinatal Consultant

A consultant has two roles in communications: off-line, managing the medical direction of the program and on-line, being available by radio or telephone to the referring physician and transport team.

Off-line duties
1. Has responsibility for the training of transport personnel and for continuous clinical review of the function and effectiveness of the communication network.
2. Works with the coordinator to develop protocols for dispatch and communications.
3. Determines mode of access to the consultation/transport system.

On-line duties
1. Is available for consultation with referring physician.
2. Determines whether transport is indicated.
3. Determines mode of transport (air or ground).
4. Determines whether any special needs (equipment or personnel, or both) are required on an individual basis.
5. Is available for immediate consultation with the transport team by telephone or radio.

*Transport Team*
In some regional programs, requests for transport are first handled by the transport team. The transport team is then responsible for documenting all patient information relayed over the telephone and communicating that information to the neonatal/perinatal consultant. The transport team may also be responsible for recommending immediate stabilization procedures to the referring physician.

Communications responsibilities of the transport team include:

Notifying the referring and receiving hospitals of the estimated time of arrival.

Relaying relevant clinical information to the perinatal consultant and clinical information and recommendations between the referring and receiving hospitals.

Providing the family with information regarding the patient's current condition, the transport, and the receiving center.

Documenting all observations, recommendations, procedures, etc., on the patient transport record.

*Referring Hospital Physician and Staff*
During the initial consultation/referral call, the referring physician is responsible for communicating all pertinent clinical information to the consultant at the tertiary care center. The American Academy of Pediatrics and the American College of Obstetricians and Gynecologists have published guidelines for information to be gathered prior to transfer of the maternal patient or the neonate [1]. Many transport programs collect this information on forms of their own design. Providing copies of these forms to the referring hospitals may assist the staff in gathering the required information. Sample forms are included in Chap. Appendices I through IV.

Staff at the referring hospital are responsible for completing all written records and sending copies of these records with the patient.

*Receiving Regional Perinatal Center*

Once the patient arrives at the perinatal center it becomes the responsibility of staff at the center to keep the family and referring physician informed of the patient's progress and outcome.

## Transport Communications

THE REFERRAL CALL

The following is a typical sequence for the referral call:

1. *Referring physician* calls via the hot line and requests transport.
2. The *perinatal consultant/transport team* receives the call. Immediate interventions are recommended and documented, the mode of transport determined, a bed located, and the transport approved. If the transport nurse is first to receive the call, he or she will consult with the perinatologist or neonatologist. If necessary, the consultant will call the referring physician back with further recommendations. When the perinatal consultant is first to receive the call, the referring physician is advised that the transport nurse or dispatcher will be either coming online or calling back for further information.
3. The *dispatcher* obtains a checklist from the sending facility (Table 4-2), and if he or she receives the initial call, locates a bed and communicates with the potential referral hospital to receive instruction regarding the most suitable vehicle and the composition of the transport team (Figs. 4-3 and 4-4). The dispatcher contacts the ambulance or helicopter and coordinates all vehicle movements.

Ideally, key conversations should be on a timed tape recorder to ensure that all of the information is obtained. If concerns or questions are raised later, these tapes can be reviewed. At the end of this information exchange, the referring facility should be given an estimated time of arrival of the transport team.

COMMUNICATIONS DURING TRANSPORT

Once dispatched, either a member of the transport team or the dispatcher should notify the sending facility of an updated estimated time of arrival and obtain a further medical report. The security department of the referring facility should be notified of both air and ground missions to ensure easy access to the facility and to provide assistance in unloading and moving equipment, holding elevators, etc. (Fig. 4-5). Members of the trans-

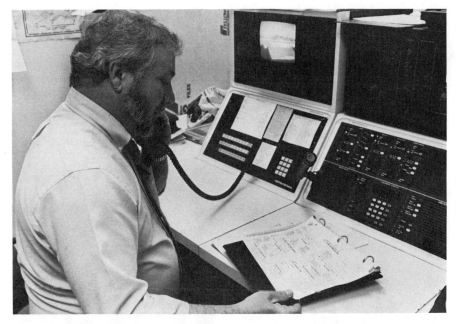

*Fig. 4-3. The referral call. Dispatcher records essential information on a check list. (Copyright © 1987, David W. Wooddell. Reproduced with permission.)*

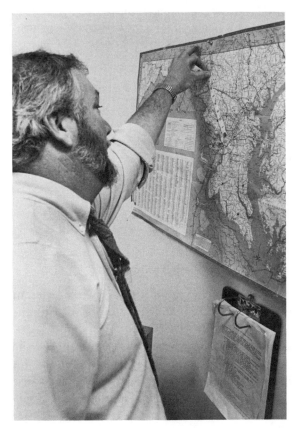

*Fig. 4-4. The dispatch center. Estimating the flying time. (Copyright © 1987, David W. Wooddell. Reproduced with permission.)*

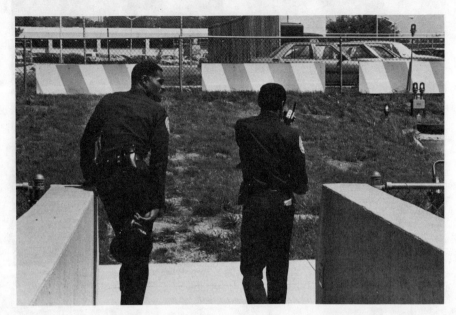

Fig. 4-5. Two special policemen stand by to assist as a transport helicopter lands at Children's Hospital National Medical Center in Washington, D.C. The Emergency Communications and Information Center (ECIC) is notified by radio that the helicopter is landing. (Copyright © 1987, David W. Wooddell. Reproduced with permission.)

Table 4-2. Basic information exchanged prior to hospital-to-hospital transfer

Name of calling individual
Call-back phone number(s) at referral hospital
Name of referring facility—address, landing zone if aircraft transfer
Number of patients to be transferred
Names of referring physician and receiving physician
Diagnosis of patient
Location of patient in referring facility
Any special equipment or personnel required
Requested time of transport (emergency, urgent, or elective)
If air transport—weather information

port team should have delineated authority; in most cases the physician or transport nurse is the individual who is ultimately responsible during the transport.

It cannot be overemphasized that the members of the transport team should be selected not only on the basis of clinical excellence but also for their interpersonal skills. The staff at the referring facility may have reservations about the transfer; transfer may have been necessitated by a complication with potential legal consequences, and the attitude might vary from extreme relief on arrival of the transport team to outright antagonism. While in the referring hospital, members of the transport team should make every effort to keep the physician and staff informed of exactly what they are doing and why they are doing it. When possible, the staff at the referring hospital should participate in the preparation of the patient for transport. This preparation may lessen any apprehension regarding the transport, provide an opportunity to educate the referring hospital staff regarding specific stabilization procedures, and ensure a smoother transfer of the responsibility for patient care.

A member of the transport team should inform the patient's family of the reason for transfer and the name of the receiving facility. A transport permit, which states the mode of transport, should be signed by the patient or responsible relative. A patient information sheet describing the transport aircraft might also be appropriate (see Chap. Appendix V). Parents of neonates who are to be transferred may be suffering from shock, guilt, and grief, as well as physical pain. The transport team must recognize this and provide information according to the parent's ability to understand. When available, families should be given printed information about the regional center, including visiting hours, phone numbers, a map or directions.

Prior to leaving the referring facility, members of the transport team should review together the plan for patient care during transport and any anticipated problems. The security department may be required again to hold elevators and ensure a smooth exit.

As soon as transport is initiated the transport team should check that the patient's status is stable and provide an entry notification (progress report) to the receiving facility (Fig. 4-6). Depending on local protocol, this notification may be done via the intensive care staff at the receiving facility or the receiving physician. If the patient remains in stable condition, an update entry notification should be made 5 to 10 minutes prior to arrival. This can be performed via the EMS communications link or by cellular telephone. This progress report should alert the security department to staff the landing zone, turn on lights, hold elevators, and so forth.

On arrival, the transport team should give a complete report to the receiving staff and ensure a smooth transition of medical care. Last, transportation records should be completed and copies retained within the transport files (for critical medical review) and in the patient's chart.

FOLLOW-UP
A member of the transport team should make an effort to speak with the patient's family as soon as possible after transfer to inform them of the

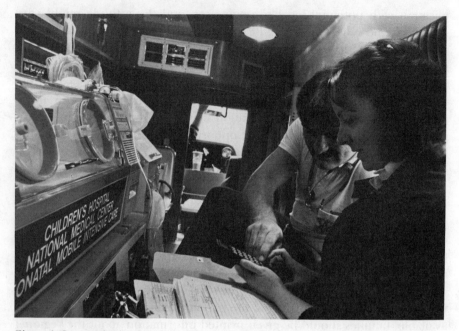

*Fig. 4-6. Communication in transit. The transport nurse provides a progress report to the receiving facility via cellular telephone. (Copyright © 1987, David W. Wooddell. Reproduced with permission.)*

clinical status of the patient on arrival and to give them further details such as the names of the physician and primary nurse caring for the patient.

The transport team should provide follow-up information to the referral facility first by telephone and later by letter. This follow-up should include information regarding any problems encountered during the transfer. Similarly, the referring hospital should inform the transport coordinator of any problems that they have encountered. It is the experience of many transport teams that constructive criticism is very helpful and may lead to needed changes in policies and procedures.

## The Limitations of the Communications Network—
## Avoiding Pitfalls
### LIMITATIONS OF OPERATIONS
Communications capability has expanded dramatically within the last few years, as microprocessors have decreased in cost. However, communications systems are usually designed to function to certain tolerances—an ex-

ample might be to provide adequate transmission to 95 percent of the area covered, 95 percent of the time. A system that provides 99 percent coverage, 99 percent of the time, might be designated for a local area. However, the cost of providing the additional coverage is frequently prohibitive.

PITFALLS IN COMMUNICATIONS
Problems with patient transport can more often be blamed on a failure in communications than on any other component of the system. Some common pitfalls include:

1. *Failure to clearly delineate roles and responsibilities*—The responsibilities of each member of the transport team should be determined and written into their job description. Strict adherence to a standard protocol must be the rule. Responsibility for a breakdown in the system can then be identified and remedial action taken.

2. *Loss of communication with the transport team*—Although not a problem with air transport (because it is Federal Aviation Administration requirement), either the dispatcher or the transport coordinator should know where the transport team is at all times and, if the transport team is overdue, have the capability to initiate a search. Mechanical breakdown of the ambulance, particularly in a rural area, can rapidly lead to secondary problems such as exhaustion of the oxygen supply to the patient. Such problems are seriously compounded if the communication system is not functional.

It should be expected that there will be times when communication cannot be effected or is subject to interference. For example, the coordinating center or the hospital may suffer a power failure. Although most hospitals and communications centers have priority, the capabilities of the communications systems in times of natural (or other) disasters should be examined and backup alternatives explored. Cellular telephones can be placed in ambulances as a backup system or, for larger areas, a mobile phone accessed through the 800 trunk system.

Future possibilities (by the 1990s) include geosynchronous satellite communications. The exact role that this communication system will play in patient transport has yet to be determined although transmission from ambulance to hospital via satellite is technically feasible [4].

Locator devices are commercially available that can relay the position of a vehicle to within 30 meters. These systems can plot and continually update the location of an air or ground vehicle. However, because of the high cost of this equipment, it is likely to be primarily used for aviation.

## References

1. American Academy of Pediatrics Committee on Fetus and Newborn and American College of Obstetricians and Gynecologists Committee on Obstetrics: Maternal and Fetal Medicine. Interhospital Care of the Perinatal Patient. In *Guidelines for Perinatal Care*. Evanston, Ill.: American Academy of Pediatrics and American College of Obstetricians and Gynecologists, 1983.
2. Bostick, J. S., Hsiao, H. S., and Lawson, E. E. A minicomputer-based perinatal/neonatal telecommunications network. *Pediatrics* 71:272, 1983.
3. *Code of Federal Regulations: Telecommunications*. Title 47 (Paut 80-End) Office of Federal Register, 1984.
4. Glass, C. J. Satellite Communications. In *Proceedings of the First International Assembly on Emergency Medical Services*. U.S. Department of Transportation. Washington, D.C.: Government Printing Office, 1982.
5. Telemetry and Communications. XV-1-XVB. In *Emergency Medical Care*. U.S. Department of Transportation. Washington, D.C.: Government Printing Office, January 1983.
6. Vogt, J. F., Chan, L. S., Wu, P. Y. K., et al. Impact of a regional infant dispatch center on neonatal mortality. *Am. J. Public Health* 71:577, 1981.

## Chapter Appendix I: Maternal Consultation Transfer Record

Date of referral call _____ Time _____
Person receiving call _____
Patient's name _____
Referring physician _____
Primary physician _____
Referring hospital _____
Person calling _____
Reason for admission _____
_____

### Maternal History

1. Age _____
2. Gravida _____
3. Para _____
4. Abortion _____
5. Weeks of gestation _____
6. Last menstrual period _____ Estimated date of confinement _____
7. Onset of contractions _____
8. Frequency of contractions _____
9. Cervical dilation _____
10. Evidence of vaginal bleeding _____
11. Rupture of membranes? Yes _____ No _____ Time _____
12. Fetal heart rate: Infant 1 _____ Infant 2 _____ Other _____
13. a. Temperature _____ b. Blood pressure _____ c. Pulse _____
14. Blood type _____
15. Referral history _____
    Relevant health problems _____
    _____

    Perinatal history _____
    _____
    _____

    Reason for transfer _____
    _____
    _____

16. Referral plan _____
    _____

17. Transported by _____
    _____

18. Assessment by _____
    Date _____

Reproduced with permission from *Guidelines for Perinatal Care*. Evanston, Ill.: American Academy of Pediatrics, Washington, D.C.: American College of Obstetricians and Gynecologists, 1983. P. 267.

## Chapter Appendix II: Patient Consultation and Transfer Sheet

---

**MARYLAND REGIONAL NEONATAL PROGRAM**
22 South Greene Street
Baltimore, Maryland 21201

History Number _____

|  | TIMES |  |  |
|---|---|---|---|
| **TEAM NOTIFIED** |  |  |  |
| Carriers Notified |  |  |  |
| Definitive Carrier Call |  |  |  |
| Carrier Arrival |  |  |  |
| Team Departure ICN |  |  |  |
| Arrive Referral Hospital |  |  |  |
| Depart Referral Hospital |  |  |  |
| Arrive ICN |  |  |  |
| Arrive Base ICN |  |  |  |
| Transport Completed |  |  |  |

### PATIENT CONSULTATION/TRANSFER SHEET

Mo___ Da___ 19___    _____         _____
                     Time of call        Name of person taking call

ICN:
1. _____ Time _____ Accepted _____
2. _____ Time _____ Accepted _____
3. _____ Time _____ Accepted _____

Patient Name _____    Patient address _____

(___ ___) ___ ___ - ___ ___ ___ ___
Patient phone number    Parents name    Insurance

REASON FOR REFERRAL CALL:
1. Prematurity    6. MAS
2. Aspiration     7. Surgical
3. RDS            8. Seizures
4. Sepsis         9. Other_____
5. Cardiac

Name of person calling    Name of referring M.D.

(___ ___) ___ ___ - ___ ___ ___ ___
Referring M.D. phone number    Name of referring hospital

_____    _____         (___ ___) ___ ___ - ___ ___ ___ ___
City of hospital    State    Referring hospital phone number

---

**INFANT INFORMATION:**

___  ___  Mo___ Da___ 19___
Sex  Race  Date of birth

_____  ___ gms  ___ wks
Time of Birth  Birth Wt.    EGA

Present Age: ___ Min ___ Hrs ___ Days

Apgars: ___     ___
        1 min.    5 min.

Type of Delivery: _____

Maternal Parity: _____

Hospital of Birth: _____

**CURRENT STATUS AT REFERRING HOSPITAL:** ___ ___ ___ Time

___•___ (C°/F°) ___ ___ ___ ___ ___ ___ ___ ___% ___% ___%
Temp (R/Ax)    Heart R.  Resp. R.   BP    Hct/Hgb  D/S   Bld. Glucose

RESPIRATORY STATUS:    Ventilator Mode: _____
                                        ETT/Bagging/IMV/Hood

| Site | Time | FiO₂ | PIP | PEEP/CPAP | Rate | PaO₂ | PcO₂ | Ph | BE |
|---|---|---|---|---|---|---|---|---|---|
| | | | | | | | | | |
| Site | Time | FiO₂ | PIP | PEEP/CPAP | Rate | PaO₂ | PcO₂ | Ph | BE |
| | | | | | | | | | |

FLUIDS:
1. _____    Skin Color _____
   Placement  Type  Amount
                                  X-Rays _____
2. _____    Blood Cultures _____
   Placement  Type  Amount
                                  Antibiotics _____

---

**POSSIBLE TRANSPORT NEEDS:**  O₂ ___  CPAP ___  IPPV ___  PERIPHERAL IV ___  UMBILICAL CATHETER ___

OTHER SIGNIFICANT DATA (Maternal, Neonatal) and Recommendations of NTN:

## Chapter Appendix III: High Risk Maternity Consultation and Referral Form

**HIGH RISK MATERNITY CONSULTATION/REFERRAL SERVICE**
MARYLAND REGIONAL NEONATAL PROGRAM—22 South Greene Street, Baltimore, Maryland 21201
Maryland Institute for Emergency Medical Services Systems

**FOR CONSULTATION/REFERRAL PHONE 578-8400**

| PERINATAL REFERRAL CENTERS | BACK-UP REFERRAL CENTERS | |
|---|---|---|
| JOHNS HOPKINS HOSPITAL | BALTIMORE CITY HOSPITAL | 396-8755 |
| 955-5850 | MERCY HOSPITAL | 332-9543 |
| UNIVERSITY OF MARYLAND HOSPITAL | SINAI HOSPITAL | 578-5192 |
| 528-6030 | ST. AGNES HOSPITAL | 368-6541 |

*THIS SECTION TO BE COMPLETED BY REFERRING INSTITUTION*

*PLEASE COMPLETE THIS FORM AND ATTACH RELEVANT CLINICAL RECORDS*

TIME OF CONSULTATION _____ TIME TRANSPORT ARRANGED _____ TIME PATIENT LEFT _____

PATIENT'S NAME _____ AGE ____ RACE _____ DATE _____

REFERRED BY _____ PHONE NUMBER _____

REFERRING INSTITUTION _____ PHONE NUMBER _____

PATIENT'S NEXT OF KIN _____ PHONE NUMBER _____

SOURCE OF PRENATAL CARE   1. Private M.D.     2. Health Dept.     3. Hospital Clinic     4. None

INSURANCE/MEDICAL ASSISTANCE NUMBER _____

### CLINICAL INFORMATION

REFERRING DIAGNOSIS _____

LMP _____ EDC _____ PARITY ___ ___ ___ ___ GESTATIONAL AGE _____

TYPE/RH _____ ALLERGIES _____ IV FLUIDS _____

MEDICATIONS WITHIN THE LAST 24 HOURS _____

MODE OF TRANSPORT:   1. Private Auto     2. Ambulance     3. Helicopter     4. Other

PATIENT ACCOMPANIED BY:   1. M.D.     2. R.N.     3. Paramedic     4. Air Trauma Tech     5. Other

### OUTCOME INFORMATION

*THIS SECTION TO BE COMPLETED BY RECEIVING HOSPITAL*

RECEIVING HOSPITAL _____ ARRIVAL TIME _____ DATE _____

ADMITTING DIAGNOSIS _____

DATE OF MOTHER'S DISCHARGE _____ DISCHARGE DIAGNOSIS _____

DISPOSITION AT TIME OF DISCHARGE:

1. Antepartum patient; discharged undelivered

2. Delivery information   Date _____   Type of Delivery   1. VD     2. C/SECT

Name of delivering M.D. _____ Attending Physician _____

BABY #1 _____ Male/Female _____ Infant to  1. ICN     2. NN
         Birthweight · Grams           Apgar 1 min   5 min

BABY #2 _____ Male/Female _____ Infant to  1. ICN     2. NN
         Birthweight · Grams           Apgar 1 min   5 min

COMPLICATIONS OF MOTHER/INFANT(S) _____
_____

DISPOSITION OF INFANT(S) AT TIME OF MOTHER'S DISCHARGE:

1. Discharged with mother 2. Remains in ICN 3. Neonatal Death 4. FDIU 5. Other _____ 6. Remains in full-term

FOLLOW-UP CARE FOR MOTHER _____
_____
_____

ORIGINAL COPY-Remains in Mother's Chart          2ND AND 3RD COPIES-Return to Transport Coordinator

## Chapter Appendix IV: Telephone Log

CHILDREN'S HOSPITAL NATIONAL MEDICAL CENTER—NICU
111 MICHIGAN AVE. N.W. WASHINGTON, D.C. 20010
202/745-5275

**TELEPHONE LOG**

ADDRESSOGRAPH

DATE:      TIME:      NAME OF PERSON TAKING CALL:

NAME OF PERSON CALLING:      HOSPITAL:      CITY:      STATE:

REFERRING PHYSICIAN:      PHONE #:

PT NAME:      SEX: M   F   U      DATE OF BIRTH:      If <24° TIME:      AGE:

GESTATIONAL AGE:      BIRTH WEIGHT:      gms      CURRENT WT:      gms

**PERINATAL HISTORY:** TYPE OF DEL.: _____ ROM: _____ hrs   MECONIUM? Y/N   APGARS: _____ 1 min. _____ 5 min. _____ other

MOM'S AGE: _____ G _____ P _____ AB _____ Complications:

Prenatal Care? Y?N

**REFERRAL HISTORY:**

**PRELIMINARY DIAGNOSIS:**

**OXYGEN DELIVERY:**

1. Nasotrach
2. Orotrach
3. Nasal prongs
4. Nasal cannula
5. Nasopharangeal
6. Hood
7. Mask
8. Trach
9. Other
10. None

**BLOOD GASES:**

| | | | | | |
|---|---|---|---|---|---|
| TIME | | | | | |
| FiO2 | | | | | |
| IMV | | | | | |
| PL | | | | | |
| P | | | | | |
| Ti | | | | | |
| pH | | | | | |
| pCO2 | | | | | |
| pO2 | | | | | |
| BE | | | | | |
| Site | | | | | |

**RECOMMENDATIONS:**

**VENT MODE:**

1. Bagging
2. Ventilator
3. CPAP
4. Other
5. None

| TUBES: | SIZE | SUCTION Y/N |
|---|---|---|
| NG | | |
| CT | | |
| OTHER | | |

**PLAN:** ACCEPT ☐
     Turn Down ☐

**ADMIT TO:** Room:
     Service:
     Attending:

**Authorized by:** _____

**VITAL SIGNS:**
Temp: _____
HR: _____
RR: _____
BP: _____

**FLUID LINES:**

| | SOLUTION | RATE |
|---|---|---|
| 1. Peripheral #1 | | |
| 2. Peripheral #2 | | |
| 3. Peripheral #3 | | |
| 4. Peripheral #4 | | |
| 5. UAC | | |
| 6. UVC | | |
| 7. Other | | |
| 8. None | | |

**NOTIFICATION:**

| | TIME | | | MODE OF TRANSPORT | ETA |
|---|---|---|---|---|---|
| Attending/Fellow | | | | 1. OUR TEAM GROUND | ☐ _____ |
| Transport Nurse | | | | 2. OUR TEAM HELI | ☐ _____ |
| Charge Nurse | | | | 3. OUR TEAM PLANE | ☐ _____ |
| Respiratory | | | | 4. OTHER TEAM GROUND | ☐ _____ |
| ECIC | | | | 5. OTHER TEAM HELI | ☐ _____ |
| Admitting | | | | 6. OTHER TEAM PLANE | ☐ _____ |

**LABS:**
Dext: _____
Hct: _____
Cxr: _____
Others: _____

**MEDS:**

**FEEDINGS:**

**COMMENTS/UPDATES:**

CHNMC 009 2

## *Chapter Appendix V: Helicopter Transfer Information Form*

---

# **Boston Med Flight** Patient Information Sheet

Patient Name: _____ Date: _____ Flight #: _____

Transferred to: _____
               Hospital                   Unit                  Phone #

_____
               Physician

**Boston Med Flight** is a critical care helicopter transport service staffed and equipped to care for the medical needs of seriously ill and injured patients while in transit between hospitals or from the incident scene to the hospital.

**Boston Med Flight** is a private non-profit corporation sponsored by eight tertiary health care centers of Boston whose locations are pinpointed on a map on the reverse of this sheet. These hospitals are prepared to accept and care for any seriously ill or injured patient. University Hospital, New England Medical Center, Massachusetts General Hospital, Massachusetts Eye and Ear Infirmary, Boston City Hospital, Brigham & Women's Hospital, Beth Israel Hospital, and Children's Hospital.

The aircraft, which flies approximately 150 miles per hour, is specially equipped with communications and medical equipment for medical emergencies. The Flight Nurse and Flight Medic, as well as the pilot, have had extensive training for **Boston Med Flight** missions. Modern technology and the skill of the crew combine to ensure that the patient receives the best possible medical care and monitoring during transfer.

If you have any comments or questions please call during business hours (9-5)Monday through Friday at 617-424-5208.

Your **Boston Med Flight** Crew,

Flight Nurse: _____

Flight Medic: _____

Pilot: _____

**BOSTON**
**Med Flight**

Peabody 1     818 Harrison Avenue     Boston, MA 02118     (617) 424-5208

# 5 Marketing an Aeromedical Transport System

Howard M. Collett

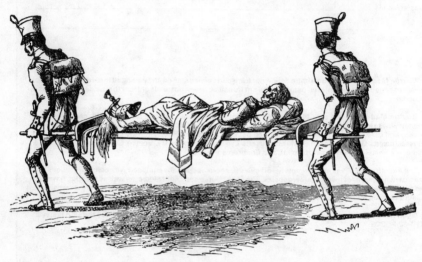

*5A. Two bearers carrying a wounded dragoon on a stretcher. Straps, which are attached to the knapsacks, receive the poles, thus assisting the hands of the bearers. They are shown walking in step, contrary to proper progression. A class 1 sick transport conveyance (conveyance borne by men). "The rule equally applies if the stretcher be carried by four instead of two men. The step must be broken by the front and rear rank men, so that the level of the stretcher may still be preserved."* (Reproduced from Longmore, T. A Treatise on the Transport of Sick and Wounded Troops. *London: Her Majesty's Stationery Office, 1869.)*

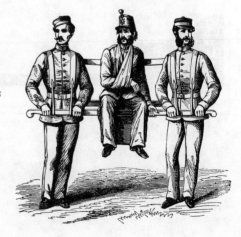

*5B. Chairstretcher, with a patient, carried by bearers marching abreast. A class 1 sick transport conveyance (conveyance borne by men).* (Reproduced from Longmore, T. A Treatise on the Transport of Sick and Wounded Troops. *London: Her Majesty's Stationery Office, 1869.)*

"In an increasingly competitive environment, hospitals are being forced to evaluate diversification into new markets in order to assure their survival." So wrote Joe B. Tye, the first president of the American Society of Hospital-Based Emergency Air Medical Services (ASHBEAMS) [3]. "Initiation of a helicopter service represents a major challenge to a hospital. The potential risk of failure associated with implementation of a helicopter service mandates that careful planning and marketing be performed," concluded Mr. Tye.

## What Is Marketing?

Marketing has been referred to as the "bells, whistles and other widgets used to attract attention" to the product or service being marketed. While this may be true for consumer goods and services, marketing has historically been a concept foreign to the medical profession. Physicians have regarded marketing (or at least advertising) as unprofessional—even bordering on unethical. It is therefore not surprising that hospital personnel have been slow to recognize that a full-scale marketing effort is required to launch a new aeromedical program. However, the health care field has become increasingly competitive in the past few years, and many hospitals have become more aggressive in their marketing efforts. One early study of an aeromedical service emphasized this point: "Inefficient marketing, public relations and physician education initially led to a slow start, but a change in program leadership finally resulted in a noticeable increase in the number of missions."

"Program leadership" is a key phrase in any discussion of aeromedical program marketing. The hospital administration developing an aeromedical service must devote the resources necessary to achieve a high degree of program use. The expense of most aeromedical services exceeds $1 million annually and, therefore, demands good management and reasonable levels of use.

The goal of the marketing effort is to provide both a forum for learning about the aeromedical program and training for optimal use of the service. The importance of marketing to the success of the program is second only to the quality of the critical care medical team. The hospital cannot park a helicopter in front and assume that its name alone will generate referrals. Even the most sophisticated medical and communications equipment will not generate missions unless users are aware of the benefits.

Marketing of a hospital-based emergency aeromedical service requires basic management tools. The careful planning, organizing, staffing, and controlling of marketing activities will lay the foundation for successful program use. The marketing strategy must be planned to overcome fears, resistance to change, and ignorance of new technology and methods of prehospital care. It must be organized to be efficient, with the ability to accomplish goals and objectives with the least expenditure of time and dollar resources. It must be staffed by a full-time coordinator capable of achieving the desired results with little or no staff or supervision. It must be constantly evaluated and assessed.

## The Marketing Plan

The outline of a marketing plan can be developed from the answers to the questions listed below:

When is it appropriate to transport a patient by air?
What are the benefits of our service?
What regional needs will the program satisfy?
Do we look professional?
Is the service readily available and convenient to use?
Who is eligible to use the service?
What is the cost?
Are the benefits worth the cost?
What is the liability of a referring agency or institution?
Is the service safe?
What protocols are required to ensure that the service is safely and optimally used?
Does our program include adequate training for all involved personnel (e.g., doctors, nurses, respiratory therapists, ground control personnel, dispatchers)?

The following goals, objectives, and methods have been suggested in a publication designed specifically for the aeromedical market [1]:

*Goals* focus planning and action efforts toward expected outcomes relating to the present and future fiscal strength and medical capabilities of the hospital. Some typical goals of a hospital-based emergency aeromedical service are as follows:

Provide rapid response critical care personnel and equipment to underserved segments of a service area.
Expand the geographical or quantitative referral base, or both, of the hospital to maximize use of hospital facilities and personnel.
Increase visibility of the hospital in the community.

*Objectives* are intermediate milestones passed while reaching the goal, with defined time limits and measurable performance criteria such as the examples below:

Awareness: Achieve a 50 percent level of program awareness in referral entities over the next 3 months.

Attitude: Achieve a favorable attitude (measured by one or more requests for aeromedical service) in 30 percent of the referral entities over the next 6 months.

Activity: Achieve a minimum of 75 flight requests during the first 3 months of the program.

*Methods* are daily or recurring activities designed to accomplish objectives. Examples are as follows:

Make five public relations flights per month to referral entities.

Make a follow-up telephone call to the referring agency within 30 minutes of patient arrival.

Mail a program newsletter to all referral entities each quarter.

Objectives and methods must be continually evaluated and modified as necessary to ensure that they are providing desired results relative to specific goals.

## Marketing Strategy

Strategy is simply defined as a plan for adapting hospital resources to achieve objectives. As the aeromedical transport concept is developed and goals and objectives are defined, hospital resources should be examined to determine capacity to meet the needs of the transport program. If available time or expertise does not permit accomplishment of one or more assigned tasks, additional assistance may be required. Such assistance may be achieved by hiring additional personnel or by the retention of public relations agencies, consultants, or other professional firms.

A general rule for the marketing strategy of an aeromedical program is that the marketing effort must be *constant* and *effective*. It must be constant because busy hospital and public safety agency staff are continually exposed to the special needs and problems of others. Transport needs constitute just a small part of their responsibilities and may be overlooked. The frequent turnover among dispatchers, department supervisors, and line personnel also produces a requirement for ongoing education. To be effective, the marketing effort must be properly directed. It is not sufficient to mail a brochure to the police chief or head of a Level I nursery and expect immediate and continued departmental support. A marketing message must be targeted to each level of the administrative and the clinical team.

Price considerations are especially complex in health care, in that only a small portion of the total cost is actually paid directly by the consumer at the time of use. It is the physician who determines what services will be used, but the physician is not obligated for payment. Such a market situation is seldom found in other industries. Although price is usually not a direct factor in determining program use, it should be remembered that the service-price relationship must be perceived to be equitable when compared to available alternatives, including both ground and other air transport services.

### Marketing Communications

Marketing plans can be as varied as the people who write them. The end result of the marketing plan is the communication of a message to the consumer or user. The specific purpose of marketing communications is to communicate the benefits of services offered to the potential users in such a way as to help them to achieve their goals while, at the same time, moving the hospital closer to its own goals.

For a hospital-based aeromedical program, users fall into two categories. The first and most obvious are the patients. However, since patients generally do not make the decision for transport, marketing efforts are targeted at referring physicians or institutions and public safety entities such as law enforcement, fire agencies, and emergency medical services (EMSs).

A basic marketing principle is that users do not buy a specific *product or service* (in this case, an aeromedical helicopter or airplane service), they buy *expectation of benefits*. In other words, they buy what the product or service will *do* for them.

The major benefit that an aeromedical service provides to a referring hospital or public safety agency is that such a program augments their existing services and capabilities, enabling them to do a better job. For a serious car crash, a ground ambulance company may be the first responder, rendering first aid and extrication. In turn, the first responders may rely on a helicopter service for critical care life support skills and equipment, coupled with a rapid transport to a trauma department at a major hospital. For a premature infant, a newborn nursery may provide initial stabilization, yet rely on a fixed-wing air service with a neonatal specialty team to transport the infant to a Level III facility. The tangible benefits of the aeromedical service to patients are that it helps reduce suffering and saves lives.

The benefits of an aeromedical program will be perceived only if properly communicated. If the marketing aspect is mismanaged or neglected, patients and their physicians will view the helicopter as an expensive, unreimbursable alternative to ground transport. Referring public safety agencies will regard the program as a competitor, a nuisance for traffic control, and an increase in their workload.


## *Target Markets*

There are several specific areas or groups (target markets) that will use an aeromedical service. Among these are hospitals, clinics, ambulance services, police and fire departments, heavy industrial complexes, major resorts and recreation areas, military bases, and former patients and employees of the sponsor hospital. However, requests for transport of a neonate or pregnant mother will almost always be generated from another medical facility.

Medical facilities can be divided into two major groups: local and distant. Both groups are potential sources for patient referrals. However, local hospitals stand apart because they may also be competing for transported patients, depending on their clinical capabilities. In addition, local hospitals will almost always transport the perinatal patient to another local hospital by ground transport.

The transport needs of local hospitals with referral services should not be overlooked. These clinical services may compete with the nursery at the hospital that sponsors the air transport program, but there may be no reason that the transport service cannot serve all facilities. Such an agreement will increase use of the transport service, thereby lowering the cost per patient. In addition, the development of competing transport services may be prevented.

Neonates are primarily physician referred to a specific facility and not to a transport service. However, a transport service at a facility offers the potential for earlier transfer of the patient (and the associated liability) from the referring hospital to the receiving hospital. The marketing potential of a transport system exists even when a clinical department relies on transport services provided by another hospital or service. The clinical departments that share the service should work with the transport service to develop standard transport protocols. The transport service and all of the involved clinical services can then be marketed together.

## Marketing Resources

Once the general marketing plan has been formulated and the target markets are identified, specific decisions must be made regarding the communication of the marketing message. A budget must be developed or revised, personnel resources identified, and formats designed to carry a clear, consistent message. Creativity should be used to prompt a positive reaction from referral entities but should not detract from the basic strategic plan.

Rapid changes in strategy can often result in a very confused consumer and should be avoided. There is usually more than one "right" way to achieve objectives. However, strong clinical aspects of the hospital should be marketed and augmented by the transport service to bring the clinical benefits and the patient together. When several alternative strategies are developed, each must be evaluated in terms of probable outcome, adverse reactions, potential risks involved, and time frames for accomplishment.

Physicians are the primary, but not the only, individuals at a medical facility who have influence over the decision to transport a patient to another hospital. Key individuals at each facility also include the hospital administrator, the medical chief of staff, the emergency department director, and emergency department nursing shift supervisors. These individuals are best contacted by their counterparts from the hospital sponsoring the aeromedical program. Since most referrals are generated by individual physicians, it is important to provide them with positive information about the transport service. Such information may best be disseminated by enlisting the efforts of influential doctors with solid professional reputations at the sponsoring hospital.

There are two forms of marketing communications: personal and nonpersonal. Personal communications include site visits, public relations flights, outreach education clinics, and telephone calls. A nonpersonal communications format usually includes brochures, form letters, and static displays. Nonpersonal formats can introduce the concept of the transport service to individuals and groups in the target market population. To be most effective, nonpersonal communications should be promptly followed by personal communications that provide the opportunity for questions and the clarification of any misconceptions.

In 1982, Aviation/Hospital Consultants conducted a marketing survey of aeromedical helicopter services to determine the most effective marketing techniques [2]. Although the survey is 6 years old, annual random follow-up surveys have revealed little change in the outcomes reported in the original study. A complete copy of the survey results was published in *Hospital Aviation* magazine (Chap. Appendix I).

The survey revealed that the most effective ongoing marketing techniques for a medical helicopter service are, in order of priority: (1) telephone follow-up by the receiving physician or flight nurse to the referring agency or hospital, (2) public relations flights to other hospitals, and (3) personal visits to other hospitals.

FOLLOW-UP

Providing immediate follow-up to the referring entity concerning the condition of a transported patient is a most successful marketing technique. Not only is this a professional courtesy but it also demonstrates pride in the program and provides positive feedback regarding the role of the aeromedical service in providing optimal patient care.

Most programs designate the responsibility for telephone follow-up to the attending transport nurse. Within 30 minutes of patient arrival, the nurse telephones the referring hospital or agency to provide details (where appropriate) of the patient's condition during transport and current procedures being performed. Some programs will ask the attending physician to make this call. In either case, the call should be made as soon as possible, followed by a written report within 48 hours.

When appropriate, the telephone follow-up technique can be used as a marketing tool when a critical patient arrives by *ground* transport. Most effective when made by a physician, such a call can be made to the referring hospital or physician, tactfully suggesting that "the next time you have a patient in a similar condition, why don't you request our critical care transport team and aircraft?"

The importance of follow-up cannot be over-emphasized. If a referring doctor or agency does not hear from the service following a transport, they may think twice before calling the next time they require patient transport.

The administrator of the hospital sponsoring the aeromedical service can play an important role in the marketing effort by telephoning or writing to the administrators of the referring hospital, commending them for their support and cooperation. This message should assure the referring hospital staff that, if possible, their patients will be transported back to the local hospital for step-down care when medically indicated. This assumes, however, that "back transfer" will not create a reimbursement problem. Such a call is in addition to, but coordinated with, the follow-up call placed by the physician or flight nurse.

Experience has shown that a reliable program of follow-up communication cannot exist without a support system. Such a system should be managed by a chief flight nurse or program director who is responsible for ensuring that follow-up communication is occurring on a timely basis. The communication can be accomplished using a transport log, a computer word-processing system, and physician dictation system. The program director or flight nurse can remind the physician that the report is due. The physician can then dictate details of patient care following a predesigned format. These details can then be transcribed onto a form letter that is designed to fit the same format. The log can then be signed off to maintain a record of task completion.

PUBLIC RELATIONS FLIGHTS AND SITE VISITS
For a new program, new clinical service, or new aircraft, public relations (PR) flights offer several advantages over other marketing techniques. The primary benefit is the "show and tell, touch and feel" aspect. Direct mail and telephone techniques can go a long way in educating referring physicians about a service, but the memories imprinted by an experience with the real thing far outweigh passive involvement.

It should be emphasized, however, that PR flights are not effective without the concurrent use of other techniques. A PR flight can be preceded by (1) a letter and program brochure explaining what the service is, (2) a telephone call to answer questions and set up an appointment for the flight, (3) a letter confirming the date, time, and location, (4) letters and telephone calls to EMS, police and fire agencies that could also attend, and (5) letters and telephone calls to members of the publishing and broadcast media.

The PR flight provides a visual inspection of the aircraft, an explanation of safety precautions, a patient loading demonstration, and the display of medical equipment carried on the helicopter. An audiovisual production regarding the service can also be presented. Other public relations materials, such as brochures, wallet cards, Rolodex inserts, and telephone stickers can be handed out prior to departure. PR flights should be followed up with a thank-you letter to all agencies involved and with telephone calls to gather feedback. The repetitive nature of these calls, letters, and visits enforces the message of the program.

A site visit is essentially the same as a PR flight, without the impact of the aircraft. The audiovisual presentation is the focus of the event. Following site visits or PR flights, attendees should be placed on the mailing list to receive the aeromedical service newsletter. The newsletter is designed to reinforce the impact of the marketing message and to provide an update on changes in program capabilities or personnel, or both.

PR flights and site visits will generate a number of questions about the service, and the aeromedical crew making the presentation must be capable of providing the answers. The following list is representative of the questions that are most commonly asked:

1. How does an aeromedical ambulance system differ from a conventional ambulance system?
2. What is the service area of the program?
3. What kinds of weather conditions prohibit flight?
4. What training is required of medical teams?
5. What training is provided by the air service?
6. Does the pilot assist with medical care?
7. What type of medical equipment is carried on board the aircraft?
8. What categories of patients can be transported?
9. Can family members accompany the patient?
10. Can the referring physician accompany the patient?
11. How is the patient's condition affected by the transport?
12. What hospitals can patients be transported to?
13. Do other hospitals in the metropolitan area offer aeromedical transport?
14. How much does the service cost, and who pays for the transport?
15. If insurance does not cover the transport charge and the patient cannot pay, is the requesting physician or agency responsible for the bill?
16. How does the aeromedical transport charge compare with a ground ambulance charge?
17. How is liability for the patient affected by the transport service?
18. Can airborne medical teams communicate with physicians or hospitals on the ground?
19. How safe is aeromedical transport?
20. What is the safety record of this particular service?

### Marketing Mature Programs

Marketing efforts for a well-established aeromedical program require a somewhat different approach from that used for new programs. While PR flights can often be conducted during the early months of a new program, increasing use will eventually limit the quantity and distance of such flights. Many existing services hold annual anniversary celebrations and make a public event out of them. Some sponsor a "patient alumni day" where former patients gather and praise the service. Special promotional materials and events are worthy of consideration. These may include participation in area disaster drills and major sporting events.

Sharing expertise is another marketing avenue for established programs. In addition to the training program for health professionals actually involved in the transport, outreach education programs for outlying hospital units and prehospital providers share clinical knowledge and generate good will.

## Conclusion

The scope and expense of an aeromedical transport program mandates marketing activity to ensure appropriate levels of use. A good marketing program requires basic management tools and strategy to effectively communicate the desired message to the proper target market. Prior analysis of the services offered and how they will be perceived is essential to the development of the marketing plan.

The marketing message must be constant and effective to reach those in other hospitals and public safety agencies who deal with patient transport on a limited basis. However, at no time must those involved in marketing a program lose sight of their responsibility to ensure that the service is used only when truly indicated and when there are no contraindications that might compromise safety (see Chap. 13).

Three methods of marketing have been identified as superior. These include PR flights, site visits, and prompt follow-up communication by telephone. The marketing plan for a mature aeromedical service may differ from that for a developing service. However, even for established programs, the requirement for ongoing effective marketing should not be underestimated.

## References

1. Collett, H. M. Hospital aviation marketing survey. *Hospital Aviation,* 2(9):8, 1982.
2. Collett, H. M. *Marketing Manual for Hospital-Based Emergency Aeromedical Programs.* Independent consulting study, 1982, Aviation/Hospital Consultants, 53 W. 1800 South, Orem, UT 84058.
3. Tye, J. B. Planning and marketing a hospital-based emergency helicopter service. *Hospital Aviation* 2(8):8, 1983.

## Chapter Appendix I: 1982 Hospital Aviation Marketing Survey

In June 1982, a marketing survey was sent by *Hospital Aviation* magazine to 43 hospital-based helicopter programs. By September 1982, 26 had responded, for a healthy 60 percent sampling. The following Table A5-1 is the format used and the response to this survey: "Which of the following marketing/public relations activities or methods have been used by your program, and what was their effect on *increasing* program utilization?"

*Table A5-1. Result of* Hospital Aviation *marketing survey*

| | Used (%) | | Effect on program utilization (%) | | | |
|---|---|---|---|---|---|---|
| | Yes | No | Significant | Moderate | Little/none | Unknown |
| PROMOTIONAL FLIGHTS | | | | | | |
| To hospitals | 96 | 4 | 60 | 24 | 4 | 12 |
| To police/fire agencies | 81 | 19 | 33 | 47 | 10 | 10 |
| To EMS agencies | 88 | 12 | 48 | 26 | 13 | 13 |
| To civic organizations | 81 | 19 | 10 | 19 | 28 | 43 |
| PROMOTIONAL VISITS | | | | | | |
| To hospitals | 96 | 4 | 60 | 24 | 4 | 12 |
| To police/fire agencies | 81 | 19 | 33 | 47 | 10 | 10 |
| To EMS agencies | 88 | 12 | 48 | 26 | 13 | 13 |
| To civic organizations | 81 | 19 | 10 | 19 | 28 | 43 |
| DIRECT MAIL (LETTERS/BROCHURES) | | | | | | |
| To hospitals | 81 | 19 | 19 | 43 | 24 | 14 |
| To police/fire agencies | 73 | 27 | 11 | 42 | 26 | 21 |
| To EMS agencies | 73 | 27 | 21 | 42 | 16 | 21 |
| To civic organizations | 23 | 77 | 17 | 17 | 33 | 33 |
| PRESS RELEASES | | | | | | |
| To TV stations | 88 | 12 | 17 | 22 | 17 | 44 |
| To radio stations | 88 | 12 | 17 | 22 | 17 | 44 |
| To newspapers | 96 | 4 | 20 | 20 | 16 | 44 |
| STATIC DISPLAYS | | | | | | |
| Fairs | 77 | 23 | 15 | 15 | 35 | 35 |
| Shopping malls | 58 | 42 | 13 | 20 | 40 | 27 |
| Athletic/civic events | 54 | 46 | 21 | 29 | 29 | 21 |
| Program open house | 62 | 38 | 13 | 19 | 37 | 31 |
| COMMUNICATIONS CENTER | | | | | | |
| Dispatcher effectiveness | 73 | 27 | 37 | 26 | 11 | 26 |
| "Showplace effect" | 50 | 50 | 31 | 23 | 15 | 31 |
| TELEPHONE FOLLOWUP TO REFERRING AGENCY | | | | | | |
| By receiving doctor | 54 | 46 | 86 | 7 | 0 | 7 |
| By flight nurse | 88 | 12 | 78 | 18 | 0 | 4 |
| By program director | 38 | 62 | 60 | 20 | 0 | 20 |

# 6

# Evaluating the Impact of Perinatal Transfer on Patient Care

Houchang D. Modanlou
Wendy L. Dorchester

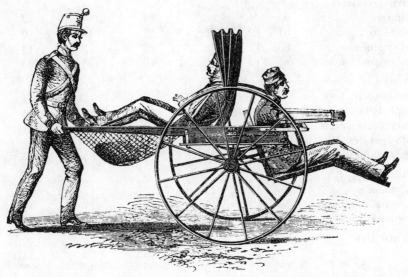

6A. Neudörfer's two-wheeled litter for the transport of one or two wounded soldiers. A class 2 sick transport conveyance (conveyance wheeled by men). (Reproduced from Longmore, T. A Treatise on the Transport of Sick and Wounded Troops. London: Her Majesty's Stationery Office, 1869.)

6B. Neudörfer's litter folded up and packed for carriage. A class 2 sick transport conveyance (conveyance wheeled by men). (Reproduced from Longmore, T. A Treatise on the Transport of Sick and Wounded Troops. London: Her Majesty's Stationery Office, 1869.)

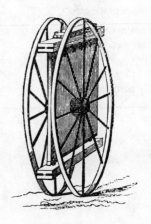

The recent health care climate has encouraged an increased emphasis on the evaluation of proposed and existing clinical programs. Concerns exist regarding the cost of health care programs, their efficacy, inequitable distribution of services, and mismanagement and waste of resources. The use of systematic databased evaluations, rooted in the epidemiological efforts at infection control at the turn of the century, has become an accepted and defined mechanism for assessing the effectiveness of health care programs [29].

Traditionally, program evaluation has been concerned with three areas: program structure, program process, and program outcome. Each of these areas contributes to a comprehensive assessment of the functions and impact of a program. In the case of evaluating a perinatal transport program, the program structure could be considered to be the organization and availability of the program. For example, is the program available to all perinatal patients within the region? Program process could be considered the actual process involved in a perinatal transfer (e.g., Does the sequence of events at the time of patient transfer occur as planned?). Program outcome is the impact or effect of the program on the target population.

Most of the published reports on the evaluation of perinatal transport systems have attempted to measure the impact of perinatal transfer on patient outcome. This approach appears to be reasonable, because patient outcome is the ultimate indicator of the effectiveness of a clinical program. However, knowledge of a program's structure and process, including cost, is also necessary to determine cost-effectiveness and cost-efficiency. In addition, the focus on a single area of evaluation fails to distinguish between the impact of the entire program versus that of a specific component. Facts that might explain the result of an outcome evaluation based on the structure or process of a perinatal transfer system are often not considered. As noted by Lipsey et al [22], "a program consists of a set of rational linkages between program activities and expected outcomes abstracted from particular behaviors in which program personnel happen to engage." Despite the limitations of this perspective, in this chapter we will focus primarily on the methods and results of evaluating the impact of perinatal transfer on patient outcome. The potential value of evaluating program structure and process will be emphasized.

## *Rationale for Evaluating a Perinatal Transfer Program*
### ENSURING OPTIMUM CARE FOR MOTHERS, FETUSES, AND NEONATES
Concerns about the efficacy of intuitively reasonable clinical programs, such as fetal monitoring, improved pregnancy outcome projects, and in-

fant feeding programs [28, 31], have produced many studies that focus on the impact of these programs on patient outcome. The intent of these outcome evaluation studies often is to document what appears to be obvious benefit; however, they may reveal that little appears to be gained from the program by patients in general or a subset of patients [28]. Published studies evaluating experiences with perinatal transfer have reported mixed outcomes, with some authors documenting significant benefit whereas others do not. These reports suggest that various regional and demographical factors, such as the availability of services in urban versus rural areas, may influence the impact of perinatal transfer on patient outcome.

Since each region has a unique set of characteristics, the systematic review of patient outcome may provide information about the types of patients that benefit most from antenatal transfer and situations in which postnatal transport of the neonate is advantageous: On-going patient outcome evaluation may help to ensure optimal care for mothers, fetuses, and neonates.

ASSESSING COST PERFORMANCE
To successfully evaluate cost-effectiveness and cost-benefit, (collectively called "efficiency"), knowledge of how the program is structured and the processes used by the program is necessary. Personnel, organization, equipment, funding sources, the institutions and communities to be served (target population) and, most importantly, the goals and objectives are elements of the program structure. Program process data includes the proportion of the target population receiving benefits from the program, the frequency of intervention (e.g., perinatal transfers), the presence or absence of marketing and educational efforts, the personnel and equipment movements surrounding a perinatal transfer, and ancillary benefits or problems such as an increased number of deliveries at the regional perinatal center (RPC). Cost-effectiveness is defined as the relative cost of achieving given interventions (e.g., cost to transport antenatally versus postnatally) in relation to program costs (e.g., the cost of an antenatal transfer system), while cost-benefit is the relationship between the cost of outcomes and the cost of the program. For example, the cost-benefit ratio might be the cost of an antenatal transfer system compared with the money saved as a result of successful tocolysis and a reduced number of premature deliveries. Much of the data required to evaluate cost is unavailable. Reports in the literature have often used length of hospitalization rather than cost to demonstrate efficiency [26]. Unfortunately, this practice fails to take into account the cost of the perinatal transfer program itself. Evaluations that include pro-

gram structure, process, and outcome could provide important information about the cost-effectiveness and cost-benefit of a perinatal transfer system. In addition, concerns over the loss of revenue, which are often expressed by referring community hospitals, could be addressed by this type of evaluation.

PROVIDING FEEDBACK

Like a complex machine, a perinatal transfer system consists of many different parts operating at various levels of competency. The movement of a mother or neonate from one facility to another can leave one set of health care givers without follow-up information about their performance levels or patient outcome. A by-product of the evaluation process is the collection of data that can serve to provide feedback to health care providers who do not see the ultimate outcome of their efforts.

Information concerning perinatal transfers is a useful educational tool and should be evaluated with the referring perinatal care team as part of a regularly scheduled outreach education program. Areas for discussion include the appropriateness of transfer, indications, feasibility, response time by the receiving team, patient preparation, modality of transfer, timeliness of feedback, as well as treatment at the RPC and outcome. Periodic, at least yearly, evaluation of the effectiveness of perinatal transport to and from each referring and receiving hospital in the regional system is recommended, with program modification as indicated.

Evaluation of the effectiveness of feedback is a difficult task because it involves perceptions of collective or individual professional behavior that are based on the assumption that the groups of professionals who interact in the system are mutually satisfied with the relationship. Based on 10 years of experience, working regularly with perinatal care givers at 20 Level I and II facilities, we have found that a successful and lasting professional relationship requires commitment, honesty, and professional integrity on both sides. The basic ingredient to initiating professional trust is the quality and behavior of the consultants from the RPC. Professional competency must be combined with tolerance, availability, and a genuine desire to work with another professional to provide the best perinatal care. Acceptance of constructive criticism and regular attendance at pertinent meetings by both parties are indirect measures of the effectiveness of a good feedback mechanism and a successful perinatal transfer system. Perinatologists and consultant neonatologists at the RPC should be aware of these facts and periodically evaluate the quality of their professional relationships with the personnel at referring Level I and II facilities.

EXAMINING THE USE OF COMMUNITY RESOURCES

Health care services within a region are a limited resource. Maximizing the appropriate use of community resources allows the greatest number of patients to be served by the health care system for the least cost. A patient transport system seeks to maximize the use of expensive technology and personnel by moving patients to a single location, the regional center. Centralization of tertiary level care prevents many hospitals from purchasing costly equipment that would be used infrequently and regional center personnel can become familiar with rarely occurring medical problems. Specifically, a perinatal transfer system allows the regional center to acquire the specialized equipment, laboratory capabilities, and personnel to effectively care for a high-risk parturient or sick neonate. The decision to transport an ill high-risk mother or a sick neonate is based on the presence of maternal and neonatal conditions for which the required care can be assessed prior to transfer. Antenatal assessment of the advantages of maternal transfer that is undertaken because the neonate *may* require special care is more complex. The transfer of stabilized pregnant women and neonates back to their referring community hospital for continued care may further optimize the use of resources [17]. The use of community perinatal resources can be monitored by an on-going evaluation process and the data collected used to produce recommendations and guidelines for program changes.

MONITORING THE PROCESS OF PERINATAL TRANSFER

Program process is the planned sequence of events involved in the perinatal transfer. Review of each of these events provides an opportunity to measure the performance of the transport/transfer team and their equipment.

The first step in the initiation of transfer by the community hospital is the communication with the RPC (or dispatch center) to arrange for transfer or consultation, or both. Performance at this step can be monitored by measuring (1) the time from the detection of a problem at the community hospital to this initial communication, (2) the amount of time from initiation of the phone call to contact with the perinatal transfer dispatcher, (3) the number of transfers refused due to lack of space, personnel, or other reasons, and (4) the availability and timeliness of telephone consultation at the RPC.

The second step in the perinatal transfer process is the response of the RPC transport team. This response can be assessed by (1) response time of the team, (2) readiness of equipment for transport, (3) availability of appropriate transportation (i.e., helicopter versus ambulance), and (4) the selection of the members of the transport team. After the transport team arrives at the community hospital, the patient must be examined and prepared for transport. How well the patient has been stabilized, the availability of laboratory reports and the medical chart, and whether the staff at the referring hospital is aware of transport procedure (e.g., clearing the parking lot for use as a helipad, and alerting personnel to hold elevators) can be assessed. The final steps in patient transport, the transit period and admitting the patient, can be monitored by examining (1) the performance of the equipment during transport, (2) the clinical skills of the transport team and adequacy of documentation, and (3) preparations at the RPC for receiving the patient.

Evaluation at each step of the perinatal transfer process provides a mechanism to enhance performance. Performance can be modified by communicating evaluation information and results to the staff at the referring hospital, the perinatal transport team, RPC staff, and equipment/instrument manufacturers.

## ASSESSING POTENTIAL ADVANTAGES AND DISADVANTAGES OF PERINATAL TRANSFER

Cordero et al. reported their experience in one Ohio region and stated that the place of birth statistically influences survival for the very low birth weight (VLBW) premature infant, and that transport of the mother to a perinatal center can significantly increase the survival of the VLBW infant [11]. A similar experience was reported from the United Kingdom [20]. The authors noted that the survival among infants transported in utero, especially those whose birth weights were between 1000 and 1999 g and whose gestational age was between 26 and 29 weeks, was significantly higher than that among infants of comparable birth weight and gestational age who were transferred after delivery. In 1978, the Liaison Committee of the British Pediatric Association and the Royal College of Obstetricians and Gynecologists recommended that mothers in danger of delivering preterm should be transferred antenatally to a center with neonatal intensive care facilities [20]. Based on experience in Maryland, Crenshaw et al. [12] recommended that all mothers who have reached 32 or fewer weeks' gestation, are in premature labor, or are anticipated to require delivery for maternal or fetal indications be transferred for delivery to a hospital with a neonatal intensive care unit. However, the rigid implementation of these recommendations could create problems at all levels of the regional system.

As noted by Kanto et al. [18], a maternal transport system leads to an increased demand for obstetric and nursery beds. This increased demand has the episodic potential to overwhelm bed capacity at tertiary level facilities. Experience [10.13, 16, 26.30] has shown that the vast majority of in utero transports are of fetuses of low gestational age, resulting in the deliv-

ery of very small infants. In our experience [26], premature labor, pre-
mature/prolonged rupture of membranes, third-trimester bleeding, and
preeclampsia/eclampsia were the indications for more than 90 percent of
acute maternal transports. About 50 percent of the mothers delivered an
infant with a birth weight of less than 1500 g, and more than 20 percent
delivered an infant weighing less than 1000 g. There has been a dramatic
increase in the survival rates for VLBW infants during the past decade, and
the average length of hospitalization has thus been prolonged. In our neonatal intensive care unit the length of hospitalization for surviving infants
of less than 1000 g birth weight is 60 to 90 days. There is a direct relationship between the increased survival of very premature infants and bed occupancy in the neonatal intensive care unit. This, in turn, may affect the
ability of the RPC to accept referred neonates.

The successful implementation of an antenatal referral and transport
system for high-risk mothers tends to yield an increased incidence of stillbirths at the RPC. Some stillbirths are referred for delivery, since the experimental drugs for the induction of labor may only be available at the
RPC. Similarly, cases involving fetuses with congenital anomalies tend to be
referred and are associated with additional physical and emotional burden
on the staff at the RPC. Data on the emotional impact of maternal transfer
on the personnel at the referring hospital are unavailable. Similarly it is
difficult to measure the emotional impact of antenatal transport on the patient and her immediate family.

Despite these negative factors there is a major advantage to antenatal
versus postnatal transfer in that the mother is in the same facility as her
offspring. Despite the unanticipated events surrounding the delivery of
her child, and depending on the experience and sensitivity of the personnel at the RPC, the emotional impact of transport on the mother can be
minimized (see Chap. 10).

## Common Methodologies Used for Outcome Evaluation

Evaluation research designs that focus on program outcome are frequently
called "impact" evaluations. This type of evaluation can be used for ongoing or new programs, or to monitor the effects of changes in existing programs (i.e., to test how well a program or intervention is producing the
intended outcome). The most common strategy used is to compare information about program participants and nonparticipants. Well-defined program goals and objectives are necessary before an impact evaluation can
begin, and these objectives must yield variables that can measure program
outcome. Identifying several program outcome variables is important to

prevent spurious association or lack of association with a single or ill-chosen outcome variable. For example, perinatal mortality is often used as an outcome variable. However, sample size or the regional mortality rates, or both, may be too small to allow meaningful interpretation of the data. Before performing an impact evaluation it is necessary to allow enough time for the intervention/program to have reached the target population.

As noted by Rossi and Freeman [29] the net effect of a program, as considered by an impact evaluation, can be described by the following equation:

$$\text{Net effect} = \begin{matrix}\text{gross outcome}\\\text{participants}\end{matrix} - \begin{matrix}\text{gross outcome}\\\text{nonparticipants}\end{matrix} \pm \begin{matrix}\text{change}\\\text{effect}\end{matrix}$$

Specifically, in assessing the impact of antenatal transfer versus neonatal transfer, the net effect on morbidity would be

$$\begin{matrix}\text{Net morbidity}\\\text{Change}\end{matrix} = \begin{matrix}\text{morbidity}\\\text{antenatal}\\\text{transfers}\\\text{(new program)}\end{matrix} - \begin{matrix}\text{morbidity}\\\text{postnatal}\\\text{transports}\\\text{(standard practice)}\end{matrix} \pm \begin{matrix}\text{change}\\\text{factor}\end{matrix}$$

The most important aspect of this comparison is to ascertain comparable participant and nonparticipant groups. These groups should be similar with respect to factors other than the program or intervention that might influence outcome. This similarity between groups should be reflected at the aggregate level. For example, the average gestational ages of the two groups should be comparable, whereas the gestational ages of any two participants and nonparticipants may differ. Aggregate similarity is facilitated by having a large sample size for each group. If a large sample is not possible, then matching individuals between the two groups is a mechanism for ascertaining risk-comparable groups. Appropriate statistical tests can control for the chance factor.

There are two major categories of impact evaluation: the qualitative/descriptive type and the quantitative/comparative type. The qualitative/descriptive impact evaluation describes only program/intervention participants or indicates differences between the participants and nonparticipants, without providing numerical comparisons between groups or making statistical inferences. Although the value of a well-executed descriptive program evaluation cannot be disputed, this type of evaluation is sometimes done because it is not possible to find comparable participant/nonparticipant groups and, therefore, it suffers with respect to internal validity. The majority of published program evaluation reports use the quantitative/comparative type of research design.

A quantitative approach implies numerical comparisons between program participants and nonparticipants and should be used only when comparable groups have been defined. Common methods used by this type of research design include randomized experiments, quasi-experiments, and pre- and postprogram implementation comparisons. These methods will be discussed and applied to the evaluation of perinatal transfer.

RANDOMIZED EXPERIMENTS
Randomization implies that every member of the sample has an equal chance of being selected as a participant or nonparticipant in the program or intervention. Randomization is performed after the sample is selected. The rationale for using a randomized experimental design is that, if the sample is sufficiently large, the groups will be comparable and the differences in outcome between the participant and nonparticipant groups will be due either to the program/intervention or to chance.

Randomized experiments to evaluate entire perinatal transfer systems are difficult to achieve. These systems are often not amenable to randomization because of ethical issues, community practice, or physician judgment, or a combination of these. However, Bourch and Wothke contend that randomization should be considered in field settings [4]. Changes within a transfer program, such as switching from ambulance to helicopter as the transport vehicle or to nurse-supervised transports, may lend themselves to evaluation using randomization.

As noted by Lipsey et al. [22] there are numerous practical difficulties inherent in the matching of a good research design to practical program circumstances. As a result the quasi-experimental designs, as categorized by Campbell and Stanley [5] and Cook and Campbell [9], have been used extensively as approximations to randomized controlled experiments.

QUASI-EXPERIMENTAL DESIGN
Clinical researchers have traditionally used classic experimental designs and shunned the quasi-experimental designs on which much of evaluation planning is based. However, as noted above, randomized experimental design often relies on assumptions about the data that may not be reasonable when assessing the impact of an entire program.

Quasi-experimental designs differ from randomized experiments because the nonparticipant/participant groups are assigned by some mechanism other than chance (randomization). Each member of the sample does not have an equal probability of being selected as a participant or nonparticipant. Often the participant group has been preselected, and the nonparticipant or "control" group is chosen to be comparable to the participants for those factors that are judged to influence the outcome variables. For example, when comparing the outcome of a new antenatal transfer program versus the standard practice of neonatal transport, the duration of hospitalization, incidence of morbidity, and days on oxygen could be chosen as the outcome variables. A "control" group of neonates transported postnatally could be selected by matching them with infants transferred in utero for those factors that could influence the outcome variables.

A disadvantage of quasi-experimental design, as compared with randomization, is that matching of the "control" group depends on knowledge about the "other factors" that can influence the program outcome variables. In the case of evaluating a perinatal transfer system, the factors that influence gross measures of patient outcome (e.g., mortality), such as birth weight, gestational age, sex, race, and plurality, are generally well known. However, for more subtle outcome variables, such as days on oxygen or the incidence of respiratory distress syndrome, it may be difficult to determine all of the contributing variables. Defining risk-comparable groups is extremely difficult when many potentially confounding variables exist.

PRE- AND POSTIMPLEMENTATION COMPARISONS
Another mechanism for performing an impact evaluation is to use pre- and postprogram implementation (PPI) comparisons. This approach is sometimes used when randomized or matching designs are not available. PPI comparisons use measurements taken prior to the program and compare them with measurements taken at a specific time after implementation; for example, comparing the low birth weight rate at community hospitals prior to the intervention of a perinatal transfer system with the low birth weight rate 2 years after program implementation. These comparisons depend on the assumption that the change in the variable, in this case low birth weight rate, can be attributed to the program and not to other events occurring during the time period. This assumption is often difficult to support. However, PPI comparisons may be the only practical evaluation method for established programs or interventions that have become the standard of care within a community.

DESIGN AND DATA COLLECTION
The value of proper evaluation research design and the adherence to the design from the onset of the program cannot be overemphasized. Experimental designs are considered "strong" if few assumptions need to be made about the groups to be compared. Randomization is the strongest experimental design, since the process of randomly assigning patients to treatment groups creates demographically similar treatment groups.

Randomization also requires consideration from the program's inception, since participants and nonparticipants must be assigned randomly. Quasi-experimental/matching designs are the next strongest experimental design, since they depend on the assumption that the groups to be compared have been well matched. This is often easier to accomplish if matching is considered early in program implementation. In spite of being the weakest experimental design involving the most problematic assumptions, pre- and postprogram implementation comparisons can be performed for existing, ongoing programs. However, defending the assumption that the program/intervention is the only agent of change may be very difficult. In an extensive review of published program evaluations, Lipsey et al. [22] concluded that evaluation begun after the program had been established for any length of time probably had a weaker research design.

These research designs, as previously mentioned, depend on the establishment of clear program/intervention goals and objectives from which outcome variables can be determined. The collection of data on program outcome variables is easier if it is an integral part of the program. These data collected on an ongoing basis facilitate the eventual evaluation of the program's impact and provide additional benefits, as described earlier under the rationale for evaluation.

Our experience with perinatal transfer data has led us to the conclusion that a central computer system enhances the collection, storage, retrieval, and statistical manipulation of these data. A computer system and the appropriate personnel can allow screen-formatted data input, data verification, storage and retrieval of large amounts of data quickly, routine reports showing progress toward program goals, and flexibility for special comparisons. The size and scope of this central computer system can be defined by the size and nature of the perinatal population to be served and the amount of data to be collected.

## Review of Evaluation Studies of Perinatal Transfer Systems

The term perinatal transfer may have different meanings depending on its use, because it combines many categories of patients at different levels of risk. For instance, in rural settings the transfer of women to an RPC for prenatal care early in pregnancy might be considered a perinatal transport, whereas in more urban settings this would be considered a referral for ongoing perinatal care. For the purpose of this discussion, an antenatal referral is defined as the referral of a pregnant patient to an RPC for ongoing perinatal care with anticipated delivery at the perinatal center. An antenatal transport involves a pregnant patient who is transported to the RPC for acute care and presumed imminent delivery. The term *transfer* combines both referral and transport.

In 1977 Merenstein et al. [24] reported their experience at Fitzsimmons Army Medical Center and noted a steady increase in the rate of antenatal transfer since 1973. Reviewing all deliveries at the two referring hospitals, the authors concluded that neonatal transport was associated with a higher-than-predicted mortality rate, whereas neonates transferred antenatally had a lower-than-predicted mortality rate and survivors had a shorter length of hospitalization. In this study, predicted mortality rates were calculated based on the mortality risk data of Lubchenco et al. [23]. This matching technique standardized mortality risk so that the antenatal and postnatal groups could be compared, although the sample size of 31 in each group was too small to allow comparisons by individual mortality risk groups. The advantage of reviewing all deliveries at the referring hospitals is that neonatal deaths among infants who were not transferred can be examined.

Giles et al. [14] in 1977 detailed an initial review of the Arizona high-risk maternal transport program and described the outcomes for infants delivered to transported mothers (excluding referrals). In this report, the authors attempted to characterize the population served by the program (program structure) by comparing the ages and ethnic backgrounds of transported women with the statewide distribution of age and race for women of reproductive age.

In 1978, improved neonatal survival through maternal transfer for Level III perinatal care was reported by Harris et al. [16] based on experiences in Arizona. Although in Arizona the RPCs are located in urban areas, much of the state is sparsely populated. The majority of the population (approximately 75%), reside in the two counties containing the state's two largest cities, Phoenix and Tucson. The population density outside these two urban counties is six persons per square mile [14]. Sixty percent of antenatal transfers in Arizona involve distances greater than 50 miles [13]. A statewide neonatal transport system was begun in 1967. The antenatal transport system was established in 1974. Harris et al. [16] reported that the neonatal mortality decreased from 17.4 per 1000 live births to 10.3 during the period from 1966 to 1973. The antenatal transfer system was established partially in response to the success of the neonatal program. It was postulated that greater reductions in neonatal mortality and morbidity could be achieved if the high-risk mother, rather than the premature or sick neonate were to be transferred to an RPC for special management of prenatal or intrapartum complications known to affect neonatal outcome. Comparing the neonatal mortality rate, again based on the intrauterine growth chart and mortality risk developed by Lubchenco et al. [23], Harris et al. [16] noted that the VLBW infant benefits more from in utero transport and birth at a perinatal center than birth in an outlying hospital and transport as a neonate to a regional center. This method of assigning neonates transferred antenatally and postnatally to expected mortality rate groups (based on birth weight and gestational age) and comparing observed mortality rate results within each expected mortality group is an excellent illustration of a quasi-experimental design. A drawback to this method, however, is the small sample size in each group that results from dividing the original sample of 239 neonates transferred antenatally and 642 neonates transferred postnatally into eight categories. Frequently the groups have to be combined in an effort to preserve an adequate sample size.

The experience at a perinatal center in Massachusetts was reported by Knuppel et al. [19] who described the outcome for 200 neonates transferred in utero. In this primarily urban center, a concurrent increase in antenatal transfers and decrease in neonatal transports was noted. The authors postulate that antenatal transfer facilitates the bonding between mother and infant.

Souma [33] reported the patient outcome after antenatal transfer to one of the five RPCs in Georgia. He noted that these transferred patients came from more than 20 different communities and that this raised concerns about the impact of the separation of the mother from her family, community, and chosen physician.

Blake et al. [3] reported on the experience with antenatal transfer from 1975 to 1977 at University College Hospital in London and noted that most of the neonates delivered weighed less than 2500 g, and that they had lower birth weight specific mortality rates than other infants born in England and Wales or infants transported as neonates. The use of birth weight specific mortality rates as a matching scheme involves the assumption that the incidences of small- or large-for-gestational-age infants in the group transferred in utero are similar to those in the population from which the birth weight specific rates have been derived.

A comparison of in utero versus postnatal transportation of high-risk neonates to the University of Alabama Hospitals was made by Harris et al. [15] for the period 1975 through 1977. The method of assigning neonates transferred antenatally and postnatally to expected mortality groups, based on birth weight and gestational age, was again employed. The results of this comparison suggested that (1) for those transferred before delivery, the neonatal mortality was significantly lower for three of the eight mortality risk groups, (2) the use of continuous positive airway pressure was less for neonates transferred antenatally, and (3) the length of hospitalization was significantly greater for the group transferred as neonates.

The maternal and infant transport program in Louisiana was described, and a comparison of antenatal versus neonatal transfer outcomes (corrected for birth weight) was reported by Levy et al. in 1980 [21]. The transport program at Ochsner Foundation Hospital in New Orleans received neonatal transports from 42 community hospitals and antenatal transfers from 23 hospitals during the study period from 1978 to 1979. The results of this review of 828 patients suggested that neonates transported in utero had a slightly better survival rate and a slightly shorter hospital stay, but neither difference was statistically significant.

Our experience [26, 27] at Memorial Medical Center of Long Beach (MMCLB), based on an exclusively urban perinatal transfer system and comparing patients who were referred with those transported antenatally, demonstrated different reasons for transfer and different outcomes. A matched-pair comparison [26] between infants transported in utero and postnatally failed to demonstrate a difference in mortality, but statistically significant differences were found for length of hospitalization, rate of cesarean section, rate of prematurity without other morbidity, and the incidence of respiratory distress syndrome. The technique of matching on an individual patient basis was undertaken to ensure comparability, with a modest sample size of 131 neonates in each group.

In an analysis of maternal transfer within a suburban metropolitan region of Chicago, Anderson et al. [1] concluded that the difference in mortality rates for antenatal versus neonatal transfer was not statistically significant for the group weighing less than 1501 g or the group that was less than 35-weeks' gestation. Significant differences were noted for length of stay and cost of hospitalization—with longer stays and greater cost among the neonates transported postnatally. A statistically significant difference was also noted in the cesarean section rate, with a higher rate of cesarean section for mothers transferred antenatally.

A 1982 report by Cho et al. [8] described the outcomes of 201 maternal transfers, compared with those for out-born neonates and infants born at the RPC. They noted the outcomes of the infants transferred in utero to be better overall than those of out-born neonates who were transported to the RPC; but no comparative statistics were provided. They reported that the highest survival rates within each of these two groups occurred for those neonates delivered by cesarean section.

Lamont et al. [20], reviewing mortality and morbidity of infants transferred in utero or postnatally to Hammersmith Hospital in London, found significantly higher mortality rates overall, higher mortality rates among certain birth weight intervals, and a higher incidence of intraventricular hemorrhage among neonates transported in the postnatal period. Based on these findings, the authors concluded that infants likely to require neonatal intensive care have decreased mortality and morbidity if transferred in utero to a center with these facilities.

In a report entitled "A regional neonatal intensive care nursery is not enough," Crenshaw et al. [12] reviewed perinatal transfer experiences at the University of Maryland Hospital. The authors found no significant differences in survival to discharge rates for neonates grouped by birth weight who were transferred antenatally versus postnatally but noted that infants transferred in utero were generally smaller than those transported as neonates. In an excellent report in 1983 by Miller et al. [25] all pregnancies in a rural Illinois region that resulted in a live-born infant with a birth weight of 1000 to 1500 g were reviewed. This technique, considering all births within the region, was designed to avoid the pitfall of examining just those neonates that are transferred antenatally or postnatally to the RPC—a potentially biased sample. The authors concluded that the survival rate for inborn infants at the RPC (antenatal transfers and "regular" RPC patients) was significantly greater than that for transported neonates, despite the fact that the mothers of the infants transported postnatally had less antepartum risk.

Using a variety of evaluation techniques, primarily creating outcome variable "risk comparable" groups based on birth weight or gestational age, or both, the programs mentioned above have concluded that perinatal transfer has a positive impact on patient outcome within their regions. This conclusion, although reasonable, suffers from problems in the evaluation research design, specifically, are the groups comparable? Common findings have included shorter lengths of hospital stay and some decreased morbidity for neonates transferred in utero versus postnatally. These two findings are subject to criticism when the selection criteria for the transported neonate are considered. As has been noted, neonates delivered prematurely at community hospitals who then exhibit a benign postnatal course are not subjected to transport. As a result, those neonates that are transported represent a unique subset. This subset would be expected to have longer hospital stays and more morbidity, since by definition they are selected because they are sicker. In contrast, premature neonates who are transported in utero are generally admitted to the intensive care nursery for observation, even if their postnatal course is uneventful. A consideration in evaluating these issues should be the length of stay and incidence of morbidity among nontransported neonates delivered at community hospitals. Another method is to consider only very small infants, for example, those with birth weight less than 1500 g, assuming that all such neonates delivered at community hospitals are transported. Miller et al. [25], as previously noted, used these techniques in a rural setting and found differences in mortality rates for inborn versus postnatally transported neonates; length of stay and neonatal morbidity were not reviewed.

When considering the cost-benefit of decreased hospital stay for infants transferred in utero versus postnatally, the cost of the anticipatory antenatal transfer of patients whose offspring do not require intensive care must also be included. On the other hand, the neonatal transport process requires more expensive equipment and highly trained personnel than does maternal transport [13].

Those authors who have reviewed cesarean section rates conclude that higher rates are found among patients transferred in the antenatal period. Williams and Hawes [34] found that delivery by cesarean section is highly associated with improved perinatal survival. This finding was also suggested by Cho et al. [8]. Some authors [1] have suggested that the complications of vaginal delivery at a community hospital may contribute to increased morbidity, length of stay, and hospital cost.

Relatively higher mortality rates among transported neonates (as compared with in utero transport) have not been confirmed by all investigators. Generally programs serving rural or large geographical areas have demonstrated mortality differences, while more urban or suburban programs have obtained inconclusive results. In contrast to some systems that exclusively serve metropolitan areas, the care options, qualifications of health care providers, and facilities may differ greatly between the RPC and rural community hospitals. The actual physical distance and time required to travel to the RPC may negatively influence such outcome variables as mortality, morbidity, and length of hospitalization. Transporting a neonate over a distance of a few miles, even at rush hour, may subject the neonate to less stress than a flight of hundreds of miles. As a result, the outcomes for neonates transferred antenatally or postnatally will tend to be more similar when distances traveled are less. If the transport distance is great, the extremely immature fetus may not be offered the chance of in utero transfer since the chance of intact survival, even at the RPC, is so small. Souma [33] indicated that, in their program, fetuses less than 26-weeks' gestation were not transported for fetal indications alone. Chance et al. [6] and Shott et al. [32] noted that transported neonates may be subjected to unqualified transport personnel and environmental difficulties that may directly affect their morbidity and mortality.

Inherent in the above observations are problems associated with the research methodology of comparative studies of high-risk infants transported in the antenatal versus the postnatal period. As mentioned above, Harris et al. [16] were the first to use mortality risk factors based on birth weight and gestational age. In our own observations [26, 27], we have employed the technique of matched pairs for birth weight and gestational age. Neither of these methods is free from concerns about biased conclusions because high-risk neonates transferred postnatally are selected for defined problems whereas those that are transferred antenatally may not have similar disease entities. In addition, despite comparable birth weight and gestational age, transported neonates may have a greater chance of receiving inadequate stabilization care during the first few hours of life prior to transport. Furthermore, transport of an ill neonate may be complicated by additional stress that may worsen existing disease processes. The matching scheme based on birth weight and gestational age may not have taken into account all of the other factors that may influence the outcome variables. Because of these and other logistic, political, and emotional problems that a fully implemented high-risk antenatal transfer program may create in a region, at the Level III perinatal center, and at the referring hospital, some [2, 7] have expressed skepticism about the wisdom of the antenatal transfer of the high-risk parturient to a Level III perinatal center.

## Summary

Optimal medical care should be regarded as a basic human right [14]. In our experience, the majority of physicians and other care givers involved in perinatal care have the goal of optimizing perinatal outcome. The results of the various investigations presented, comparing antenatal with postnatal transfer, are inconclusive. They generally indicate positive benefits from antenatal transfer, however, these studies are fraught with methodological concerns. The evaluation of the impact of a perinatal transfer system on patient outcome is confounded by numerous variables, some of them specific to each individual region. These include the quality of medical care, demographical and geographical characteristics of the region and care facilities, and socioeconomic patterns. Extrapolating the results from one region to another is difficult. Collecting data from an entire region, instead of a single RPC, addresses many of the concerns regarding the validity of previous impact evaluations, such as the outcomes of nontransported premature infants delivered at community hospitals. Carefully reviewing the program process should allow more meaningful comparisons; for example, do neonates suffer from cold stress during transport? The overall cost of the transport program must take in to account the cost of both perinatal transport to a regional center and the transfer back of the growing neonate or stabilized parturient to the community hospital. Evaluation of the impact of a perinatal transfer system and its efficiency should be considered an important aspect of both planning and maintaining a perinatal transport program.

## References

1. Anderson, C. L., et al. An analysis of maternal transport within a suburban metropolitan region. *Am. J. Obstet. Gynecol.* 140:499–504, 1981.
2. Auld, P. Maternal transport is not the answer (editorial). *Perinatol.-Neonatol.* Vol. 2, No. 2, 1978. Pp. 8, 50.
3. Blake, A. M., Pollitzer, M. J., and Reynolds, E. O. Referral of mothers and infants for intensive care. *Br. Med. J.* 2:414–416, 1979.
4. Boruch, R. F., and Wothke, W. (eds.). Seven Kinds of Randomization Plans for Designing Field Experiments. In R. F. Boruch and W. Wothke (eds.), *New Directions for Program Evaluation-Randomization and Field Experiments.* San Francisco: Jossey-Bass, 28 95–113, 1985.
5. Campbell, D. T., and Stanley, J. (eds.). *Experimental and Quasi-Experimental Designs for Research.* Skokie, IL: Rand McNally, 1966.
6. Chance, G. W., O'Brien, M. J., and Swyer, P. R. Transportation of sick neonates, 1972: An unsatisfactory aspect of medical care. *Can. Med. Assoc. J.* 109:847–851, 1973.
7. Chiswick, M. L. Perinatal referral: A time for decisions. *Br. Med. J.* 285:83–84, 1982.
8. Cho, S., et al. Outcome of 201 Maternal Transports Compared with Newborn Transports and Infants Born at the Tertiary Center. *Birth Defects: Original Article Series* March of Dimes Birth Defects Foundation. 18:199–201 3A, 1982.
9. Cook, T. D., and Campbell, D. T. (eds.). *Quasi-Experimentation Design and Analysis Issues for Field Settings.* Skokie, IL: Rand McNally, 1979.
10. Cooke, R. W. In utero transfer to specialist centers. *Arch. Dis. Child.* 58:583–584, 1983.
11. Cordero, L., Backes, C. R., and Zuspan, F. P. Very low birth weight infant I. Influence of place of birth on survival. *Am. J. Obstet. Gynecol.* 143:533–537, 1982.
12. Crenshaw, C., et al. Prematurity and the obstetrician: A regional neonatal intensive care nursery is not enough. *Am. J. Obstet. Gynecol.* 147:125–132, 1983.
13. Giles, H. R. Maternal transport. *Clin. Obstet. Gynecol.* 6:203–213, 1979.
14. Giles, H. R., et al. The Arizona high-risk maternal transport system: An initial view. *Am. J. Obstet. Gynecol.* 128:400–407, 1977.
15. Harris, B. A., et al. In utero versus neonatal transportation of high-risk perinates: A comparison. *Obstet. Gynecol.* 57:496–499, 1981.
16. Harris, T. R., Isman, J., and Giles, H. R. Improved neonatal survival through maternal transport. *Obstet. Gynecol.* 52:294–300, 1978.
17. Jung, A. L., and Bose, C. L. Back transport of neonates: Improved efficiency of tertiary nursery bed utilization. *Pediatrics* 71:918–922, 1983.
18. Kanto, W. P., et al. Impact of a maternal transport program on newborn service. *South. Med. J.* 76:834–837, 1983.
19. Knuppel, R. A., et al. Experience at a Massachusetts perinatal center. *N. Engl. J. Med.* 300:560–562, 1979.
20. Lamont, R. F., et al. Comparative mortality and morbidity of infants transferred in utero or postnatally. *J. Perinat. Med.* 11:200–203, 1983.

21. Levy, D. L., Noelke, K., and Goldsmith, J. P. Maternal and infant transport program in Louisiana. *Obstet. Gynecol.* 57:500–504, 1981.
22. Lipsey, M. W., et al. Evaluation: The State of the Art and the Sorry State of the Science. In D. Cordray (ed.), *New Directions for Program Evaluation—Utilizing Prior Research in Evaluation Planning,* San Francisco, Jossey-Bass, 27:7–28, 1985.
23. Lubchenco, L. O., Searls, D. T., and Brazie, J. Neonatal mortality: Its relationship to birth weight and gestational age. *J. Pediatr.* 18:814, 1972.
24. Merenstein, G. B., et al. An analysis of air transport results in the sick newborn II. Antenatal and neonatal referrals. *Am. J. Obstet. Gynecol.* 128:520–525, 1977.
25. Miller, T. C., Denserger, M., and Krogman, J. Maternal transport and the perinatal denominator. *Am. J. Obstet. Gynecol.* 147:19–24, 1983.
26. Modanlou, H. D., et al. Perinatal transport to a regional perinatal center in a metropolitan area: Maternal versus neonatal transport. *Am. J. Obstet. Gynecol.* 138:1157–1164, 1980.
27. Modanlou, H. D., et al. Antenatal versus neonatal transport to a regional perinatal center: A comparison between matched pairs. *Obstet. Gynecol.* 53:725–729, 1979.
28. Peoples, M. D., Grimson, R. C., and Daughtry, G. L. Evaluation of the effects of the North Carolina Improved Pregnancy Outcome Project: Implications for state-level decision making. *Am. J. Public Health* 74:549–554, 1984.
29. Rossi, P. H., and Freeman, H. E. (eds.). *Evaluation: A Systematic Approach* (2nd ed.) Beverly Hills, CA: Sage Publications, 1982.
30. Sachs, B. P., et al. Neonatal transport in Georgia: Implications for maternal transport in high-risk pregnancies. *South. Med. J.* 76:1397–1400, 1983.
31. Schramm, W. F. WIC prenatal participation and its relationship to newborn medicaid costs in Missouri: A cost/benefit analysis. *Am. J. Public Health* 75:851–857, 1985.
32. Shott, R. J. Regionalization: A time for new solutions. *Pediatr. Clin. North Am.* 24:651, 1977.
33. Souma, M. L. Maternal transport: Behind the drama. *Am. J. Obstet. Gynecol.* 134:904–910, 1979.
34. Williams, R. L., and Hawes, W. E. Cesarean section, fetal monitoring and perinatal mortality in California. *Am. J. Public Health* 69:864–870, 1979.

# III

# Legal, Ethical, and Psychological Aspects of Patient Transport

# 7 The Hospital Administrator's Perspective

Dennis C. Brimhall

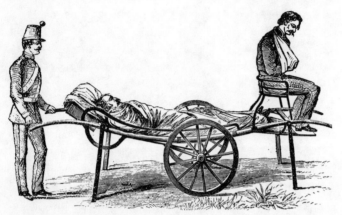

*7A. Evan's hand-wheeled litter. A type 2 sick transport conveyance (conveyance wheeled by men). ". . . Not approved on examination by a board of army medical officers in April 1855 in London."* (Reproduced from Longmore, T. A Treatise on the Transport of Sick and Wounded Troops. *London: Her Majesty's Stationery Office, 1869.*)

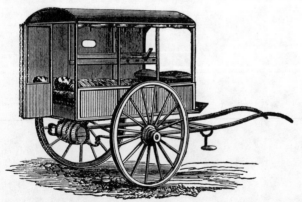

*7B. The Coolidge sick transport cart. A type 2 sick transport conveyance (conveyance wheeled by men). "The 'Coolidge' carts were found to be too frail for the rough roads on which they were employed . . . the excessive elasticity of the springs, the body of the cart being tossed about to such an extent in consequences as to add greatly to the sufferings of the patients transported in it."* (Reproduced from Longmore, T. A Treatise on the Transport of Sick and Wounded Troops. *London: Her Majesty's Stationery Office, 1869.*)

In the early 1970s the federal government began providing funds to improve the nation's emergency medical services. One of the initial targets of these funds was ambulance vehicles and services. As is generally the case with this type of funding, federal standards were created that had to be met before the funds were awarded. Funding led to standards, standards to common expectations, and expectations to monitoring of standards and the potential for legal action against those not meeting the standards.

About the same time that the ambulance services of the country began to upgrade, the concepts of perinatal transport emerged. Although the coincidental development of sophisticated emergency medical service (EMS) and perinatal transport services may have been serendipitous, perinatal transport benefited from better EMS ambulance services.

## The Uniqueness of Perinatal Transport

Within the generic classification of patient transport systems there are two basic types. Each has different legal profiles and issues.

The first type provides the primary response to an emergency situation, for example, the scene of an accident. These programs are generally not hospital based. Their operating philosophy is one of very quick response and the provision of essential medical care until the patient can be treated at the closest medical facility. Emphasis is placed on speed and ability to provide primary level emergency care to patients with a wide variety of clinical problems.

The second type of patient transport program is exemplified by perinatal transport and is more complex. This type of program is designed to transport critically ill patients from one institution to another.

There are important differences between traditional EMS transport and perinatal transport. These differences relate to the service and to the equipment, personnel, and operation (Table 7-1).

First, most of the perinatal transport programs in the country are hospital based. This means that perinatal transport programs must deal not only with regulations and laws pertaining to EMS but also with those applicable to hospital systems.

Second, most perinatal transport programs use a different type of personnel from that found in typical EMS ambulance operations. Whereas EMS ambulance programs frequently use emergency medical technicians (EMTs, paramedics), most perinatal transport programs use nurses, physicians, respiratory therapists, and other hospital personnel. Most of these perinatal team members function in expanded roles so that they are per-

*Table 7-1. Some aspects of a perinatal transport service that differ from a general emergency medical service*

Teams are usually hospital based
Provides interstate service
Few specific state or local statutes or regulations
Requires highly specialized personnel and equipment
Specifically designed for the transport of very ill patients
Transport team is under direct physician supervision

forming tasks and procedures on transport that may be beyond the scope of their "in-house" role.

Third, because it is unique and relatively new, the body of regulations and laws currently applicable to EMS ambulance programs have not yet been formally adapted to perinatal transport. In addition, a body of regulations has not yet been developed that is solely applicable to perinatal transport. Thus perinatal transport programs currently enjoy a relative degree of freedom from regulation. As is true with most freedoms, however, this creates both benefits and liabilities.

Fourth, because perinatal transport programs often service large areas, transport teams are faced with the issue of practicing their skills in more than one state. Because licensing laws vary in different geographical settings, a unique set of regulatory issues arises.

Fifth, a perinatal transport system is designed to transport critically ill patients, as opposed to providing convenience or courtesy transports. These patients have complex medical problems that require sophisticated equipment, personnel, and operating structure.

Sixth, although some perinatal transport programs are part of existing EMS transport systems, most of the perinatal teams include a physician or are under the very close direction of a physician at the receiving hospital, or both. This intense physician involvement in the transport creates a relationship between the receiving hospital and the patient.

## Authorization and Protection

There are two basic principles underlying the authorization for the transport team to perform their duties. The first is that the administration of the employing institution (which is ultimately responsible for the acts and omissions of the transport team) has authorized a properly trained team to act, and has generally assumed the responsibility for their actions. The institution should determine that the transport team members have appropriate training and experience to perform in their roles, and that there is adequate supervision for the team.

Protocols should be developed that identify exactly what the transport team member can and cannot do. It is important for the transport program, whether using team members in traditional or expanded roles, to receive appropriate endorsement from the governing medical body within the institution and for the transport team members to know precisely what latitude they have been granted. This institutional authorization gives the team legitimacy as it functions and provides a legal "parent" to stand behind.

The second authorizing principle is that the transport team is operating at all times under the direction of a supervising physician. As the transport and most associated procedures can only be performed on a direct physician's order, physician interaction is essential for authorized performance of the team's duties and responsibilities. The involvement of the supervising physician is part of the administrative supervision of the sponsoring hospital.

In principle, protection for the transport team is achieved in two ways. First, the teams must render "correct" care within the course and scope of their employment. This correct care implies appropriate selection, training, and experience of the team members as determined by a responsible physician director. For quality assurance, the participants in the transport program, including representatives of the hospital administration and any independent contractors, should meet on a regular basis to review program function and performance.

The second protecting principle is that as long as the transport team members are performing within the course and scope of their employment, the accepted principles of law establish that the employer is ultimately responsible for the acts and omissions of its team (employees). This principle should provide for the coverage of the transport team under the malpractice insurance policy of the sponsoring institution.

### Out-of-state Transports

An issue that is frequently raised concerns licensure of transport team members when they perform their duties outside their home state. This is a difficult issue to address because state laws vary so dramatically throughout the country. In some areas, states have approved reciprocal relationships regarding licensure or have endorsed special provisions for transport teams crossing state lines. However, this is not generally the case. When this issue was raised with the Utah State Attorney General for the University of Utah

Hospital transport teams (these teams work in portions of seven states), the response included the following statement: "I do not believe the licensure problem with respect to nurses working out of Utah is a serious one so long as the nurse is licensed in the state of her (or his) residence, that is, the state of Utah where she (or he) is employed." Whether or not this philosophy would be applicable to other transport situations in other states is unclear, but it may provide some guidance. Competency, rather than licensure, is usually the focal point in malpractice litigation.

## A Model for Determining Responsibility for Patient Care

The responsibility for perinatal transport can change during the transport because of the changing level of interaction between the referring and receiving hospitals (see Chap. 8). Figure 7-1 is a graphical representation of the changing levels of responsibility for patient care. The vertical axis represents the level of responsibility of the transport team/receiving institution versus that of the referring institution. The horizontal axis represents the definitive transport events.

Point A represents the point in time when the transport request is received by the referral institution. Simply by publishing a telephone number and promoting the program, the referral institution incurs some responsibility. The referring hospital is looking for help from a transport program

Fig. 7-1. Changing levels of responsibility for patient care

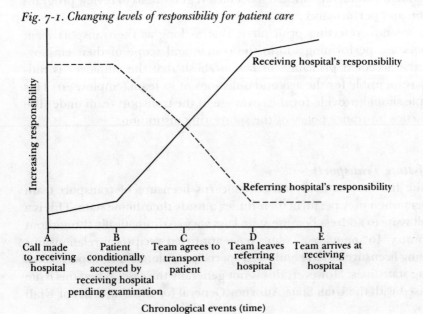

that has indicated an ability to provide help in the form of patient transport to a facility that has the capability to provide the required specialized care. At this time, the referring institution still has almost all of the responsibility for the patient. They may have reduced their legal responsibility somewhat, however, by recognizing that their hospital cannot provide the level of care necessary for the patient and by calling the transport program.

Once a call is placed to the receiving institution and the patient is conditionally accepted for transport (point B), instructions are provided regarding the further care and preparation of the patient for transport. At this point the receiving institution and the transport team begin to assume more responsibility for the patient. This responsibility increases as the receiving institution provides more advice and as the referring hospital begins to act on that advice in the belief that the transport team is en route and will arrive within a given time period.

When the transport team arrives at the referring institution and begins "hands-on" care in preparation for transport, the responsibility for the patient is shared (point C). The transport team is providing advice, care, and some equipment but the referring hospital is providing environment, equipment, and some personnel. Although a definitive determination of responsibility during this time may be difficult, it is wise for the transport team to think and act as though they have the greatest share of the responsibility. This should be done in a tactful manner.

When the transport team leaves the referring institution with the patient, they accept most of the responsibility (point D) for the care of the patient on behalf of the receiving institution. At the point that the transport team arrives back at the receiving hospital it has virtually total responsibility for the patient; a remaining area of responsibility for the referring institution is that associated with having arranged for a properly trained and equipped transport team to move the patient to an institution that can provide the necessary medical care (point E).

## *Interpersonal Skills and Legal Responsibility*

One of the common challenges associated with the transportation of patients from one institution to another involves the interaction of the team members with professionals at the referring institution. Although in many cases there is an acceptance that the transport team has expertise above that available at the referring institution, this may not always be true. The transport team may begin to stabilize and prepare the patient for transport only to find that individuals at the referring institution disagree with the type and timeliness of that care.

Although this may appear to be more of a public relations matter than a legal issue, it has legal overtones concerning the determination of who is in charge of the patient care. The transport team may feel that it is under the direction of its medical director, yet find itself receiving instructions from the patient's private physician at the referring hospital. Thus, the team is placed in an untenable position.

The best method for avoiding such dilemmas is for the team members to remain uninvolved in any conflict over patient care, and to refer any questions raised by professionals at the referring institution directly to the physician supervisor of the transport team at the receiving hospital. The transport team should facilitate such communication and avoid being caught in the middle. Once the referring and receiving physicians arrive at a consensus, the transport team can receive instructions directly from their supervising physician and proceed appropriately.

In any conflict over timeliness or modality of care with a referring physician or institution, the team should seek and follow the advice from its own institution and physician supervisor.

It may be intuitively obvious that derogatory statements should not be made about the quality of care given at the referring institution either to staff at that institution or to the patient's family. Many malpractice cases are initiated by a disgruntled family after an unsatisfactory interpersonal experience with a health care provider. The transport team should avoid any confrontation that might permit the referring institution to inappropriately accuse the transport team or the receiving institution of negligent care.

## The Medical Record

The role of the medical record in a quality of care matter is very significant. Despite the complexity of modern medical charting, there are a few simple guidelines to ensure that the transport record fulfills both its patient care purposes and any ultimate legal requirements.

It will take some efforts to eliminate the effects of a comment made in the record or to establish facts not noted in the record. The record serves a clinical function and a legal function; it must be accurate and objective. Entries should document actions taken by the team on behalf of the patient, as well as those observations of change in the patient's condition that led to those actions. If the patient's temperature drops, this observation should be documented, and the action taken by the team (e.g., increasing the temperature in the incubator) should be noted. This "paper-trail" type of charting does not require voluminous entries but does effectively document the patient's clinical course and the responses of the transport team.

It is essential to avoid long time lapses between entries. Standard protocols should dictate that regular observations be recorded, even if the patient's status has not changed. Most institutions have effective charting guidelines and standards that provide adequate protection for the team and for the patient. A transport is an extraordinary event, the level of detail in the patient's medical chart should reflect this.

## Program Safety

The hospital administration has a key role to play in the safety program for a patient transport service [1]. In addition to the perceived and actual legal responsibility, the administration must be strongly and visibly supportive of the safety aspects of the program to ensure that safety remains a top priority with all transport personnel. The responsibilities of the hospital administration include [2]:

1. Establish regular safety meetings with all personnel involved in patient transport.
2. Ensure compliance with safety directives.
3. Show visible support for the safety directives.
4. Discourage the "speed at all costs" attitude.
5. Support attendance at operational management and safety seminars.
6. Become familiar with recognized published guidelines.

## Conclusion

A safe and well-managed transport program involves the hospital administration, the hospital staff, and the transport team. An efficient, effective, well-documented program will minimize hospital-patient conflicts and litigation.

## References

1. Honaman, C. J. Safety and the hospital administrator. *Hospital Aviation*, 5, February 1987.
2. Second Opinion: Reducing the Risks of Accidents (editorial). Vol. 6: No. 2. *Hospital Aviation*, 12, February 1987.

# 8 Legal Issues in Medical Transport

## Harold M. Ginzburg

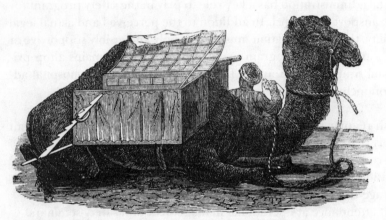

8A. Larrey's Egyptian camel-litter. The litter is open and ready to receive a patient. A class 3 sick transport conveyance (conveyance borne by animals). ". . . While two wounded men could be easily placed in the panniers on its two sides by making the camel sit down for their reception, in accordance with the ordinary habit of the animal when being loaded with baggage." (Reproduced from Longmore, T. A Treatise on the Transport of Sick and Wounded Troops. London: Her Majesty's Stationery Office, 1869). (Originally published in Memoires de Chirurgien Militaire et Campagnes de D. J. Larrey, tome i. Paris, 1812.)

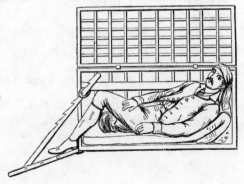

8B. Larrey's camel-litter. One side is removed to show the position of a wounded man who has been placed in it following an amputation above the knee. (Reproduced from Longmore, T. A Treatise on the Transport of Sick and Wounded Troops. London: Her Majesty's Stationery Office, 1869).

The transport of a pregnant woman or a neonate in acute life-threatening distress requires the cooperation and integration of the services of more than one medical facility and possibly several different transportation systems. The application of the concepts of command (leadership), communication, and coordination are the critical components that ensure optimal medical care and the safety of all participants in a transport and treatment system [13]. Failure of any of these critical elements may result in less than optimal care and the initiation of a malpractice claim.

The federally enacted Emergency Medical Services Systems Act of 1973 provided for the development of hospital-to-ambulance communication systems and the regional categorization of hospital facilities and services [13]. The act defined an emergency medical services system as one that

provides for the arrangement of personnel, facilities, and equipment for the effective and coordinated delivery, in an appropriate geographic area, of health care services under emergency conditions (occurring either as a result of the patient's condition or of natural disasters or similar conditions), which are administered by a public or not-for-profit, private entity that has the authority and the resources to provide effective administration of the system [44].

This act, although later repealed in 1981, provided the basis for hospitals to formally develop outreach capability using their health care providers and equipment in conjunction with medical transport vehicles. The act established requirements for manpower, training, equipment, transfer of patients, hospital emergency care, record keeping, review and evaluation of services, and patient information. As a result of this act, hospitals no longer waited for critically ill patients to be delivered to them; organized and sophisticated emergency treatment services extended beyond the walls of the institution.

The regionalization of perinatal care has increased the number of neonatal and maternal transports from local hospitals to tertiary facilities. Intertertiary neonatal transport is also increasing because there is limited access to scarce medical resources such as extracorporeal membrane oxygenation (ECMO) or organ transplantation [11]. Intertertiary transport may involve moving an extremely critically ill patient by ground and air ambulances across multiple state boundaries.

Although the emergency transport of neonatal and obstetric patients has decreased the overall patient morbidity and mortality, such activities have not been without cost. Each year helicopter flight crews and medical care teams and their patients are killed or maimed in flying accidents. More frequently, optimal medical care is not achieved because of the inappropriate selection of patients for transport, undertrained or inadequately supervised transport team members, inordinate delays in the arrangement for transportation, transport in unfavorable weather conditions, and the inability to maintain patient stability within the transport environment. The patient outcome in such circumstances is often predictable; the legal remedies are often dramatic.

Some of the basic legal considerations relating to patient transport are

1. The duty to act—when does the health care professional–patient or hospital–patient relationship commence?
2. What is the hospital's responsibility and liability for medical transport and subsequent treatment?
3. What are the relevant legal principles that may arise in transporting neonates?
4. What are the relevant issues in informed consent?

An understanding of legal principles is analogous to an understanding of basic public health and preventive medicine principles. The use and understanding of preventive medicine principles help protect the community; the use and understanding of legal principles help protect the health care provider.

### *The Duty to Act—Determination of When the Health Care Professional–Patient or Hospital–Patient Relationship Commences*

A duty is a legal and ethical responsibility [21]. There is no legal duty for a physician or a hospital to accept a patient for care or to even provide emergency medical care. However, if the hospital represents itself as a public hospital providing emergency care, and the community has come to expect such care, the hospital cannot arbitrarily deny such services to a patient [23].

In medical transport care it may be legally argued that the duty to transport the patient, pending an examination by the transport team at the referring hospital, commences at the time the oral agreement (contract) for assistance and transport is made between the referring hospital and the transport team dispatcher. The individual who dispatches the transport team should be an attending physician at the receiving facility since he or she is accepting responsibility and liability for the transfer and medical care of the perinatal patient and the safe transport of all others involved in the transport, including any accompanying relatives of the patient.

The referring hospital is reliant on the services of the transport team; if the team does not arrive when expected and the infant suffers, legal liability may be an issue. If the medical transport team dispatcher determines that the weather conditions are uncertain, the referring hospital should be informed that they will have to make contingency plans for patient management and transport. If alternative travel arrangements are not organized and a helicopter dispatched in marginal weather conditions fails to reach its destination, while the patient awaiting transport suffers because of the delay, the patient may have a cause of action for negligence.

Once care commences there is a duty to provide that care at a particular standard or level [39]. Once the health care professional/hospital–patient relationship is established, there is a legal and moral obligation not to abandon the patient [17]. However, a referral hospital transferring an infant to another institution does not abandon the patient when it places the neonate in the hands of the transport team. The patient becomes the responsibility of the transport team (and by inference the receiving hospital) once a member of the transport team examines and prepares the patient for transport. If the transport team (after examining the patient and preferably after consultation with the attending physician at the receiving hospital) determines that transport is not an appropriate course of action, the patient remains the responsibility of the referring hospital. The referring hospital cannot order a transport team to transport a patient. A hospital can be held liable for negligently transferring a patient when such a transfer aggravates the patient's condition or increases the possibility of death [36]. In circumstances in which it is determined that transport is inadvisable, the transport team may provide recommendations for care and treatment but may not actually perform any procedure for the referring hospital without express approval of the attending physician at the receiving hospital. That is, the transport team must convey their intentions not to transport the patient to their attending physician at the receiving hospital and receive permission to assist the staff at the referring hospital for a very limited period of time. An extended stay at a referring hospital potentially affects availability for the transport of other patients.

The transport team becomes the health care provider when it stabilizes and transports the patient. The transport team has a duty to the patient; there is no duty to the referring hospital. However, a follow-up report to the referring hospital after the completion of the transport is sound medical practice and a wise political action.

## Hospital Responsibility and Liability
The principle that the hospital is legally responsible for the medical and nursing care provided by its health care providers, independent of a pa-

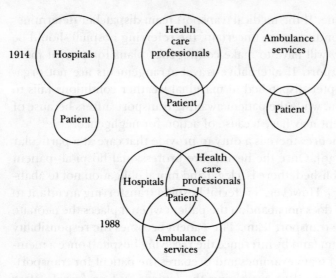

*Fig. 8-1. Changing patterns of responsibility/liability.*

tient's ability to pay for such care, is a relatively recent concept (Fig. 8-1).
Historically, hospitals were protected from legal liability. This theory, articulated in 1914 by the New York Court of Appeals in *Schloendorff v. Society
of New York Hospitals,* ruled that a hospital could not be held liable for the
negligence of its physicians and nurses in the treatment of patients, specifically for the alleged unconsented surgical operation performed within its
structure (failure to obtain a proper informed consent) [32]. In that decision, Judge Cardozo stated that the hospital was perceived to be nothing
more than a "workshop" for the physicians. The hospital administration
was perceived as a management team that merely rented space; provided
utilities; arranged for service amenities such as food preparation and distribution and waste disposal services; and acted as an employment agency for
technicians, nurses, and physicians. Physicians and nurses were considered
to be independent contractors with the hospital; they were not perceived to
be directly supervised by the hospital.

An additional finding of the *Schloendorff* case was that the hospital was
held not to be responsible for the negligence of the nurses and physicians,
even if they were employees, because "one who accepts the benefit of a
charity enters into a relation which exempts one's benefactors from liability
to the negligence of his servants in administering the charity" (independent
of whether or not the patient is paying the hospital for services rendered)
[32]. This doctrine of charitable immunity was deemed to be sufficient for
patients to be unable to sue for damages. Both of these judicial concepts

were maintained for four decades before hospitals began to be treated as coequal defendants in medical malpractice (negligence) litigation, independent of the financial ability of the patient [22]. In 1957 in *Bing v. Thunig,* the concept of charitable immunity was definitively rejected [4]. One reason for the rejection of this concept was the court's observation that, with the existence of insurance, the hospitals could protect themselves from financial disaster. The court believed that medical malpractice suits would, therefore, not threaten the economic existence of hospitals.

Immediately after the conclusion of World War II, the Hill-Burton federal program began to provide loans and grants to hospitals for construction and renovation of hospital facilities and to increase public access to hospitals [31]. One of the requirements for receipt of the Hill-Burton funds was the adoption of hospital licensure laws. With the new licensure laws came the realization and acceptance that a hospital, as an independent institution and not as a work place for physicians, had specific duties and responsibilities to its patients. By the end of the 1960s, the doctrine of charitable immunity had been rejected by almost all states [29]. At present, in addition to hospitals and physicians, the individual employees of the hospital such as nurses, house officers (interns, residents, and fellows) and technicians can be held personally liable for their own acts of malpractice or negligence that cause injury to a patient [33].

Today's courts are unlikely to limit hospital responsibility to medical care given within the four walls of the institution; care provided by the medical transport team can be perceived as an extension of care provided in the receiving hospital [13]. The medical transport team must determine that the patient is sufficiently stable for transport, that the patient is an appropriate candidate for transport, and whether it is safe and prudent for their patient(s) (and themselves) to board the transport vehicle and be transported to the receiving hospital. The responsibility for these decisions ultimately rests with the medical team dispatcher, the attending physician at the receiving hospital.

The medical transport team members may be held to a different standard of care while stabilizing and caring for a neonate aboard a helicopter, as compared to when they are performing similar tasks in a newborn intensive care unit. Regardless of the standard of care, if they exercise poor judgment, have an equipment failure, or otherwise act in a negligent manner, they (and the referring and receiving hospitals) may be subjected to a law suit for medical malpractice [29].

The receiving hospital may be found vicariously liable for the actions of the medical transport team under the doctrine of corporate negligence: Employers are responsible for the actions of their employees [12]. The referring hospital may also be found liable under an ostensible agency theory, that is, since the patient has no means of determining whether a given physician who is practicing in a hospital is an employee of that hospital, and since patients go to hospitals to receive treatment, any action by a physician who appears to be practicing in the hospital is that hospital's responsibility [38]. Thus, if a member of the medical transport team errs in a hospital, the hospital will almost invariably be held accountable for that action [15].

The hospital administration is an integral component of the delivery of medical care services; it and health care providers are partners and have equal responsibility in the provision of medical care and treatment [9]. The medical staff is perceived as an integral part of the hospital [45]. In addition to state case law and regulations, the federal government, by promulgating the *Medicare Conditions of Participation for Hospitals,* articulates in detail standards governing the institutional relationships of hospitals and physicians [25]. The hospital is held to have a duty of care (legal responsibility) for the welfare of a patient under state and federal law. If hospital-provided services are found to be deficient, the hospital may be found legally responsible and financially liable for damages. Thus, the hospital is as liable for ensuring that the medical equipment being used aboard a chartered medical transport vehicle is in satisfactory condition as it is for keeping its steps free from ice after a winter snow storm.

The federally enacted National Labor Relations Act was amended in 1974 to extend jurisdiction of the National Labor Relations Board (NLRB) to "health care institutions" [43]. Health care workers are thus afforded the opportunity to assert a concerted effort (defined as two or more persons acting together to achieve a common goal) to improve their working conditions; retaliatory actions by hospitals (termination) are considered to be in violation of this federal law [26]. Patient care issues such as inadequate or unsanitary facilities, deficient emergency room and admission policies, and nursing staff shortages are "inextricably intertwined" with staff "working conditions." Thus, an ambulance driver cannot be discharged for refusing to operate an ambulance that lacks essential emergency equipment. The court ruled that "Inadequate medical equipment can affect a health care provider's ability to properly care for a patient. To the extent that an employee's duties relate to providing patient care, therefore, a lack of necessary medical equipment affects both the patient's welfare and the working conditions of the health care provider" [30]. Thus, there is federal (and state) protection for health care workers who express their concern about safety issues in their work place. They can object to placing themselves or their patients at risk.

The dispatching hospital may be liable for injuries to members of the transport team while they are engaged in the transport. Many hospitals have not developed specific position descriptions for physicians and other health care professionals, which include an explanation of the potential risks involved in the transport of patients. Just as a patient should be provided information before agreeing to a procedure, a staff member asked to engage in an activity that increases his or her personal risk should be made aware of those risks and be allowed to freely decide whether to participate in the activity. It is highly advisable for hospital administrators to develop a plan to deal with the expenses that may result from their staff being injured during a transport. To minimize potential liability in the case of a transport-related accident, hospital administrators should consider obtaining special life insurance and disability insurance for members of the transport team.

Hospitals are held to a minimum standard of care as defined by the Joint Commission on Accreditation of Hospitals (JCAH) [19]. The hospital governing body and the hospital administration must conduct themselves in a manner that provides high-quality patient care. This goal includes the determination that all medical and nursing personnel are qualified for their assigned duties. The quality assurance program that each hospital establishes and maintains may be an effective means for reviewing and evaluating patient care given by individual members of the medical staff within the hospital, but it does not always examine those components of patient care that occur beyond the physical boundaries of the hospital building. The hospital administration owes the patient a duty to use due care not only in the operation and management of the hospital, but also in the selection of medical transport contractors. Failure to adequately and appropriately monitor all aspects of patient care and treatment, including the transport of patients to the facility (even if the transport team is not under the direct control of the hospital), may result in legal liability.

The author is unaware of any hospital in the United States where the suitability and relative safety (for both the patient and the transport team) of the transport vehicle selected for each medical transport is routinely reviewed with the hospital administrator (see Chap. 13). Further, there are currently in the United States neither standardized qualifications nor certification for civilian physicians and nurses involved in the transport of critically ill neonates.

The court concluded in *Tonsic v. Wagner* that a hospital could be found negligent under the principles of respondeat superior for not devising adequate rules and regulations to govern the procedures followed by its operating room personnel [37]. Thus, current case law holds that a hospital can be held negligent and legally responsible if it has not developed and implemented an ongoing policy for monitoring and updating all treatment protocols, patient precaution protocols, and rules and regulations designed for the safety of the patients and staff. This principle was applied in *Air Shields, Inc. v. Spears,* a case involving an infant who developed retrolental fibroplasia as a result of prolonged exposure to an excessive partial pressure of oxygen [2]. The hospital was held liable for the negligent medical treatment protocol that was formulated by the medical staff.

In addition, a hospital can also be found to be negligent in the delivery of medical care if its own rules or regulations are breached. A hospital has a duty to "make a reasonable effort to monitor and oversee the treatment which is prescribed and administered by physicians practicing at the facility" [5]. The hospital is also responsible for ensuring that it is adequately staffed with the proper mixture of health care professionals to provide the services that it offers and for ensuring that, when appropriate, consultants participate in the care and treatment of patients. The court determined in *Darling v. Charleston Community Memorial Hospital* that the hospital has an obligation to ensure that appropriately qualified health care professionals are available [9]. It is reasonable to assume that this principle applies to any health care services provided by a hospital, including medical transport services. After all, the contract for the transport commences within the hospital and is provided by hospital personnel for the ultimate benefit of the patient (and hospital).

### The United States Legal System and Health Care

Health care workers need to understand those aspects of the legal system that directly affect their ability to deliver optimal medical care. There is no single legal system in the United States. Each state (and the District of Columbia, Puerto Rico, and the possessions of the United States) has their own legal system for matters that involve their residents. The federal system applies to those matters that are specified within the Constitution. Interstate transport is a federal matter; patient transport within a given state may be governed solely by state law. Patient transport across state lines involves both state and federal law.

An aircraft, because it has the potential to fly across state borders, must be inspected and maintained according to federal regulations; pilots are subject to Federal Aviation Administration (FAA) regulations. Ground ambulances are licensed and inspected in a single state. Ambulance drivers are licensed by a state, usually the state in which the ambulances are physically located when they are not in use. Health care providers (physicians, nurses, emergency medical technicians) may be licensed in more than one state;

they must be licensed in the state in which they maintain their primary office or place of employment. The authorities in most states are not concerned about whether a health care provider who enters the state solely to transport a patient to another health care facility is licensed in that state: however, they are concerned that the individuals involved in the transport are competent to perform their job.

An individual who enters a state, regardless of the reason, may be subject to that state's laws. If a driver is involved in an accident, he or she is subject to the laws of the state in which the accident occurred, not to those of the state that issued the driving license; this legal principal applies to medical transport vehicle operators as well [16]. Failure to obtain informed consent may result in litigation in the state in which it was inadequately obtained or in the state to which the patient was transferred.

Patients and their guardians may initiate medical malpractice litigation in the state in which they reside, the state in which the alleged negligence occurred, the state in which the hospital is located, or the state in which the physician resides. If the patient-plaintiff can show that their residence is in a different state from that of the defendant-hospital and defendant-health care provider, then the plaintiff can commence the litigation in a federal court, because the matter involves diversity of jurisdiction. The defendant can request that the matter be removed to the federal court system for a similar reason [42]. Most plaintiffs prefer state courts, especially if the defendant is from a different state. Some state courts are known for their large awards to plaintiffs, whereas others are known to be more sympathetic to defendant-health care providers.

The legal system is divided into two broad areas. Civil litigation is based on the need to correct or remedy a wrong between one individual (corporation or partnership) and another. Criminal prosecution is instituted to correct a wrong against the community. In a civil litigation matter (or case) the plaintiff is the party bringing the lawsuit and alleging the wrong; it is filed against the party (defendant) who is accused of causing the damage. In a criminal prosecution the plaintiff is the government (local, state, federal) alleging that the community has been harmed by the action or inaction of a party (also known as the defendant).

Plaintiffs may sue for an injury that occurred as a result of negligence or a tort (physical or mental harm), or both. Since the criminal court will not usually award monetary damages to the victim of a crime, and since the standard of proof for conviction is "beyond a reasonable doubt" (quantitatively this can be conceptualized as at least 95% certain), plaintiffs usually will prefer to sue for injuries resulting from a tort in civil court. In civil litigation monetary damages may be awarded and, if the injury was determined to be egregious, then punitive damages could also be assessed against the defendent. The standard of proof in civil litigation is the "preponderance of the evidence" or the "more likely than not" standard; it is a "superiority of weight" test that requires that in order for the plaintiff to be successful, 50.1 percent of the evidence must weigh in his or her favor [18]. Thus, the preponderance of the evidence rule is a threshold test [24]. Either the plaintiff proves that the damages were more likely to have been caused by the defendant agent than by any other source and is, therefore, entitled to full compensation, or he or she fails to meet the burden of proof and is entitled to nothing [28].

NEGLIGENCE
*Professional Negligence*
Negligence "is conduct, and not a state of mind" [35]; "involves an unreasonably great risk of causing damage" [35]; and is conduct "which falls below the standard established by the law for the protection of others against unreasonable risk of harm" [34]. Professional negligence, or medical malpractice, is a special instance of negligence. The medical profession is held to a specific minimum level of performance based on the possession, or claim of possession, of "special knowledge or skills" that have been accrued through specialized education and training. For negligence to be proved, the following elements must be present [20] (Fig. 8-2):

1. There must be a *legal duty* owed by the defendant to the plaintiff.
2. There must be a *breach* or violation of that duty, usually an unreasonable act or *unacceptable standard of care.*
3. There must be an *injury* to the plaintiff that directly results from the breach of the duty or the unreasonable act or unacceptable standard of care.
4. There must be proof (at a more likely than not or 50.1 percent standard) that the health care provider's act was the *proximate cause* (it was reasonably foreseeable that the act in question would cause the injury that resulted) of the injury and the breach of the duty.
5. The damages that occurred must be *quantifiable* (e.g., the future costs of treatment or lost productivity, or both).

The most difficult element to prove is whether or not the standard of care was adequate. The plaintiff usually must provide expert witnesses to establish what a prudent health care provider in similar circumstances might have done. A "conspiracy of silence" may have existed in prior years

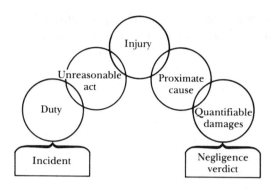

Fig. 8-2. The elements of negligence. There must be an unbroken chain for a successful verdict in favor of the plaintiff. If any link is not proved, the plaintiff will lose the case.

[1]. Today, there are many "experts" willing to testify anywhere about anything.

*Res Ipsa Loquitur*

There are circumstances in which no expert witness is required to corroborate the finding of negligence. The doctrine of res ipsa loquitur essentially means that "the thing speaks for itself." Under such circumstances the negligence is inferred from the act itself, that is, proof from circumstantial evidence. In the classic case, *Ybarra v. Spangard,* a patient was well prior to being anesthetized for an appendectomy, and when he woke up he had an injured arm [40]. Clearly, he could not determine how his arm was injured; the operating room and recovery room staff either could not or would not explain who might have caused the injury. The court found for the injured plaintiff, without the introduction of any expert witnesses, because

1. The plaintiff had not done anything that in any way could have contributed to the injury.
2. The injury could not have occurred unless someone was negligent.
3. The instrumentalities (hospital staff and physicians) that allegedly caused the injury were at all times under the control of the defendant hospital.

MEDICAL TORTS AND CONTRACTS

Civil matters resulting in litigation generally are either contract disputes or torts. A contract dispute occurs when two or more parties have entered into an agreement and one or more parties believes that the terms and conditions of the agreement, either an oral contract or written contract, have not been met. It is important to appreciate that, in a court, oral contracts have the same weight as written contracts. The general purpose for bringing a contract dispute to the attention of the judiciary is to achieve a satisfactory resolution. This usually results in the payment of monetary damages.

A personal tort is an injury to a person or his or her reputation or feelings that directly results from a violation of a duty owed to the plaintiff (in medical malpractice cases this is usually the patient) and produces damage. The remedy, after the nature and extent of the damages have been proved to the court (judge, with or without jury) by a preponderance of the evidence, is usually the award of monetary damages.

Battery is a tort; it is an intentional and volitional act, without consent, that results in touching that causes harm (e.g., the touching of a patient's body without consent). A technical battery can occur when there is no actual harm but touching occurred without consent. Patient transport, with a beneficial outcome but without an informed consent, may be considered battery.

### Informed Consent

Informed consent requires that sound, reasonable, comprehensible, and relevant information be provided by a health care professional to a competent individual (patient) for the purpose of eliciting a voluntary and educated decision by that patient about the advisability of permitting one course of clinical action as opposed to another [41]. Physicians and other health care providers are held to have a fiduciary duty to their patients. Such a duty exists when one individual relies on another because of the unequal possession of information. The failure to obtain proper informed consent may result in the defendant-physician or defendant-hospital being sued for battery in some states or for negligence in others.

According to the battery theory, the defendant is to be held liable if any deliberate (not careless or accidental) action resulted in physical contact. The contact must have occurred under circumstances in which the plaintiff-patient did not provide either express or implied permission and the defendant-health care provider knew or should have known the action was "unauthorized." However, if the scope of consent is exceeded, then a claim of battery is proper. The plaintiff in *Mohr v. Williams* consented to have her right ear operated on [27]. During the procedure the surgeon determined that the right ear was not sufficiently diseased to require surgery, but the left ear required surgery. Since the patient was already anesthetized, the surgeon performed the operation. The operation was a success, but the patient successfully sued for battery. The court held that there was no informed consent for an operation to the left ear. It is not necessary for injury to occur for damages to be awarded, demonstration that there was unpermitted touching is sufficient. In this instance, the court found that there was no medical emergency that would threaten the plaintiff-patient if the surgery were not immediately commenced. If there were evidence of a medical emergency, the court's decision might have been significantly different.

Failure to specifically identify the risks that accompany a surgical procedure can also result in a successful claim of battery. In *Canterbury v. Spence* the plaintiff-patient successfully proved that he was not informed of the risks attendant in the surgical procedure and that had he known them he would not have given permission [6]. The court held that the physician has a duty to disclose all reasonable risks of a surgical procedure, and since he failed to perform that duty, the court held him liable for damages to the patient. Thus, the court held that the concept of informed consent may be more appropriately replaced with the concept of educated consent. The court also articulated an objective standard that could be used in legal cases involving informed consent. This objective standard is based on what a reasonable person in circumstances similar to that of the patient would have decided if he or she had been provided with an adequate amount of information. Thus, the central issue in a battery is whether an educated, effective, or valid consent was given for the actual procedure that was performed.

Most families do not question the need for air transport or the qualifications of those involved in such activities. However, the emotional circumstances surrounding the need for a maternal or neonatal transport, especially an air transport, may preclude the patient or relatives from carefully considering alternative transport systems or the hazards of air transport. Informed consent forms should reflect that the patient or the parents (in the case of a neonate) were informed of the risks and alternatives to the recommended mode of transport.

The unavailability of a neonate's parent in a life-threatening circumstance should not preclude therapeutic action. Just as informed consent is imputed to an unconscious accident victim who has a life-threatening condition that requires surgery, such rational behavior can be imputed to the "absent parent." However, in such circumstances, consultation with the hospital administration is recommended.

When an operation is for the benefit of a minor, the decision to proceed usually belongs to the parent or legal guardian. The failure of the parent to consent to blood transfusions (even if the refusal is based on sincere religious convictions such as those held by Jehovah's Witnesses) or other routine procedures for a small child, that are clearly medically indicated and required for the maintenance of life, can be overridden by petitioning the court for the appointment of a temporary legal guardian [3]. If the parents are unavailable and a reasonable attempt has been made to contact them, then continuing to withhold the emergency treatment because of the failure to obtain consent may be the basis for malpractice liability [7].

A physician is not required to disclose every possible risk to a patient for fear of being guilty of battery [14]. The court in *Cooper v. Roberts* held that "[t]he physician is bound to disclose only those risks which a reasonable man would consider material to his decision whether or not to undergo treatment" [8]. Thus, the court stated that such a standard creates no unreasonable burden for the physician. However, the physician must disclose risks that are material and feasible alternatives that are available. The information should be provided in a manner that reflects the emotional and educational status of the patient or, when the patient is a neonate, the neonate's parents [6]. In *Davis v. Wyeth,* the court held that any medical complication or risk that has a probability of occurring with a frequency of greater than 1:1000 should be included in the informed consent [10].

Is the informed consent of the mother more substantive than that of the father, assuming that the father is both the biological and legal father? It is one of the ironies of the law that a teenage unwed mother has the ultimate legal responsibility for the care of her child, unless the court is petitioned for custody. She is considered an emancipated minor. In contrast, a nonpregnant teenager who is living at home and attending school does not have the legal ability to make decisions about her own medical care.


## Summary

In the final analysis, the determination of whether a lawsuit will be filed against a health care provider and a medical institution is based on one or more of the following issues:

1. Whether the patient or his or her legal guardians or parents were dissatisfied with the medical care
2. Whether the patient was injured, had an untoward medical event, or was led to believe that the outcome would be better than that achieved
3. Whether the medical records are complete and adequately and factually document all events

Health care providers involved in transporting patients need to practice defensive medicine. Defensive medicine is nothing more than a conscious effort to recognize that transporting patients is an inherently dangerous enterprise. There are dangers from litigation for negligence, but there are also physical dangers associated with the transport itself. Nothing more tragic and ironic can happen to a health care provider than to be killed in a transport accident and have his or her estate sued for negligence for the failure to provide adequate care to the patient.

## References
1. Agnew v. Parks, 33 Cal. Rptr. 465, 343 P.2d 118 (1959).
2. Air Shields, Inc. v. Spears, 590 S.W.2d 574, 578 (Tex.Civ.App. 1979).
3. Application of President of Georgetown College, Inc., 331 F.2d 1000 (D.C. Cir.), cert. denied, 377 U.S. 978 (1964).
4. Bing v. Thunig, 2 N.Y.2d 656, 143 N.E.2d 3 (1957).
5. Bost v. Riley, 44 N.C. App. 638, 269 S.E.2d 621 (1980).
6. Canterbury v. Spence, 464 F.2d 772 (D.C. Cir. 1972), cert. denied, 409 U.S. 1064 (1972).
7. Chayct, N. L. *Legal Implications of Emergency Care.* New York: Appleton-Century-Crofts. P. 102.
8. Cooper v. Roberts, 286 A.2d 647, 650 (1971).
9. Darling v. Charleston Community Memorial Hospital, 33 Ill.2d 326, 211 N.E.2d (1965); cert. denied, 383 U.S. 946 (1966).
10. Davis v. Wyeth, 399 F.2d 121 (9th Cir. 1968).
11. Donn, S. M. Intertertiary neonatal transport. *Perinatol.-Neonatol.* 11:35–50, 1987.
12. Early v. Bristol Memorial Hospital, 500 F. Supp. 35 (E.D.Tenn. 1980).
13. *The Emergency Medical Services Systems Act of 1973,* Pub. L. No. 93–154.
14. Getchell v. Mansfield, 260 Or. 174, 489 P.2d 953 (1971).
15. Grewe v. Mt. Clements General Hospital, 273 N.W.2d 429 (Mich. 1978).
16. Hess v. Pawlowski, 274 U.S. 352 (1927).
17. The hospital-physician relationship, 50 *Wash. L. Rev.* 385 (1975).
18. Jackson v. Johns-Mansville Sales Corp., 727 F.2d 506, 516 (5th Cir. 1984).
19. *Joint Commission on Accreditation of Hospitals. Accreditation Manual for Hospitals,* 1986.
20. Keeton, W. P. *Prosser and Keeton on the Law Torts* 164-8 (5th ed. 1984).
21. Id. at 356.
22. Lewis, S. M., and McCutchen, J. R. *Emergency Medicine Malpractice.* New York: Wiley, 1986.
23. Mancini, M., and Gale, A. *Emergency Care and the Law* 50 (1981).
24. McCormick, C. *McCormick on Evidence,* section 339 (2nd ed. 1972).
25. *Medicare Conditions of Participation for Hospitals,* 42 C.F.R. 403 et seq. (1985).
26. Misercordia Hospital Medical Center v. NLRB, 623 F.2d 808 (2nd Cir. 1980).
27. Mohr v. Williams, 104 N.W. 12 (S. Ct. Minn. 1905).
28. Morgan, E. *Basic Problems of Evidence* 24 (4th ed. 1963).
29. Mulholland, The evolving relationship between physicians and hospitals, 22 *Tort & Ins. L. J.* 295-311 at 296 (1987).
30. NLRB v. Parr Lance Ambulance Service, 723 F.2d 575, 578 (7th Cir. 1983).
31. Pub. L. No. 79-725 (1946), as amended by Pub. L. No. 83-482 (1954), Pub. L. No. 88-443 (1964), and Pub. L. No. 91-296 (1970).
32. Schloendorff v. Society of N.Y. Hospitals, 105 N.E. 92 (Ct. App. N.Y. 1914).
33. Schwartz, S., and Tucker, N. *Handling birth trauma cases* 38 (1986).
34. *Second Restatement of Torts,* section 282.

35. Terry, Negligence, 29 *Harv. L. Rev.* 40 (1915).
36. Thompson v. Sun City Community Hospital, 141 Ariz. 1, 688 P.2d 647 (1983), aff'd in part, rev'd in part, 142 Ariz. 597, 689 P.2d 605 (1984).
37. Tonsic v. Wagner, 458 Pa. 246, 329 A.2d 497 (1974).
38. Walker v. Winchester Memorial Hospital, 585 F. Supp. 1328 (W.D.Va. 1984).
39. Wilmington General Hospital v. Manlove, 54 Del. 15, 174 A.2d 135 (1961).
40. Ybarra v. Spangard, 25 Cal. App.2d 486, 154 P.2d 687 (1944).
41. Zebarth v. Swedish Hospital Medical Center, 81 Wash. 2d 12, 499 P.2d 1 (1972).
42. 28 U.S.C. 1332.
43. 29 U.S.C. section 152(14).
44. 42 U.S.C. section 300d-4.
45. 51 *Fed. Reg.* 22,010 (June 17, 1986).

# 9

# *Bioethical Issues Surrounding the Transport of Neonates*

Anne B. Fletcher
John J. Paris

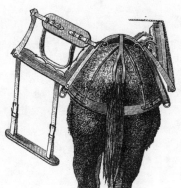

*9A. British cacolet open for use and packed for travel. A class 3 sick transport conveyance (conveyance borne by animals). This type of cacolet or "chair stretcher" was used in the battle of Fair Oaks, May 31, 1862. They "were used only on the first day of battle, proving utterly unserviceable."* (Reproduced from Longmore, T. A Treatise on the Transport of Sick and Wounded Troops. *London: Her Majesty's Stationery Office, 1869).*

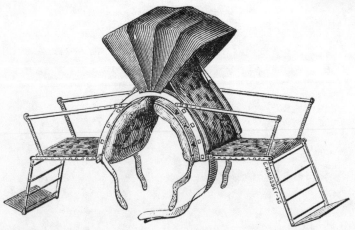

*9B. Cacolet of Lawrence, Bradley, and Pardee. A class 3 sick transport conveyance (conveyance borne by animals). "It combines an unusual degree of the undesirable qualities of weight weakness and inconvenience."* (Reproduced from Otis, G. A. A Report to the Surgeon General on the Transport of Sick and Wounded by Pack Animals. *War Department, Surgeon General's Office, Circular No. 9, March 1, 1877. Washington, D.C.: Government Printing Office, 1877.)*

An infant boy was born on April 9, 1982 in Bloomington, Indiana with a tracheoesophageal fistula. If his only medical problem had been the fistula, he would have been immediately transported to a hospital capable of performing pediatric surgery. Since he also had Down's syndrome, the family and the attending physician agreed not to treat his surgical problem. He was not transported and he died. A few months later the federal government mandated that the Department of Health and Human Services issue the so-called Baby Doe Regulations, which established strict criteria related to the care and treatment of seriously ill newborns [1]. Although in 1986 the Supreme Court denied access to medical records under the Baby Doe Regulations, some of the same criteria are laid out in the 1984 amendment of the Child Abuse and Treatment Act [2].

Transport is an essential component of regionalized emergency perinatal care. The technology and highly skilled personnel necessary for the successful transport of low birth weight, premature, or critically ill neonates have transformed a once simple ambulatory service into what is now virtually a portable neonatal intensive care unit (NICU). As with other technological advances in the medical field, there are concerns that it not be applied inappropriately to those who cannot derive any benefit. Concurrent with advancing technological sophistication, transport has become increasingly costly. These developments force us to critically scrutinize the ethical issues surrounding transport: (1) Do the criteria established in the Baby Doe Regulations and Child Abuse Amendment apply to infant transport? (2) Is there always an obligation to transport an infant? (3) Should costs of transport ever be considered in the treatment of an infant? (4) How should decisions be made about the appropriateness of transport?

## The Baby Doe Regulations and Child Abuse Amendment— Do They Apply?

The most recent Baby Doe Regulations, published on April 15, 1985, and the Child Abuse Amendment of 1984 state that all infants with life-threatening conditions should not have medically indicated treatment withheld (including *appropriate* nutrition, hydration, and medication) when, according to the treating physician's reasonable medical judgment, this treatment would be effective in ameliorating or correcting all such conditions [1, 2]. Exceptions to this requirement to provide treatment may be made when (1) the infant is chronically or irreversibly comatose, (2) the treatment would only prolong dying and not be effective, and (3) the treatment would be futile or inhumane.

Although there is no specific reference to transport in these documents, the requirement that the physician provide the treatment that in his or her medical judgment would offer a reasonable expectation of correcting a life-threatening condition, including "referral to tertiary institutions," makes it clear that transport is regarded as part of the medical care of the patient. As such, the use of transport is to be assessed and provided as would any other component of the medical care of seriously ill infants. It should not be used when, in the reasonable medical judgment of the physician, the treatment would be virtually futile, or would serve merely to postpone or prolong the dying process. Thus, there is not only no requirement but also no impetus in the regulations for community hospitals or those lacking NICU facilities to transfer infants with Potter's syndrome, lethal forms of dwarfism, anencephaly, or any other invariably fatal diagnosis. Infants with such dismal prognoses can be cared for appropriately, and their dying made as easy as possible for the family, in the local hospital. If such diagnoses are recognized early, then transport, which would only add the trauma of distance and delay to the inevitability of dying, need not and ought not be imposed as an additional burden on the infant and the family.

The regulations similarly make it clear that there is no attempt by the federal government to "intimidate" local physicians into transferring seriously ill neonates to tertiary care facilities when, in their judgment, such a transfer is not necessary for the proper care of the child.

Further, there is no requirement that any infant need undergo or a parent consent to any "experimental" treatment to preserve the life of an infant. This standard applies to all patients: No one is obliged to undergo an experimental procedure to preserve his or her life. The choice to do so is entirely that of the parent (or surrogate). If elected, such treatment can be terminated whenever the parent determines that the burdens of the therapy outweigh the actual benefits.

Under the regulations, the same norm applies to treatments that, though not experimental, offer only a "slim chance" of benefit to the patient. Such treatments, though they may be agreed to by the parent, fall outside the parameters of "medically indicated treatment." As such they may be elected or declined by those who speak for the infant without any violation of the patient's rights or the physician's duty. Consequently, transport, although it may be accepted by parents, is not mandated by the regulations or the traditions of medical ethics.

### Which Infants Should Be Transported?

All hospitals involved with the delivery of babies should have explicit written policies for delivery room practices, special care nurseries, and transport teams. The following mnemonics should assist in formulating these policies:

1. ACUTE (*A*cute, *C*ritical, *U*nexpected, *T*reatable, and *E*asily diagnosed). Infants included in this group are those with prematurity and hyaline membrane disease; small preterms (800–1250 g); term or preterm infants with sepsis, pneumonia, or meningitis; and infants with surgically correctable malformations. Without question, these infants should be cared for in or transported to an acute care hospital capable of treating such patients.

2. UNSURE (*UN*known disease, *SU*spected *RE*sponse). This group includes preterms weighing less than 800 g, infants with severe birth asphyxia, and any infant with an unexplained disease or syndrome that requires further diagnostic efforts. Within this group there will be a significant number of infants for whom the response to treatment will be unpredictable. These infants should be given full medical care until the diagnosis is made or the response is clear. Decisions to omit treatment or not to transport should not be made precipitously for this class of patients.

3. KNOT (*K*nown, *NO*t *T*reatable). Although only small numbers of infants fit into this category, treatment decisions for this group frequently take a disproportionate amount of time. Neonates with anencephaly should not be transported unless the child is a potential transplant donor, and even this indication for transport is controversial. Infants with trisomies 13 and 15 should likewise not be transported if there are facilities for accurate diagnosis and appropriate care in the local institution. When distance is not prohibitive, the suspicion of the presence of a lethal disorder is high but not certain, and diagnostic facilities are not available locally, an on-site consultation by a specialist from the tertiary center is a feasible and appropriate alternative to transport.

Extremely low birth weight infants (< 600 g) who are not resuscitated and left to die and severely asphyxiated infants (Apgars 0,0) with little or no response after 20 minutes of resuscitation should, if possible, be kept at the hospital of birth until they die.

It is particularly important when dealing with the very low birth weight infant to remember that it is better to initiate treatment immediately than to delay treatment until the infant can be weighed. It is also better to initiate treatment and then monitor to determine whether the infant responds than it is to presume nonviability, leave the infant unattended, and find unexpected gasping an hour later. A late resuscitation serves no purpose and leaves the care giver (and the infant) with monumental problems. When anticipating low birth weight it is better, if possible, to communicate with the mother or parents before delivery to work out a realistic plan for future management of the infant.

Many physicians believe that it is easier not to begin treatment than it is to stop it once begun. Others believe there is no moral difference between not starting and stopping. Both statements may be true, but there are two consequences that must be considered: (1) if care is never initiated, an infant will *almost* certainly die without having had a chance, and (2) if not resuscitated initially, but with delayed spontaneous breathing and subsequent resuscitation, the infant may live but with significant and avoidable damage. As a rule of thumb: "When in doubt, do; when unable to diagnose, transport." It might also be advisable to transport the child with inherited, untreatable disease or marked physical deformities if the medical personnel at the local hospital are not equipped to handle the parental response to such a personal tragedy. Similarly, it may be advisable to transport when parents of a second child with an inherited, untreatable disease need the support of familiar personnel in the tertiary institution.

One of the dilemmas facing care givers is whether or not to transport late second trimester abortuses. Not a year passes in our neonatal intensive care unit without a caller asking, "This was to have been an abortion, but the infant weighed 800 g and is now breathing. What should we do?" While the laws in various jurisdictions may vary with regard to the age of viability, and it is frequently difficult to make an accurate prenatal assessment of weight and postnatal gestational age, the abortus should be treated as any other premature delivery. If there is a possibility of viability, it is better to resuscitate immediately than to wait and find that the infant eventually breathes spontaneously. However, if a very small infant is not resuscitated initially and a call comes to the referral hospital long after there is reasonable chance of salvage, it is better not to transport. The child should be kept comfortable at the local hospital.

Finally, there are times when a transport team arrives at the referring hospital and finds an infant too sick to transport and already in the dying process. Further care would not only be costly but also futile. After discussing the condition of the infant with both the referring and receiving attending physicians, the parents should be told as humanely as possible that there is no further medical intervention that can save the child. The parents should be encouraged to hold the child if they wish and, with the support of the staff, comfort the infant as best they can.

## Cost of Transport—an Ethical Issue?

Despite the existence of private insurance coverage and public assistance programs that, to date, have covered a large portion of the cost of newborn care, the emergence of cost constraints is forcing health care providers to reassess the enormous expense of newborn care. Transport costs, particularly those for back transfer, are frequently not covered by health insurance. To date, tertiary hospitals have been able to assume some of the costs of ground transport. Likewise some Level II hospitals have been willing to pay the cost of return transport, because they were benefiting from the further hospitalization of the infant.

A ground transport usually ranges in price from $500 to $1100. Air transport by helicopter or fixed-wing aircraft is far more costly, ranging from 1500 to $5000 per trip. Most parents cannot afford to pay such costs, and hospitals are reluctant or refuse to absorb these large losses. In some instances, especially when there is great distance to be traveled and rural services are sparse, the state will subsidize the transportation costs. However, particularly when the therapy is experimental, such as heart transplant, or not widely available, such as liver transplants or extra corporeal membrane oxygenation (ECMO), the hospital may insist on "up front" payment of the airfare before the patient is transferred. To date, these transports have been paid for by the parents, local fundraising, or private philanthropy. As technological advances become more common, good will may fail. Cost containment and constraint will increase, and pressure will be exerted to restrict treatment to those who can pay for it. How the medical profession responds to such pressures—especially when the salvageable life of a baby lies in the balance—will be a test of our priorities.

## Making Decisions Regarding the Appropriateness of Transport

Establishment of the following will facilitate making ethical decisions: (1) delivery room policies regarding resuscitation, (2) policies on prenatal and postnatal communication with parents, (3) criteria for maternal transport, (4) criteria for infant transport, (5) easy availability of consultation with appropriate personnel at a tertiary care institution, and (6) criteria for not transferring infants.

If these essential components are in place and operational, they will help avoid the mishaps and misunderstandings that occur when decisions are deferred until a moment of crisis. The decision makers will not necessarily all be in the same hospital, but the principal physicians, the parents, the nurses, and the members of the transport team should be in communication with one another. These participants must be certain that they have all the necessary facts at hand; they must know the interests and the concerns of all parties; and they must be consistent in the implementation of the decision. Whatever decisions are made, the rationale for them must be fully documented in the medical record.

Finally, it must be remembered that medical transport bears an associated morbidity for both the patient and the members of the transport team. The ethical decision making involved in determining whether or not to transport a patient must include both a consideration of the benefits to the patient and the risks to the members of the transport team. Thus, it would be ill advised and unethical to knowingly dispatch an air transport team in adverse weather conditions, regardless of the potential benefits to the patient.

## References

1. Child Abuse and Neglect Prevention and Treatment Programs; Final Rule. 50 *Fed. Reg.* 14, 878 (April 15, 1985) (45 CFR 1340).
2. Child Abuse Prevention and Treatment Act and Child Abuse Prevention and Treatment and Adoption Reform Act Amendments. *Cong. Rec.-Senate* (June 29, 1984). P. 58951.

# 10

# Psychological Aspects of Perinatal Transport

Susanne Bennett
Elisabeth K. Herz
Nancy M. Nagel

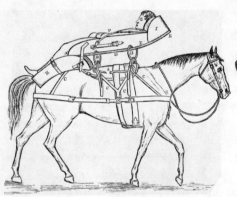

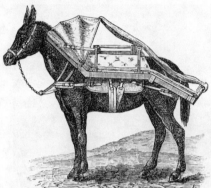

*10A. Thistle's single litter for horse or mule. A class 3 sick transport conveyance (conveyance borne by animals). This litter was first used in the Florida campaign, 1836. (Reproduced from Otis, G. A. A* Report to the Surgeon General on the Transport of Sick and Wounded by Pack Animals. *War Department, Surgeon General's Office, Circular No. 9, March 1, 1877. Washington, D.C.: Government Printing Office, 1877.)*

*10B. British army mule-litter with pack-saddle. A class 3 sick transport conveyance (conveyance borne by animals). "A litter on one side and cacolet on the other." (Reproduced from Longmore, T. A* Treatise on the Transport of Sick and Wounded Troops. *London: Her Majesty's Stationery Office, 1869.)*

The transport of a mother or her neonate to a tertiary care center can be viewed as a medical and psychological crisis. The transfer affects the mother and father, other family members, her obstetrician and pediatrician, and the hospital care givers. The level of stress produced and the response to stress are conditioned by the perceived severity of the medical situation, as well as personality factors and the social environment of the family. This review is based on the combined clinical experience of the authors in dealing with the psychological impact of perinatal transport, in addition to semistructured interviews with families and obstetricians.

The literature contains very little information regarding the psychological impact of patient transport. However, there is an abundance of literature on related topics, such as "crisis theory" (including the developmental crisis of pregnancy), and the emotional impact of neonatal loss, prematurity, and birth defects. Our understanding of crisis theory has derived from the psychoanalytic theory of traumatic neuroses [9, 10], the understanding of developmental crises [8, 17], and the classic study of bereavement by Erich Lindemann [16]. In recent years, David Kaplan and Edward Mason [12] have introduced the concept that giving birth to a premature infant should be viewed as causing an "acute emotional disorder" that results from the individual's efforts to cope with a threatening event for which she is not psychologically prepared. The studies of Gerald Caplan [5] have further explored the theory that the patterns of parental response to the crisis of premature birth can have a significant impact on future mental health.

Pregnancy itself may be viewed as a developmental crisis [1, 3, 4]. It is a vulnerable period for parents, during which the mother goes through many physical changes, and they both may experience emotional changes. If, in addition to the normal emotional responses, the mother and father must face a potential threat to the pregnancy, feelings of anxiety, helplessness, guilt, anger, and loss can result. They are suddenly faced with the loss of "the perfect pregnancy" and "the perfect baby."

The attachment process that occurs between the parents and fetus [13] is critical to the impact on the parents if the pregnancy is threatened. During gestation, the mother has been experiencing a growing attachment to her imagined baby, fantasizing with varying degrees of intensity about who and what her baby will become. After the first detectable fetal movements, she begins to experience the fetus as a separate individual. Many mothers and fathers assign a personality or sex to their unborn child, based on their interpretations of the fetal movements. As one mother said, "I projected myself onto this child."

When a baby is born prematurely, or when an immediate transfer to a neonatal intensive care unit (NICU) is required for an acute illness, the normal attachment process is interrupted. Some mothers of very premature babies may not have had their pregnancies confirmed or may not have recognized fetal movement. They have not had time to anticipate and prepare for their baby as a separate individual. As a result, the mother of a premature baby may not be prepared for emotional attachment to her infant. Since she has not had the opportunity to fully accept the reality that the baby is a separate person, her interest and love is still primarily invested in herself. The mother of a sick full-term infant has had the complete term gestation during which to anticipate her imagined child, but the period of actual acquaintance with her newborn is interrupted. In both instances, mothers feel an acute sense of guilt and ask "Why is this happening to my poor baby?" or "Why is this happening to me?" There is often obsessive concern with actions that the mother took or did not take, which she fears may have caused the interruption in the pregnancy, illness, or birth deformity in the baby [18]. She frequently experiences a severe blow to her self-esteem and feels a sense of failure because she is not able to produce a healthy baby or protect her infant from harm. Her own sense of failure may be compounded by feelings of disappointment, confusion, despair, and anger toward the staff at the referring hospital who she may perceive as having failed to provide all the care that her infant required. One mother describes her experience: "I had had no problems in my pregnancy and had lots of fantasies about delivery and the first few moments of birth. Then my baby was wrenched from me and they sent him away. It felt like he had been extracted. The first few days I was in total shock. I was alone and felt like I wasn't a mother. I cried and cried, and it was impossible to integrate what had happened."

In the past 5 years the frequency of transport between tertiary care centers has increased [6]. This increase is caused by the development of new treatment techniques such as extracorporeal membrane oxygenation (ECMO). Intertertiary neonatal transport magnifies the emotional problems experienced by the parents. The sense of separation is exacerbated by the significantly greater distance that is usually imposed. The parents may not have the financial resources to allow them to be near their infant and may have to place their faith blindly in the health care team at the receiving hospital. Communication may be limited to telephone calls. In addition, the parental expectations of a "miracle cure" from the new technology involved may place a significant strain on the parent-physician relationship.

## *The Emotional Impact of Transport*

### THE REFERRING OBSTETRICIAN

The family's emotional reaction to maternal transport will greatly depend on the smoothness of the transfer, which in turn depends on the frame of mind of the referring and receiving obstetricians. It can be difficult for an obstetrician to relinquish the care of a patient by arranging for her antenatal transfer to a tertiary care center. The patient presumably chooses an obstetrician in whom she has confidence. The obstetrician becomes the primary physician for many women, and the bond is further strengthened by the frequent visits for prenatal care. However compelling the reasons for transfer, it may remain difficult for the referring obstetrician to disappoint the patient in her expectation for continued care. This situation is especially frustrating in cases in which the referring physician is perfectly capable of handling the obstetrical complication—but the transfer is required for the sake of the premature child.

Statistics show that premature rupture of membranes or premature labor, or both, are the indications for the majority of antenatal transfers [14]. Some studies have shown an impressive advantage, comparing in utero versus neonatal transport, the former in terms of neonatal mortality and morbidity [7, 11, 15] (see Chaps. 6 and 14). The obstetrician's decision to transfer the mother is, therefore, predominantly determined by the fact that the care of her infant is beyond the capacity of the referring institution. Some obstetricians consider maternal transfer a breach of confidence with the patient, and they feel let down by an institution that does not provide an NICU. The physician may also feel that his or her professional capability is placed in question by the need for maternal transfer. The current litigious atmosphere in our society also contributes to a defensive approach to patient care. However, in an acute obstetric crisis the referring physician may be relieved to refer the patient for tertiary care.

The administrative aspects of maternal transfer are frequently frustrating. The referring obstetrician who has made the decision to ask for help expects a prompt response. However, the admitting protocol at the receiving institution may require reiteration of reasons for transfer to a hierarchical medical and administrative system. Frustration creates anger, which is aggravated when the referring obstetrician perceives that the appropriateness of maternal transfer is questioned by staff at the tertiary care center.

Frequently the transport team is headed by a physician who is junior to the referring obstetrician. The transport physician is obligated to reevaluate whether the patient is stable enough for transfer, to retake the medical history, to fill out the transferal forms, and, if necessary, to take steps to stabilize the patient for transfer. Friction may develop between the obstetrician, who feels scrutinized, and the transport physician, who acts according to established protocol. To avoid counterproductive conflict, both physicians should have sensitivity to the issues involved in maternal transfer and the recognition that the common goal is to achieve optimal care for the mother and child. It is of considerable help if the referring obstetrician has previously met the obstetric consultant that will care for his or her patient and knows the protocol for maternal transfer.

The most delicate task for the referring physician is to find the right balance between being an "alarmist" and giving unrealistic hopes. This balance can be achieved by telling the mother what to expect but avoiding being so specific that she is confused when an alternative treatment is chosen by the new team. A delicate professional dilemma arises if a patient wishes to remain under the care of the tertiary care center. The reasons for her decision need to be carefully evaluated and discussed with her. It is important to encourage her to talk with her referring physician about the factors leading up to her choice and to find an appropriate closure for their doctor-patient relationship.

## THE CONSULTING OBSTETRICIAN/PERINATOLOGIST

The current high incidence of obstetrical malpractice litigation has led to the concern that community hospitals will attempt to "dump" high-risk patients at the tertiary care centers. Staff at the referral center may feel that they have to carefully investigate the appropriateness of a transfer, especially from an unfamiliar source. The referring obstetrician may present an over-optimistic prognosis to the mother, creating unrealistic expectations for the outcome at the tertiary care center. Furthermore, the receiving obstetrician is often not aware of information that has been given to the mother about her obstetrical problem and probable further clinical management. It is difficult for the new team to deal with a medical crisis when the patient is highly apprehensive and doubts the validity of the reevaluation and proposed treatment.

Temporary privileges extended to the mother's obstetrician may best serve her emotional needs. However, this solution is frequently not feasible for her physician and can create problems at the tertiary care center. The obstetrician on temporary privileges has to operate in unfamiliar surroundings. He or she may become overextended and, therefore, have to relinquish some of the care. This situation may create inconsistencies in the clinical approach, confuse the patient, and lead to conflict over who is in charge of her care.

The better the patient is psychologically prepared by her obstetrician, the easier it will be for her to transfer her trust to the new professional team. The effectiveness of the new team will be enhanced if the referring physician indicates to them what information has already been presented to the patient.

OTHER HOSPITAL PERSONNEL

Involvement in the delivery and stabilization of the infant often results in a bonding between the mother-baby dyad and the staff. They have gone through the initial crisis of birth together and when the infant then requires transfer to a different facility, the staff frequently has mixed emotions. Feelings may range from disappointment to a sense of failure at being unable to provide for all of the infant's needs. At times there may be some jealousy or resentment toward the tertiary care center and a reluctance to let the baby go. The staff has feelings of anxiety and concern for the infant and lacks a sense of completion. Similar to the mother, whose bonding process is prematurely interrupted, the staff too may feel the pangs of separation. A transport that occurs after negative staff-family interactions may also leave the staff of the referring hospital with some feelings of resentment.

THE MOTHER AND FAMILY

There are many variables that affect the emotional impact of maternal and infant transfer on the family (Table 10-1), and it is helpful to examine these in detail.

*Type of Transfer—Planned versus Acute*

The events surrounding the transfer of the mother have a significant impact on how she is able to cope emotionally. If she has already been hospitalized at her local hospital with, for example, elevated blood pressure, and

*Table 10-1. Variables that affect the emotional impact of maternal and infant transfer on the family*

Type of transfer—planned versus acute
Medical indication for transfer
Previous pregnancy experience
Marital strife
Family support systems
Maternal age
Maternal cognitive abilities
Precrisis personality traits of family members
Cultural and religious factors
Economic factors

then needs transfer, she has had some time to adjust to her condition. However, she has had an opportunity to develop relationships with the medical and nursing staff and may find it difficult to give these up.

Transfer that is precipitated by a more emergent situation, for example, premature labor, tends to be more harried, confusing, and frightening. There is less time to prepare emotionally, and the patient may feel overwhelmed and out of control. Most transports involving neonates are acute and result in an intense crisis for the family.

### Medical Conditions for Which Transfer Is Indicated

In the majority of cases, the mother is transported so that appropriate care can be provided for her fetus. The mother then focuses on her fears and apprehensions for the baby and begins to readjust her fantasy wish for the perfect baby. If, however, she is transported because of her own clinical condition, her fears are compounded. She must not only cope with the possibility of a premature or abnormal infant but also with a threat to her own health. Frequently mothers will later describe feelings similar to those experienced by patients with "posttraumatic stress syndrome." That is, they may have reactions consisting of explosive outbursts of anger, flashbacks, and nightmares alternating with a numbing sensation and the loss of a sense of control over their destiny. They may feel driven repeatedly to go over events in their minds and "reenact" what happened to them when they were critically ill.

Benfield et al. [2] reported that the results of an "anticipatory grief questionnaire" given to mothers and fathers of transported infants did not appear to be associated with severity of infant illness. In our experience, however, the emotional impact of neonate transfer does vary according to the diagnosis and prognosis. The resulting reaction will depend on the level of attachment that has taken place between the mother and fetus and the lifelong implications for the family. Certain diagnoses, particularly birth defects and genetic disorders, tend to have a more damaging effect on parental self-esteem. Thus, the family may be very emotionally fragile and communication may be difficult.

The longer the baby remains at the hospital of birth prior to transfer, the more difficult the separation will be for family and staff. However, if the first hospitalization has been a negative experience for the family, they may be relieved by the transfer but have unrealistic expectations for the tertiary care center.

### The Mother's Previous Experience with Pregnancy

If the mother has had previous uncomplicated pregnancies, she may wonder why this one is different. If she has had similar previous experiences, she may be angry that it is happening again, especially if she has lost high-risk pregnancies in the past. Mothers become especially anxious and worried at the gestational point in the present pregnancy when they had problems in a previous pregnancy.

If this pregnancy was not a planned one, or if there was ambivalence about the pregnancy, the mother may feel guilty about the current problems. She may attribute the current problems to "bad" thoughts or feelings she has had during the pregnancy. She may also feel guilty about things she perceives she has done wrong during the pregnancy (e.g., worked too hard, had sexual intercourse, or had a fight with her partner or husband).

When an older mother experiences problems with her pregnancy, especially a first one, she may have a harder time coping because of limitations on child bearing years.

### The Mother's Support Systems

Is the mother single and alone, single and emotionally connected to the father, or married? Is the marriage stable? Is there extended family? Does the mother have a network of friends or religious community? If the mother perceives that she will have an ongoing support system at the new hospital, she will be better able to adjust to the thought of transfer.

If the mother has other small children and does not have the support of an extended family, she may suffer significant emotional distress related to the care of her other children at home, and how they will adjust to her absence.

When the mother is transported to another hospital prior to delivery, she is separated from family, friends, and community. At times, the transfer takes the mother many miles from her home community, which makes it difficult for family members to visit. Friends, community organizations, and religious contacts are suddenly much less available to her. This situation can increase feelings of isolation and anxiety.

Babies transported out of the mother's city or immediate locality present special considerations for the family and for the new staff trying to communicate with the family. The greater the distance, the more isolated and anxious the mother may feel.

### The Mother's Cognitive Capabilities

Is she able to understand why she is being transported and what will happen at the new hospital? Any indication of intellectual impairment that may affect the mother's ability to understand what is happening and to make decisions for herself or her child should be noted and appropriate support provided. In cases with significant intellectual impairment, an assessment should be made to determine whether a guardian *ad litem* should be appointed.

### The Mother's Age
Is this an older mother, who may have feelings of guilt because she believes her age has affected her baby's chances of normality or survival? Or is she an adolescent, and if so, how mature? Adolescents have particular needs because of the developmental crises of adolescence [8], in conjunction with the crisis of transport. They may have special problems in relating to authority figures regarding their baby or in fully understanding the complexities of the situation.

### The Precrises Personality of the Parents
A mother who has any type of mental illness or personality disorder will have more difficulty dealing with the crisis of transfer. The effectiveness of mechanisms that she has used in past crises are a good indication of how she will cope with the current crisis. Parents who present with a mental illness, depression, anxiety disorder, or other serious personality disorder will also have a more difficult adjustment to the transfer of their baby. A recent death in the family, particularly if the individual died in an intensive care unit, makes transport of their baby to an NICU a very threatening and frightening experience.

### Cultural and Religious Factors
Is the mother from a culture that believes that each pregnancy should run its own natural course and, therefore, does not agree with medical intervention? Is a maternal transport considered "too heroic?" There may be a belief that some pregnancies are "not meant to be" and that "God knows best." Some cultures view the birth of a less-than-healthy infant with much more horror than others and may not understand or agree with medical measures taken, such as transport, to save a critically ill or damaged neonate.

### The Economic Variables
If there are financial difficulties, extended stay in a hospital may seem overwhelming to the parents and their families. Parents may be especially worried about the cost of a helicopter or jet, or the cost of a tertiary care center. They must consider not only the cost of hospitalization, but also transportation costs for family visits, extra child care costs while mother is away and cost for telephone calls. If a significant distance is involved, there may be a fear that they cannot afford to travel to see their infant.

*Table 10-2. Methods for reducing the emotional impact of
prenatal transport on the mother and referring hospital staff*

MOTHER
Communicating medical information clearly and concisely
Identifying care-takers at the receiving hospital
Allowing husband or other to accompany the mother during transport
Facilitating visiting by family and friends
Identifying emotional and cognitive problems, and providing early intervention
REFERRING HOSPITAL STAFF
Using preestablished, rapid, and clear lines of referral
Using established protocols for pretransport stabilization of the patient
Involving the referring obstetrician in stabilization and pretransfer decisions
Allowing the referring obstetrician medical privileges at the receiving hospital
Providing frequent feedback information on patient progress

## *Optimizing Maternal Transports*

To minimize the negative emotional responses to maternal transport, measures should be taken to aid the mother, the obstetrician, and the family
(Table 10-2). The most important of these measures is clear, concise communication between the involved parties. Plans and procedures for medical
management should be clearly communicated to the patient, family, and
referring obstetrician. Each step of the process, from diagnosis to medical
management at the new hospital, should be explained in as much detail as
time will allow. The name of the receiving obstetrician at the new hospital
should be given to the mother. All of these measures help the patient to
feel more in control of the situation. If possible, the patient should be accompanied in the ambulance by her husband or partner. When feasible,
the midwife, nurse, or obstetrician might accompany her also. One patient
reported that her experience was vastly improved when her obstetrician
chose to ride in the ambulance with her; she felt comforted and safe knowing he was there.

When possible, the referring obstetrician should be accorded temporary
privileges at the new hospital. If this is not possible, the obstetrician should
continue to contact the patient by phone until she returns for follow-up
care. This communication minimizes disruption of the patient-physician
relationship. Follow-up contact between referring and receiving obstetricians will contribute to their collaboration, as well as greatly reassure the
patient. It also facilitates a smoother transition when the patient ultimately
returns to her physician's care.

While at the referral hospital, the mother should obtain clear, concise
communication about her condition and medical management. The spe-

cific medical/nursing team members who will be caring for her should be identified as soon as possible after admission. It is helpful for the unit social worker or, if indicated, the consulting liaison psychiatrist to visit soon after arrival to encourage the mother and other family present to verbalize their feelings about the transfer. The social worker will be available for both emotional support and to help with practical matters.

Family and friends should be encouraged to visit when feasible. Rules and regulations regarding visitation might be loosened somewhat if the hospital is a great distance from the patient's home. When possible, financial assistance for costs incurred in visiting (e.g., for parking or bus service) might be offered to the family.

### Optimizing Infant Transport

As is the case for maternal transport, there are measures that can be taken to ease the emotional trauma of a neonatal transport (Table 10-3). Of primary importance is open communication between the staff at the referring hospital and the family regarding the need for a transfer. It is helpful for the referring pediatrician to explain the baby's medical problems clearly and why a transfer to a tertiary care center is necessary. The family should be told that their pediatrician will remain informed of their baby's condition for purposes of follow-up care.

Prior to transporting the infant, it is important for the parents to see and touch their baby. Leaving a photograph of the baby with the parents (Fig. 10-1) continues the acquaintance process and provides comfort after the baby leaves.

*Table 10-3. Methods for reducing the emotional impact of neonatal transport on the parents and family*

---

Communicating reasons for transfer clearly and concisely

Allowing contact with infant prior to transport

Providing materials that describe the NICU (including important telephone numbers and names)

Providing emotional support to the parents after their baby has left the referring hospital

Calling to update parents and staff on the condition of the infant on arrival at the receiving center

Encouraging parents to express their emotions and to call the NICU

Encouraging other family members to visit the infant when parents are unable

Providing a photograph of their infant to parents who cannot visit

Identifying emotional, cognitive, and socioeconomic problems early and providing appropriate intervention

---

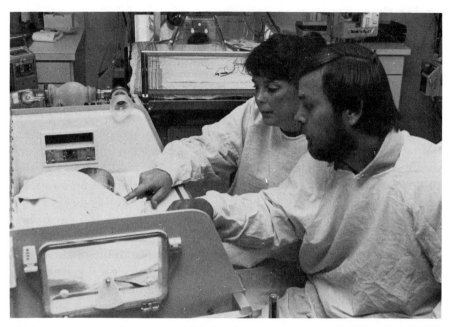

*Fig. 10-1. Parents communicating with their infant prior to transport. The infant in the picture is not critically ill and his mother is ambulatory. It is important to take the infant to the mother if she is nonambulatory. Even the sickest neonate can be touched gently through the portholes in the incubator.*

As soon as possible after admission of their infant, parents should be informed of the names of the pertinent staff at the tertiary care center, including the attending physician, primary nurse, and social worker. Many parents are initially overwhelmed by the large numbers of staff at an NICU. Careful explanation of the roles of the individual personnel in the nursery and the lines of authority is also helpful. It is especially difficult for parents to understand the roles of residents, fellows, and attending neonatologists in a teaching hospital, or the difference between a neonatal nurse practitioner, a staff nurse, or a primary nurse. A photograph of the tertiary care center and an informational letter or pamphlets about the hospital and the NICU policies are also helpful, as well as directions to the facility. Parents should be given telephone numbers and encouraged to call at any time.

In addition to visiting their baby and receiving information, the parents should be encouraged to express emotions because this outlet can provide an initial step in the adjustment to the crisis. It also enables the staff to assess their needs and level of understanding. After departure of the baby, personnel at the referring hospital should be sensitive to loneliness and grief. Many parents find it comforting to be able to talk to a nurse, social worker, chaplain, or family member at this time. Most mothers prefer to be in a private room, away from the newborn nursery, although a minority have indicated that they are comforted by seeing other women with their babies. Offering a choice of room location shows sensitivity and allows the mother some degree of control over her circumstances [2].

The first few days after the transport are important for assessing and stabilizing the family, as well as the baby. Personnel at the tertiary care center should reach out to the family, particularly the mother who is still hospitalized. She needs to hear from the attending physician or resident, as well as the primary nurse, so that she can be informed of the baby's medical progress and can begin to establish some level of trust in the new staff. It is helpful for the social worker to talk with the mother at this time, to try to prepare her for her first visit and to initiate a relationship for providing emotional support.

The parents need to be reassured that "bonding" with their baby will not be disturbed and that the separation does not have to have serious damaging effects on their relationship with the baby. Parents should be encouraged, when feasible, to touch and communicate with their baby, and to bring in toys and pictures. If the mother is interested in breast-feeding, this should be encouraged. If the baby is too sick to breast-feed, breast-pumping and storing the breast milk should be explained. Everything possible should be done during these first few days to help the mother establish a role with her infant and to continue the attachment process, since the patterns established in the first few days or weeks often set the tone for the remainder of the hospitalization.

Reaching out to the father and an extended family is a vital step in stabilizing the crisis [2]. Fathers often feel torn between trying to comfort the mother and trying to be with the baby. Understanding his conflict and exhaustion and involving him fully in the communication process are essential in establishing a relationship with the family unit. In addition, the significance and influence of grandparents should not be underestimated. Although it is not appropriate to relay specific medical information to the extended family without the parent's permission, it is important to be sensitive to their concerns and help them to feel welcome in the nursery. If the mother wishes, the extended family should be encouraged to visit the baby in her absence. The social worker or other staff members should also ensure that the family has a place to stay if they are from out of town and that they have maps and directions to the hospital. Providing financial aid to those who cannot afford the expense of long-distance travel, phone calls, meals, and parking is also helpful.

If it is apparent that the mother is unable to comprehend information or to be involved and make decisions because of serious cognitive impairment or mental illness, then a guardian *ad litem* may have to be appointed for the baby. This action is sometimes necessary even if there is extended family involved because of the legalities of informed consent. In such cases, extended family members should be encouraged to assume a nurturing role with the baby and to understand the medical decisions, although a court-appointed guardian is making the decisions regarding informed consent.

It is both considerate and beneficial for the NICU staff to provide interim and follow-up information to the referring hospital. This information exchange enables the referring staff to give appropriate support to the mother who remains their patient and alleviates their feelings of lack of closure. Sensitivity to the needs of the referring staff is often overlooked but is essential to ensure a smooth transition of care and a good working relationship between the hospitals in the future.

## Summary

In summary, maternal and infant transfer can be viewed as a psychosocial as well as a medical crisis, affecting the family, obstetrician, and other staff. How the family copes with this crisis depends not only on the type of transfer (planned or acute) but also on a variety of psychosocial variables, such as support networks, mental functioning, coping styles, financial resources. We have outlined some methods to decrease the psychological trauma of transport and to ensure the best possible benefit from patient transfer. Further research in this area should help to enhance support services to patients, families, and staff.

## References

1. Benedek, T. Parenthood as a developmental phase. *J. Am. Psychoanal. Assoc.* 7: 389–417, 1959.
2. Benfield, D. G., Leib, S. A., and Reuter, J. Grief response after referral of the critically ill newborn to a regional center. *N. Engl. J. Med.* 244:975–978, 1976.
3. Bibring, G. Some considerations of the psychological processes in pregnancy. *Psychoanal. Study Child* 14:113–121, 1959.
4. Bibring, G. L., Huntington, T. F., and Valenstein, A. F. A study of the psychological processes in pregnancy and of the earliest mother-child relationship. *Psychoanal. Study Child* 16:9–72, 1961.
5. Caplan, G. Patterns of parental response to the crisis of premature birth. *Psychiatry* 23:365–374, 1960.
6. Donn, S. M. Intertertiary neonatal transport. *Perinatol.-Neonatol.* 11:35–50, 1987.

7. Elliott, J. P., O'Keefe, D. F., and Freeman, R. K. Helicopter transportation of patients with obstetric emergencies in an urban area. *Am. J. Obstet. Gynecol.* 143: 157, 1982.
8. Erikson, E. H. *Childhood and Society.* New York: Norton, 1950. P. 228.
9. Fenichel, O. *The Psychoanalytic Theory of Neurosis.* New York: Norton, 1943.
10. Freud, S. Mourning and Melancholia. In J. Strachey (ed.), *The Standard Edition of the Complete Psychological Works of Sigmund Freud,* 14. London: Hogarth Press, 1957. Pp. 239–258.
11. Harris, B. A., Jr., Wirtschafter, D. D., Huddleston, J. F., et al. In utero versus neonatal transportation of high-risk perinates: A comparison. *Obstet. Gynecol.* 57:496, 1981.
12. Kaplan, D. M., and Mason, E. A. Maternal reactions to premature birth viewed as an acute emotional disorder. *Am. J. Orthopsychiatry* 30:537–547, 1960.
13. Klaus, M., and Kennell, J. *Maternal-Infant Bonding.* St. Louis: C. V. Mosby, 1976. Pp. 1–15, 99–166.
14. Knox, G. E., and Schnitker, K. A. In-utero transport. *Clin. Obstet. Gynecol.* 27(1):11, 1984.
15. Levy, D. L., Noelke, K., and Goldsmith, J. P. Maternal and infant transport program in Louisiana. *Obstet. Gynecol.* 57:500, 1981.
16. Lindemann, Erich. Symptomatology and management of acute grief. *Am. J. Psychiatry* 101:141–148, 1944.
17. Rapoport, L. The State of Crisis: Some Theoretical Considerations. In H. Parad (ed.), *Crisis Interventions: Selected Readings.* New York: Family Service Association of America, 1965. Pp. 22–31.
18. Solnit, A. J., and Stark, M. H. Mourning and the birth of a defective child. *Psychoanal. Study Child* 16:523–537, 1961.

# IV

# *Technical Aspects of Patient Transport*

# 11 The Transport Environment

Carl L. Bose

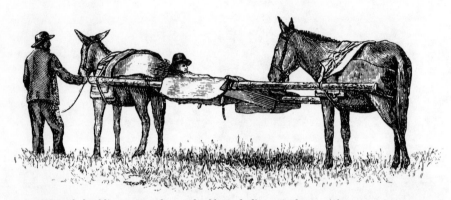

*11A. Wounded soldier conveyed on a double mule-litter. A class 3 sick transport conveyance (conveyance borne by animals). Assistant Surgeon Munn, in transmitting the photograph above remarked: "The litter with two mules, long in use, I believe to be inferior to the travail. When animals move at an uneven pace, the result is disastrous to the harness and to the patient." (Reproduced from Otis, G. A.* A Report to the Surgeon General on the Transport of Sick and Wounded by Pack Animals. *War Department, Surgeon General's Office, Circular No. 9, March 1, 1877. Washington, D.C.: Government Printing Office, 1877.)*

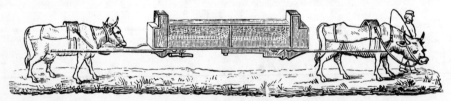

*11B. Bullock litter. A class 3 sick transport conveyance (conveyance borne by animals). "Rodlich (Aachen 1815) has proposed to suspend a large litter for two or more wounded between two oxen, . . . but he considers this expedient unlikely to be of general application, since the movements of oxen are very slow." (Reproduced from Otis, G. A.* A Report to the Surgeon General on the Transport of Sick and Wounded by Pack Animals. *War Department, Surgeon General's Office, Circular No. 9, March 1, 1877. Washington, D.C.: Government Printing Office, 1877.)*

The needs of perinatal patients, even those who are critically ill, are often clearly identified by providers in community hospitals. Appropriate therapy is usually initiated by the referring hospital personnel to the limits of their capabilities. Care provided by the transport service, therefore, should be either a continuum of that therapy or an improvement on it. In either case, the principles of care during transport are not different from the principles of inpatient care. The only differences arise from the unique features of the transport environment. Therefore, providing appropriate patient care during transport demands that personnel understand the principles of inpatient care, understand the unique features of the transport environment, and be prepared to adapt to that environment.

Although ground transport services now provide sophisticated vehicles and equipment and highly trained personnel, many of the environmental handicaps of the early years of patient transport still exist. Also, as air transport has become more common, patients and personnel are confronted with a host of additional hazards.

The following features may distinguish the transport environment from that of the inpatient care unit:

excessive noise
vibration
improper lighting
variable ambient temperature and humidity
changes in altitude
confined space
limited support services

In this chapter I will discuss the impact of each of these environmental features on the patient, the care providers, and the transport equipment. General methods of adapting to these environmental handicaps will also be discussed.

### Excessive Noise
Sound levels in neonatal intensive care units (NICUs) have been extensively investigated. Shenai recorded sound levels in a NICU under three conditions: inside a transport isolette with the portholes open, inside a transport isolette with the portholes closed, and outside the transport isolette [15]. In the NICU, sound levels varied between 58 and 70 dB and were not different inside or outside the isolette, regardless of porthole closure. The range in levels was attributed to the addition of various monitoring and patient

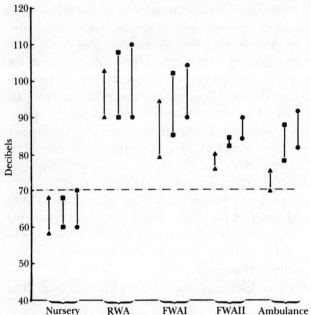

*Fig. 11-1. Sound levels in various transport vehicles (RWA = rotary-winged aircraft, FWA = fixed-winged aircraft) and in the nursery. Levels were measured inside a neonatal transport isolette with the portholes closed (condition I), inside the isolette with the portholes open (condition II), and outside the isolette (condition III). (▲ = condition I; ■ = condition II; ● = condition III.)* (From Shenai, J. J. Pediatr. 90:812, 1977.)

care equipment. Bess et al. quantitated the relative contribution of life support equipment [2]. They found that the standard equipment required for the care of critically ill infants, such as ventilators, infusion pumps, and manual ventilation bags, contributed from 8 to 25 dB to baseline sound levels, mainly in the low- and high-frequency ranges. Further, they observed that impulse signals generated by striking the isolette or by opening and closing the isolette doors resulted in peak sound levels as high as 140 dB.

Shenai also made measurements in a variety of transport vehicles, including a ground ambulance, a rotary-winged aircraft, and two types of fixed-winged aircraft. Sound levels were invariably and significantly higher in all types of vehicles (Fig. 11-1). The highest sound levels were recorded in rotary-winged aircraft, and these levels were not attenuated significantly by closure of the isolette portholes. Campbell et al. reported similar, but somewhat higher, sound levels in a variety of transport vehicles [3]. Thus, transport personnel, adult patients, and neonates in transport isolettes are all exposed to sound levels in the 80 to 110 dB range during transport. Levels at the lower end of this range correspond to the level of noise produced by a barking dog, whereas levels at the upper end would be heard while operating a lawn mower.

Relatively brief exposure to the high sound levels encountered during transport has unknown effects on patients. It is unlikely that brief exposure has any permanent effects on adults. However, neonates and particularly preterm infants may be more susceptible. Changes in heart rate and peripheral vasoconstriction may occur at levels as low as 70 dB, while disturbances in sleep cycles are observed at slightly higher levels [7]. Sound levels as high as those observed in transport vehicles may have more profound effects. High-tone hearing loss is commonly reported among the graduates of NICUs. This handicap is not necessarily attributable to exposure to noise during the neonatal period. A number of other factors, such as the use of potentially ototoxic drugs, intracranial hemorrhage, and birth asphyxia, may also contribute. However, the potential contribution of excessive sound levels, particularly the extremely high impulses resulting from isolette manipulations, must be considered.

Perhaps the greatest hazard in caring for critically ill patients in an environment with high noise levels is the inability to use the sense of hearing to assess the patient. For example, auscultation of the heart and breath sounds is difficult, and auscultative determination of blood pressure is usually unreliable. Communication between care providers or between care providers and adult patients may be difficult. Finally, prolonged exposure to excessive noise may rapidly fatigue transport personnel and diminish their efficiency.

Hearing loss, particularly in the high-frequency range, is a problem encountered by helicopter pilots who have acquired a large number of flight hours. Presumably, there is a direct relationship between time of exposure and hearing deficit. Whether hearing loss is a significant problem among medical transport personnel is unknown. Because of this potential risk, many programs require that all personnel have annual hearing tests. These tests will identify changes in auditory acuity outside of the conversational range that might not be apparent without testing.

Fortunately, there are ways to minimize the impact of excessive sound levels. Adult patients can wear ear plugs, and malleable, sound insulating material can be placed in the ears of neonates. The retrofitting of the rotary-winged aircraft for aeromedical use should include the use of sound-insulating material that will reduce noise exposure for both personnel and patients. Aircraft should also be equipped with communication earphones for transport personnel so that they are further insulated from high sound levels but can still communicate with one another. Finally, transport equipment should include electronic monitors for physiological variables that might be evaluated by auscultation in the inpatient setting, such as blood pressure transducers and heart rate monitors. Most of these monitors are equipped with visual as well as audible alarms.

## Vibration

Vibration levels to which patients and personnel are exposed during transport have been investigated in only a limited fashion. Campbell et al. measured vibration inside an isolette transported in three types of vehicles: ground ambulance, rotary-winged aircraft, and fixed-wing aircraft [3]. Vibration was measured in the vertical and one horizontal axis. Vibration acceleration magnitude ranged from 0.4 to 5.6 m/sq sec. The highest levels were measured in rotary-winged aircraft and the lowest in fixed-winged aircraft (Fig. 11-2). Greatest vibration was experienced during the takeoff and landing of aircraft. Shenai et al. observed somewhat higher levels that were greatest in the low-frequency (3–18 Hz) range [16].

The effects of these vibration levels on patients and care providers are uncertain. However, there is experimental data to suggest that these effects may be considerable. Low-frequency, high-amplitude vibration causes alterations in peripheral nerve conduction and an associated drop in body temperature in rhesus monkeys [6]. Adey et al. reported electroencephalographical changes in healthy adult volunteers exposed both to vibration and to modest increases in gravitational forces that suggest the potential for diminution in the seizure threshold [1]. Anesthetized dogs exposed to horizontal vibration demonstrate a drop in mean arterial pressure and an increase in heart rate [4]. Similar exposure does not appear to have the same effect on healthy awake adult human volunteers. These studies do not demonstrate conclusively that vibration causes significant physiological disturbances in transported patients. However, if adverse effects do occur, patients with underlying pathology, particularly premature infants whose cardiovascular autoregulatory mechanisms are poorly developed, appear most likely to be affected.

The effects of vibration on care providers are probably less profound but may be of equal importance. The International Organization for Standardization has established recommendations for limiting exposure to vibration based on estimations of when vibration exposure is likely to cause reduced comfort and reduced efficiency [12]. Reduced efficiency may result from auditory and visual fatigue or more obvious somatic complaints such as headache or motion sickness. Transports of the duration experienced in

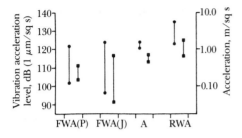

Fig. 11-2. *Vibration levels measured in the vertical and one horizontal axis in an infant incubator during transport in various vehicles (FWA[P] = fixed-wing propeller aircraft, FWA[J] = fixed-wing jet aircraft, A = ambulance, RWA = rotary-winged aircraft). (From Campbell et al. Am. J. Dis. Child 138:969, 1984.)*

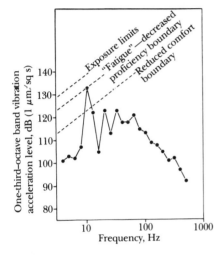

Fig. 11-3. *Typical vibration levels that might be encountered during horizontal flight in a rotary-winged aircraft (indicated by solid line). The hatched lines indicate the predicted effects on healthy adults from 1 hour of exposure to those levels. (From Campbell et al. Am. J. Dis. Child 138:969, 1984.)*

many perinatal regions, particularly in rotary-winged aircraft, frequently result in exposures likely to result in reduced comfort and sometimes in fatigue and decreased efficiency. Figure 11-3 depicts vibration exposure during a typical transport in a rotary-winged aircraft. The estimated effects are indicated by the hatched lines. Repeated exposures may also have an additive effect. That is, personnel who perform repeated transports with brief intervals between them are probably more likely to suffer the effects of vibration than those who experience less frequent exposure.

These potential effects should be appreciated by transport personnel and their supervisors. Every attempt should be made to limit exposure. Staffing patterns should consider the potential hazard of repeated exposure. Also, the evolution of patient care equipment, particularly neonatal isolettes, should include devices to attenuate vibration.

The potential impact of motion sickness cannot be overstated. The most overt form of motion sickness is accompanied by nausea, increased salivation, sweating and often vomiting. These symptoms obviously impair the ability of personnel to perform their duties and may be totally incapacitating. A variety of medications are available to treat or prevent this severe form of motion sickness. Unfortunately, most have at least some sedative effect in addition to the desired pharmacological effect. Some personnel have reported that skin adhesive applicators that contain scopolamine (Transderm Scop, CIBA Pharmaceutical Co.) prevent motion sickness without significant sedative side effects.

A more subtle, but perhaps more common and equally important, manifestation of motion sickness has been termed the sopite syndrome [9]. The symptoms associated with this syndrome include drowsiness, yawning, disinclination for work, either mental or physical; and lack of willingness to participate in group activities. These symptoms often accompany the more overt symptoms of motion sickness or may be the sole manifestation. The sopite syndrome is more likely to occur in isolation when the evoking stimulus is just above an individual's limit of susceptibility or after a long period of exposure during which adaptation has resulted in the disappearance of the more overt symptoms of motion sickness. The symptoms associated with the sopite syndrome are often ignored or attributed to physical or emotional fatigue. It is extremely important that these symptoms be recognized as a manifestation of motion sickness so that they can be managed accordingly. Considerable research into discovering therapies for the treatment of the sopite syndrome has been conducted by the military [9]. Their investigation suggests that a combination of medications, including an anticholinergic (such as scopolamine) or an antihistamine in combination with a stimulant (such as amphetamine or ephedrine), will result in the greatest benefit.

The propensity to develop motion sickness is highly individual. Fortunately, after repeated exposure most affected individuals adapt to the stimulus that evokes motion sickness, so that symptoms either become mild or disappear. Some individuals have also used biofeedback techniques to control symptoms. However, the unfortunate individuals who are highly susceptible and cannot successfully manage symptoms must seriously consider their eligibility for the transport team.

Although the effects of vibration on patients and personnel are either theoretical or difficult to quantify, the effects on transport equipment are well known. In a high-vibration environment, monitor artifact is a common phenomenon. The digital readout on heart rate monitors often bears no relationship to the patient's ventricular rate. In this setting, the oscilloscope tracing may be more reliable because transport personnel may be able to visually distinguish artifact from real electrical impulse. Although there is considerable variation between individual cardiorespiratory monitors regarding their resistance to the effects of vibration, none is immune to these effects. Selection of a model for transport should consider this particular feature, especially if transport will be conducted in rotary-winged aircraft.

Other monitors are usually more resistant to the effects of vibration. For example, blood pressure transducers are relatively unaffected by the usual vibration levels experienced during transport. If heart rate monitoring is impossible, visual inspection of an arterial pressure waveform on the monitor oscilloscope provides a moment-to-moment estimation of ventricular rate.

Another effect of vibration is damage to equipment. Monitors deteriorate much more rapidly when used for transport, compared with their longevity in inpatient units. Preventive maintenance of transport equipment must be on an accelerated schedule compared with other patient care equipment (see Chap. 12). Calibration should also be performed much more frequently than is recommended by manufacturers. Finally, premature obsolescence of equipment must be anticipated when long-term budgets for transport programs are constructed.

### Improper Lighting

Inadequate lighting is a problem encountered in many vehicles not specifically outfitted for the care of critically ill patients. These patients often require careful examination or the performance of invasive procedures in transit. In either case, adequate illumination of all or part of the patient may be critical. Standard ambulances usually provide auxiliary lighting in the patient care area, but this lighting rarely permits extra illumination of designated areas. Aircraft that are not specifically retrofitted for medical use generally have totally inadequate lighting for medical care.

Programs that use vehicles dedicated exclusively for transport activities can circumvent this problem by preparing all vehicles with appropriate lighting. The patient care compartment should be illuminated with an average of 40 candlepower in the area where the patient will be located [13]. Directional, high-intensity lighting can then be added to provide additional illumination for the performance of procedures. It should be possible to screen the patient care area from the driver or pilot compartment so that light will not disturb the vehicle operator during night travel, and to shield the infant's eyes with a neutral density filter or eye shield [8].

Several neonatal isolettes contain a light source inside the isolette box. These are usually low-wattage lights that shine directly on the infant from very close range. Because the distance between the source and the patient is short, illumination is usually quite good for areas in direct line with the source. However, since the source can rarely be located to illuminate the

whole infant, shadowing or differential illumination often occurs. Therefore, these internal light sources often cause more problems than they
solve. The selection of an isolette based primarily on the availability of an
internal light source is probably not wise. In the absence of an electrical
source in the ambulance battery-powered lights can be clamped to the
transport isolette module for emergency use.

Although an inadequate amount of light is a fairly common problem in
transport vehicles, too much light is encountered in some. Ground vehicles
usually have few or no windows in the patient care area, so that too much
light from outside is rarely a problem. Aircraft, however, often contain
many windows. On bright days, when there is little cloud cover, these aircraft may be flooded with light. Excessive light may interfere with examination of a patient, but it is more likely to cause discomfort and fatigue of the
care providers. Manufacturers have recognized the potential discomfort
from excess light and have installed tinted glass in many aircraft. This glass
is certainly a benefit to most passengers but may compromise the ability of a
medical attendant to use subtle changes in the patient's color as an evaluation tool. For example, it may be difficult to identify a neonate who becomes
cyanotic in a vehicle with windows that are tinted blue. Transport vehicles
that do not have windows directly adjacent to the location of the patient
obviate this problem and are preferable.

### Variable Ambient Temperature and Humidity
The body temperature of adults, even critically ill patients, is rarely affected by the range of ambient temperature in a hospital, and adults can
usually be protected quite easily from the wider range of temperatures encountered during transport. Hypothermia in neonates, however, is often a
very significant problem with grave consequences. Neonates, particularly
premature infants, have a very narrow range of thermal neutrality compared with that of adults. In addition, they must often be left unclothed
during critical care. In the NICU a neutral thermal environment is provided by maintaining a reasonably high ambient air temperature and caring for critically ill infants in a convection-heated isolette or under a radiant
warmer. Constant high ambient temperatures cannot be ensured during
transport. Several isolettes have been developed specifically for transport.
Most use convection heat; one uses radiant heat. Except under unusual circumstances, these isolettes provide a thermal environment comparable to
that provided by isolettes in the NICU.

The difficulty in maintaining a neutral thermal environment for a neonate during transport arises from increased opportunities for heat loss. Neonates lose body heat by four mechanisms: conduction, evaporation, convection, and radiation. Heat loss by conduction and evaporation does not present special problems in the transport setting. Heated isolettes prevent conductive heat loss. Evaporation from the infant's body surface to a greater degree than is encountered in the NICU usually does not occur during transport. However, excessive convective heat loss can be a problem. The infant may inadvertently be exposed to drafts of air that are often at temperatures well below the neutral thermal range. This problem can be minimized by heating the air in the transport vehicle to the limit of the comfort range of attendants. The isolette should not be opened unless absolutely necessary. Even then, entry should be through the portholes. One manufacturer has created an isolette that includes a plastic bag insert into which the infant is placed. This insert further isolates the infant from convective losses.

Radiation is perhaps the most common mechanism for heat loss during neonatal transport. In the NICU, the isolette in which a neonate is placed can be isolated from cold surfaces (e.g., windows or outside walls). In transport vehicles all walls are exterior walls. Although the air within the vehicle can easily be heated, it is often difficult to adequately warm the walls and windows. In addition, it is impossible to position the patient a significant distance from exterior surfaces. Neonates can rapidly radiate substantial portions of their relatively small heat energy reservoir to the much larger inanimate mass of these cold surfaces and in cold weather radiant heat losses during transfer between vehicles or between vehicle and hospital may be considerable. This problem can be formidable for care providers and can only be minimized, not eliminated. When isolettes do not use radiant heat, all areas of the infant's body to which easy access is not essential should be covered. If necessary, selected areas of the isolette can be covered to create an additional barrier between the infant and the cold surface. This problem may also be minimized by new isolette models that incorporate a double wall.

### Changes in Air Humidity

Decreased humidity is another potential stressor. Cool air loses its ability to hold moisture. After 2 hours of flying in a fixed-wing plane, the humidity may drop as low as 5 percent. All oxygen administered on the plane should be humidified, and obstetric patients who cannot take liquids every hour should have intravenous fluids for flight.

## Changes in Altitude

Change in altitude during transport presents problems only in very limited situations. The change must be of sufficient magnitude, usually in excess of 5000 ft, and the change must occur in a relatively short period of time. Virtually the only time when a transported patient is likely to be affected is during rapid ascent in an unpressurized aircraft.

There are three primary effects of change in altitude. With increase in altitude air temperature decreases, partial pressures of gases decrease, and total atmospheric pressure decreases. Air temperature drops by an average of about 3°F for each 1000 ft of altitude change. A fall in ambient air temperature of this magnitude rarely represents a significant problem for attendants, because most aircraft are adequately heated. However, lower air temperatures may accentuate the radiant heat loss encountered by premature infants when the transport isolette must be positioned near a poorly insulated exterior wall or window.

Gases expand as the surrounding atmospheric pressure drops and are compressed as it increases. Fluids, however, are relatively noncompressible and nonexpandible. The human body contains both fluid- and gas-filled spaces. However, because the vast majority of these spaces are fluid filled, the human body is relatively resistant to changes in atmospheric pressure. Gas-filled spaces that are in continuity with the atmosphere are also relatively unaffected by changes in atmospheric pressure. As these gas-filled spaces expand or compress, they merely equilibrate with the surrounding atmosphere (e.g., the total volume of gases in the lungs remains unchanged during rapid ascent).

The body's tolerance to changes in atmospheric pressure is primarily dependent on gas contained in spaces not in continuity with the atmosphere. Atmospheric pressure changes little over time at any given ground altitude. However, during a substantial change in altitude, atmospheric pressure may change to a degree such that gases in closed spaces may expand significantly. For example, ascent from sea level to the following altitudes may result in the indicated expansion of gases [5]:

| ALTITUDE | EXPANSION FACTOR |
|----------|------------------|
| 5000 ft  | 1.2 ×            |
| 10,000 ft | 1.5 ×           |
| 18,000 ft | 2.0 ×           |

Healthy humans have few gas spaces that are not in continuity with the atmosphere. However, many diseases, particularly respiratory diseases of the newborn, result in gas trapped in closed spaces. Gas contained in the thorax resulting from an untreated pneumothorax will expand during ascent because this gas is not in continuity with the atmosphere. The magnitude of expansion of this gas may not be clinically significant during the change in altitude encountered during a typical aeromedical transport; except in the most critical cases who have no ventilatory reserve. Gas in the thoracic cavity can be easily vented to the atmosphere by placement of a thoracostomy tube. Gas within tissue, however, may create a hazard as a result of even modest expansion, and this gas is usually impossible to vent to the atmosphere. Pulmonary interstitial emphysema may cause significant compromise of ventilation and become life-threatening as a result of change in altitude. Gas trapped in the bowel wall in necrotizing enterocolitis may rupture into the peritoneal cavity as a result of modest expansion. Similarly, gas in the cuff of an endotracheal tube may expand and cause necrosis of tracheal mucosa. (It is recommended that these cuffs be filled with saline for air transport purposes.)

The expansion of gases in closed space during transport is usually a very manageable problem (Table 11-1). When significant ascent is anticipated,

*Table 11-1. Prevention of problems during air transport*
*of the sick newborn caused by pressure changes during ascent*

GAS EXPANSION
1. Insert orogastric or nasogastric tubes open to air in every infant
2. Avoid use of cuffed endotracheal or tracheostomy tubes
3. Ensure that chest tubes, endotracheal tubes, and other artificial vents are patent
4. Suction airway well prior to transport and during transport as needed
5. Reevaluate frequently for presence of extrapulmonary air
   a. Carry a portable transillumination device
   b. Have a needle thoracentesis set available
6. Request that, if possible, the pilot fly at a lower altitude for an infant with trapped gas
DECREASED PARTIAL PRESSURE OF OXYGEN
1. Before leaving the referring hospital
   a. Ensure that the infant is as optimally oxygenated as possible (ideally with $PO_2$ > 60 mm Hg)
   b. Correlate arterial $PO_2$ measurement with cutaneous $PO_2$ or $O_2$ saturation monitor reading
   c. Check placement and stabilization of the endotracheal tube
2. En route
   a. Use a cutaneous monitor for $PO_2$ or oxygen saturation for all patients requiring oxygen or assisted ventilation (along with frequent careful assessment of the color of skin and mucous membranes)
   b. Increase $FiO_2$ as needed to maintain cutaneous $PO_2$ >50<100* or $O_2$ saturation >95<100*

*These limits may not be appropriate for some conditions (e.g., congenital cyanotic heart disease, persistent pulmonary hypertension).

Table 11-2. Theoretical relationship between atmospheric pressure and the
partial pressure of oxygen in the atmosphere and in the alveolus at varying altitudes

| Altitude above sea level (ft) | Atmospheric pressure (mm Hg) | Atmospheric partial pressure of oxygen (mm Hg) | Alveolar partial pressure of oxygen (mm Hg) |
|---|---|---|---|
| 0 | 760 | 160 | 110 |
| 2000 | 707 | 148 | 99 |
| 4000 | 656 | 138 | 88 |
| 6000 | 609 | 128 | 78 |
| 8000 | 565 | 119 | 69 |
| 10,000 | 523 | 110 | 60 |
| 12,000 | 483 | 101 | 52 |

Adapted from Ferrarra, A., and Harin, A. Emergency Transfer of the High-Risk Neonate. St. Louis: C. V. Mosby, 1980.

efforts should be made to vent closed-space gas to the atmosphere prior to beginning transport. When venting is not possible, ascent should be limited as much as is feasible. Aircraft pilots are usually quite willing to assist within the limits imposed by safe aircraft operation. Pressurized aircraft can also eliminate the hazard of expansion of gases. The pilot must cooperate in this effort by pressurizing the cabin to an altitude comparable with that of the referral hospital.

The partial pressure of all gases in the atmosphere decreases as altitude increases. The most important gas for perinatal patients and their care providers is, of course, oxygen. Table 11-2 depicts the theoretical decline in the partial pressure of oxygen in the atmosphere and in the alveolus at increasing altitude. In healthy humans, the partial pressure of oxygen in arterial blood is directly proportional to the partial pressure of oxygen in the alveolus. Healthy adults can tolerate rapid ascent to altitudes up to 12,000 ft for short periods of time without side effects. Higher altitudes are tolerated by those who have first acclimated to high altitude. Ascent to altitudes above 12,000 ft can result in significant hypoxemia or cause a variety of symptoms commonly referred to as "altitude sickness." For that reason, air travel above 12,000 ft in unpressurized aircraft is unsafe and prohibited by the Federal Aviation Administration unless supplemental oxygen is provided (FAR part 135.89). Newborns are more likely than adults to develop hypoxemia as the alveolar partial pressure of oxygen falls during ascent. Although the usual alveolar arterial difference in partial pressure of oxygen in adults is about 10 mm Hg, the difference in newborns is about 25 mm Hg. Therefore, modest diminution in alveolar oxygen partial pressure will result in hypoxemia in the newborn.

Patients with respiratory diseases are less likely to tolerate ascent without consequences. Those with marginal blood oxygenation at ground level may experience hypoxemia with even modest changes in altitude. Patients who are particularly susceptible are those whose disease includes gas diffusion defects. Respiratory distress syndrome is an example of such a disease. Treatment of diffusion defects is dependent on creating a large oxygen gradient from alveolus to pulmonary capillary. Diminution in the partial pressure of oxygen in the alveolus decreases the magnitude of the gradient and will result in diminished partial pressure of oxygen in the blood.

Increase in the fraction of inspired oxygen delivered to transported patients will usually compensate for any diminution in the partial pressure resulting from altitude ascent [11, 14]. When patients are already receiving 100 percent oxygen this increase is not possible. In these situations, pressurization of the aircraft or flight at low altitude are alternate maneuvers. Patients who are being mechanically ventilated may also benefit from manipulations of the ventilator that improve blood oxygenation (e.g., increase in mean airway pressure). At the very least, the blood oxygenation of patients with respiratory diseases, particularly those with marginal oxygenation who are transported by air, should be constantly monitored during transport so that the impact of altitude change can be accurately assessed.

### Confined Space

One of the obvious handicaps of the transport environment is the confined space in which to care for the patient. The usual area of the patient care compartment in a standard ambulance is about 47 sq ft. The same space in most civilian aeromedical helicopters ranges from about 22 to 36 sq ft, depending on the make and model. The utility of this limited space is further compromised by the necessity of using a portion of the area for stationary seating for personnel. The area available in transport vehicles compares with 80 sq ft of floor space recommended for the care of critically ill neonates in NICUs and 100 and 350 sq ft recommended for labor and delivery rooms, respectively [10]. The height and total volume of the working space are also important to consider when choosing a vehicle to transport critically ill patients.

Access to the patient is often further compromised by the requirement that personnel must remain seated and restrained while the vehicle is in motion. This requirement should not be amended under almost any circumstances. The net result is often that only one attendant has reasonable access to the patient.

Care for maternal patients in this environment is extremely limited. The mother's medical problems can usually be adequately managed, but delivery of the infant may be a catastrophe. Neither the mother nor the attendant can be positioned ideally for a well-controlled delivery. Few vehicles are large enough to transport the mother, an isolette, attendants, and the equipment necessary to care for both the mother and an infant. The confined space of the transport environment, therefore, limits the population of maternal patients who should be transported to those with little or no likelihood of delivery en route.

Although well below the standards for inpatient care, the confined space of the transport environment does permit the provision of neonatal intensive care. This care is usually limited to that which can be provided by a single care provider. Manipulation of the patient usually exposes the infant to the hazard of convective heat loss. Invasive procedures may be more difficult because of increased vibration levels and inadequate lighting. Therefore, every effort should be made to avoid situations in which manipulation of the patient will be required.

### Limited Support Services

In addition to the handicaps of the physical environment, transported patients do not have the benefit of the support services for inpatient care. Sophisticated monitoring devices have been miniaturized in recent years, so this handicap has been minimized to a great extent. For example, it is now possible to monitor blood oxygen saturation, transcutaneous partial pressure of oxygen and carbon dioxide, partial pressure of oxygen in arterial blood, and pressure in virtually any vessel into which a catheter can be placed. The inability to directly analyze blood gases is no longer a significant handicap. Radiography is perhaps the only critical support service not available in the transport environment.

Although most transport services use knowledgeable and highly skilled personnel as patient care providers, the assistance of specialists is usually not directly available during transport. Unless unusual problems develop, this handicap is inconsequential. In fact, the current sophistication of communication equipment permits direct voice contact between transport personnel and specialists at virtually any time during a transport.

### Principles of Care Related to the Handicaps of the Transport Environment

An appreciation of the handicaps of the transport environment and the development of plans to minimize the impact of these handicaps are necessary for one to provide optimal care during perinatal transport. Although the manner in which each program adapts to the features of their vehicles, geography, and patient population will be unique, certain general principles apply. Suggested guidelines include:

1. *Properly prepare the transport vehicle.* Transport vehicles should be carefully selected based on the expected needs of the entire patient population that will use the vehicle. The interior of the vehicle should be prepared to best simulate the inpatient environment. This preparation should include attention to the provision of a satisfactory thermal environment, particularly for neonates. High-intensity, directional lighting should be placed in appropriate locations. Seats for personnel should be situated for maximum access to the patient.

2. *Carefully assess and appropriately stabilize the patient prior to transport.* The extent of assessment and treatment of a patient prior to transport and the appropriate amount of time devoted to this preparation will depend entirely on the problems of the patient and the reason for transport. Many maternal patients are transported for the sole purpose of delivering the infant at a regional perinatal center. Stabilization prior to transport of these patients should focus primarily on determining the likelihood of delivery en route. Lengthy stabilization beyond this assessment cannot usually be justified. Most neonates, by contrast, have diseases that can be adequately managed by a skilled, properly equipped transport team. Once the team is in attendance, the most critical and unstable period of care will be during transit between hospitals. Therefore, stabilization with precise identification of all emergent problems is usually mandatory.

3. *Electronically monitor as many physiological parameters as possible.* Perinatal patients, particularly neonates, are often transported during the most dynamic phase of their disease. The milieu of transport may add to their instability. Monitoring to ensure the success of therapy is therefore absolutely critical.

Because of excessive noise and vibration in transport vehicles, usual evaluation techniques that rely on auscultation, and to some extent the sense of touch, are unreliable. Therefore, evaluation by physical examination should be replaced as much as possible by electronic monitoring. For example, the following parameters should be monitored in all critically ill neonates:

Body temperature
Heart rate
Respiratory rate
Blood pressure
Transcutaneous $PO_2$ or oxygen saturation

In some patients, it may also be advisable to monitor transcutaneous $PCO_2$ and central venous pressure.

4. *Anticipate deterioration.* "Always anticipate the worst" is sage advice to transport personnel. Preparation of the patient for transport should include the initiation of all appropriate monitoring techniques with which to identify deterioration and a contingency plan to support the patient in the event that deterioration occurs. For example, placement of an umbilical arterial line with a pressure transducer may be necessary in a neonate with unstable blood pressure.

In practical terms, stabilization of the patient in preparation for transport often means more aggressive prophylactic intervention than might be indicated in the inpatient setting. For example, the decision to intubate and mechanically ventilate a neonate is usually based on the degree of impairment of oxygenation and ventilation or on the severity of apnea. The threshold for intervention should be somewhat lower for infants who will be transported. When the patient has a tracheostomy, the tube should be changed before flight. The tracheostomy should be postoperative 24 to 48 hours. A spare sterilized tracheostomy tube of the appropriate size should be sent with the patient.

5. *Assist hospital-based personnel in understanding the unique features of the transport environment.* To properly prepare a patient for transport, personnel in a referring hospital must have at least a basic understanding of the features that distinguish the transport environment from the inpatient setting. With this understanding, they are more likely to obtain appropriate diagnostic tests and perform all necessary invasive procedures. Without this understanding, community hospital personnel may evaluate and treat the patient appropriately for continuing care as an inpatient but may not properly prepare the patient for transport. Time-consuming stabilization will then have to be performed by the transport team, often to the detriment of the patient. In these circumstances, referral hospital personnel are also less likely to understand the necessity for the additional intervention provided by the transport team. This misunderstanding can cause resentment on the part of community hospital personnel and may result in overt confrontation. The content of outreach education programs should deal with this issue during instruction on stabilization of patients in preparation for transport. In addition, transport personnel should make every effort to explain why they are performing diagnostic tests or therapeutic procedures in the event that the need for this intervention is not obvious to hospital-based personnel.

## References

1. Adey, W. R., Winters, W. D., Kado, R. T., et al. EEG in simulated stresses of space flight with special reference to problems of vibration. *Electroencephalogr. Clin. Neurophysiol.* 15:305, 1963.
2. Bess, F. H., Peek, B. F., and Chapman, J. J. Further observations on noise levels in infant incubators. *Pediatrics* 63:100, 1979.
3. Campbell, A. N., Lightstone, A. D., Smith, J. M., et al. Mechanical vibration and sound levels experienced in neonatal transport. *Am. J. Dis. Child* 138:967, 1984.
4. Clark, J. G., Williams, J. D., Hood, W. B., et al. Initial cardiovascular response to low frequency whole body vibration in humans and animals. *Aerospace Med.* 38:464, 1967.
5. Ferrarra, A., and Harin, A. *Emergency Transfer of the High-risk Neonate.* St. Louis: C. V. Mosby, 1980. P. 40.
6. Floyd, W. N., Broderson, A. B., and Goodno, J. F. Effect of whole-body vibration on peripheral nerve conduction time in the rhesus monkey. *Aerospace Med.* 44:281, 1973.
7. Gadeke, R., Doring, B., Keller, R., et al. The noise level in a children's hospital and the wake-up threshold in infants. *Acta Paediatr. Scand.* 58:164, 1969.
8. Glass, P., Avery, G. B., Subramanian, K. N. S., et al. Effect of bright light in the hospital nursery on the incidence of retinopathy of prematurity. *N. Engl. J. Med.* 313:401, 1985.
9. Graybiel, A. and Knepton, J. Sopite syndrome: a sometimes sole manifestation of motion sickness. *Aviat. Space Environ. Med.* 47:873, 1976.
10. *Guidelines for Perinatal Care.* Evanston, IL: American Academy of Pediatrics and American College of Obstetricians and Gynecologists, 1983. Pp. 17, 19, 30.
11. Henry, J. N., Krenis, L. J., and Culting, R. T. Hypoxemia during aeromedical evacuation. *Surg. Gynecol. Obstet.* 136:49, 1973.
12. *International Standard* (2nd ed.) (ISO No. 2631-1978). Geneva: International Organization for Standardization, 1978.
13. Patient compartment illumination. *Federal Specifications for Ambulance KKK-A-1822B.* Washington, D.C.: National Automotive Center, General Services Administration, 1985. Para 3.8.5.1.
14. Saltzman, A. R., et al. Ventilatory criteria for aeromedical evacuation. *Aviat. Space Environ. Med.* 958, 1987.
15. Shenai, J. Sound levels for neonates in transit. *J. Pediatr.* 90:811, 1977.
16. Shenai, J. P., Johnson, G. E., and Varney, R. V. Mechanical vibration in neonatal transport. *Pediatrics* 68:55, 1981.

# 12        *Biomedical Aspects of Neonatal Transport*

Robert P. Howard
Oswaldo Rivera

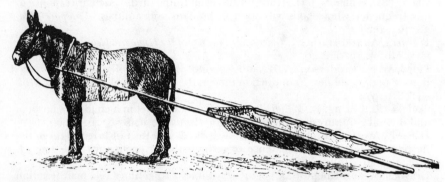

*12A. Greenleaf's combined hand and horse litter hitched to a mule (From a drawing by Dr. Greenleaf). A class 4 sick transport conveyance (conveyance drawn by animals). "On October 27, 1876 Dr. Greenleaf contributed to the Army Medical Museum a model of this combined hand and horse litter, which is numbered 804 in section vl Army Medical Manual."* (Reproduced from Otis, G. A. A Report to the Surgeon General on the Transport of Sick and Wounded by Pack Animals. *War Department, Surgeon General's Office, Circular No. 9, March 1, 1877. Washington, D.C.: Government Printing Office, 1877.)*

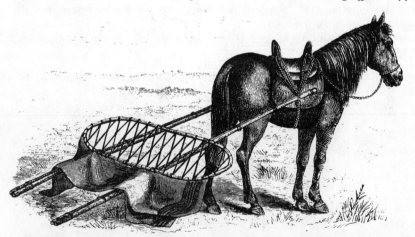

*12B. Dakota Indian litter. A class 4 sick transport conveyance (conveyance drawn by animals). (Reproduced from Otis, G. A.* A Report to the Surgeon General on the Transport of Sick and Wounded by Pack Animals. *War Department, Surgeon General's Office, Circular No. 9, March 1, 1877. Washington, D.C.: Government Printing Office, 1877.)*

The infant transport system is a complex combination of modern medical instrumentation. During the past decade, patients requiring transport during the neonatal period are increasingly of lower gestational age and are more critically ill. Thus, the transport unit is expected to provide many of the acute therapeutic and monitoring capabilities that are typically available in the neonatal intensive care unit (NICU). Hence, a more descriptive name for an infant transport system might be a neonatal mobile intensive care unit (NMICU).

The NMICU should be designed with the capability to maintain the most critically ill infant. Such a system typically consists of a transport incubator, a physiological monitor, one or more intravenous pumps, a ventilator system with on-board oxygen and air supplies, and an electrical power system that provides for either AC or DC operation. This instrumentation should be integrated into a configuration that is sufficiently lightweight and compact to fit into a variety of vehicles including ambulances, helicopters, and fixed-wing aircraft. In addition, all instrumentation controls and indicators should be easily accessible to transport personnel, even while their mobility is limited by seat belts.

Designing one system to meet the specific needs of every infant transport program is a difficult, if not impossible, task. Because of this design problem and the small market for this type of system, manufacturers are reluctant to manufacture them. Of the few commercially available systems, most are designed for less-than-critical patients. Consequently, many transport programs have either modified these commercial systems to meet their needs or have designed their own systems using commercially available medical instrumentation as building blocks. Examples of such custom systems are shown in Figs. 12-1 and 12-2.

### Building Blocks

INCUBATOR

The focal point of the NMICU is the incubator or heating system. It is the largest single component and, therefore, has a significant impact on the final configuration of the transport unit. The purpose of the incubator is to provide a neutral thermal environment in which the infant's body temperature is maintained with minimal metabolic energy expenditure. The environmental requirement will vary with the size and condition of the patient [1] (see also Chap. 11).

Heat transfer (or heat loss) can occur in several different ways:

1. Conduction is the transfer of heat between two adjacent solid objects. For example, heat conduction occurs between the infant and the mattress.

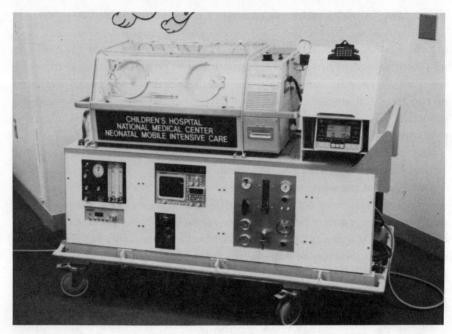

*Fig. 12-1. Custom NMICU for ambulance transport. Features include incubator; physio-logical monitoring; ventilator with airway pressure and oxygen monitoring; transcutaneous oxygen and carbon dioxide monitoring; on-board oxygen cylinders, air compressor, and suction pump; and from one to four IV syringe pumps.*

Heat transfer by conduction will be determined by the conductivity of the mattress material; it is also proportional to the area of contact between the infant and the mattress, as well as to the thermal gradient between them. Typically, only 1 percent of the infant's heat production is lost through the mattress [1].

2. Convection is the transfer of heat between a solid object and the air around it. Heat is transferred from the infant's skin to the surrounding air. The heated air then moves away and is replaced by cooler air that is again heated by the infant. Convective heat loss increases with increased air flow over the infant but will decrease as the temperature gradient between the infant and the air decreases.

3. Evaporation is similar to convection but results from the diffusion of gas molecules transporting water vapor rather than energy. The skin surface of preterm infants has very low resistance to the passage of water, hence evaporative heat loss in these patients can be very significant. One g of water lost by evaporation represents a heat loss of 580 calories at 37°C

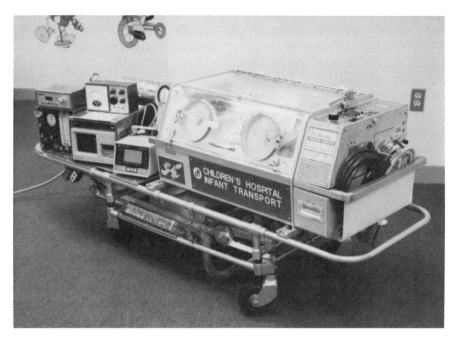

*Fig. 12-2. Custom NMICU for air transport. Features include incubator, physiologic moni-toring, ventilator with airway pressure and oxygen monitoring, transcutaneous oxygen and carbon dioxide monitoring, on-board oxygen and air cylinders, and from one to four IV syringe pumps.*

[1]. Heat loss by evaporation is proportional to the air velocity over the in-fant and is inversely related to the level of humidity in the surrounding air.

4. Radiation is the transfer of infrared energy between solid objects. All objects with temperatures between 0 and 100°C emit infrared radiation, re-sulting in thermal energy transfer [1]. In the incubator environment, this radiant energy transfer occurs between the infant and the walls of the incubator.

All of the mechanisms of heat loss described above occur simultaneously in the incubator environment. The incubator's design should make it pos-sible to balance these thermal transfers in a way that minimizes the overall heat loss from the patient. Most commercial incubators heat their enclosure by forced convection (i.e., warm air is circulated around the infant). In single-walled incubators, about 64 percent of nonevaporative heat loss from the infant occurs through radiation, while the balance is lost to con-vection [2]. Single-walled incubators are characterized by cooler walls and higher compartmental temperatures, whereas double-walled incubators have warmer walls and lower compartmental temperatures. In a double-walled incubator, the radiant heat loss from the infant is decreased, but the convective heat loss is increased [2].

Evaporative heat loss can be very significant in preterm infants, and most incubators provide a method for humidifying the patient compartment. The advantage of decreased evaporation in a humidified environment, however, must be weighed against the increased possibility of bacterial contamination, especially with *Pseudomonas* species [2].

Incubator performance will vary significantly with the manufacturer and is the most important factor to consider when purchasing a unit. The incubator's temperature regulation may be very different when operating in a cold environment from when operating in a warm one (e.g., winter versus summer). Several commercial systems, which performed perfectly in a warm environment, were unable to maintain the required internal temperature levels when subjected to winter conditions. The potential function of an incubator in winter can be pretested in the summer months using a large refrigerator or freezer as a simulated environment.

Another factor to consider is the temperature "map," or distribution within the patient compartment. How and where is the heat generated, how is it distributed, and where is the control temperature measured? For example, one system that was mapped yielded temperatures in excess of 39°C at the mattress while temperature indicators in the upper level of the patient compartment read temperatures below 37°C. In this particular instance, a large heating element was located directly below the patient mattress and transferred a significant amount of heat to the mattress by conduction and radiation [unpublished data]. As another example, many of the earlier forced convection incubators have a glass thermometer mounted at, or near, the top of the patient compartment. It is important to realize that, since hot air rises, this thermometer may register higher temperatures than those actually present at the level of the patient.

Although the primary purpose of the incubator is to maintain the temperature of the infant, it is equally important that it provide an environment that minimizes the patient's exposure to external noise and vibration and protects the patient in the event of a vehicle accident. Vibration can be minimized by shock mounting the incubator to the transport frame. The use of 4- to 5-inch diameter wheels will reduce the bouncing that occurs when rolling over thresholds or uneven sidewalks.

It is important to provide a restraint to keep the patient from bouncing around the incubator compartment in the event of a vehicle accident. Suitable restraint can be accomplished very easily with disposable Velcro

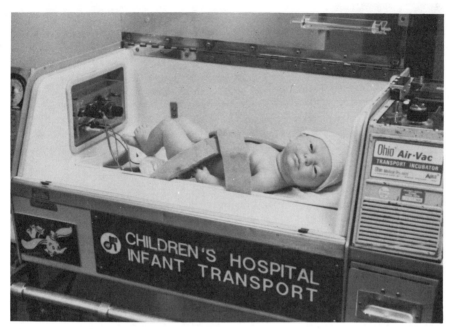

*Fig. 12-3. Simulation of infant restraint mechanism.*

straps. If used properly, they can secure the patient without limiting access (Fig. 12-3).

PHYSIOLOGICAL MONITOR

Another important building block is the physiological monitor. It should be capable of monitoring and displaying heart rate and ECG wave; respiration rate and wave; systolic, diastolic, and mean blood pressure measurements; blood pressure wave; and patient temperature. The monitor should also operate on battery as well as AC power. These requirements have been met by the Spacelabs 413 monitor (Spacelabs, Inc., Redmond, Wash.) (Fig. 12-4). This monitor is 7.5 inches high (with the optional digital module) × 9 inches wide × 13 inches deep and weighs only 18 lb. It was developed in the early 1970s by Tektronix and, because of its small size, rugged construction, and high reliability, it has been the monitor of choice for most transport applications. Unfortunately, Spacelabs discontinued manufacturing of the 400 series monitors in 1987. To date, a suitable replacement has not been identified.

Several attempts have been made to incorporate microprocessor technology into transport monitoring. The result has been a series of new monitors overloaded with trend and data storage capabilities, which are almost twice the size and the weight of the Spacelabs 413. However, the future

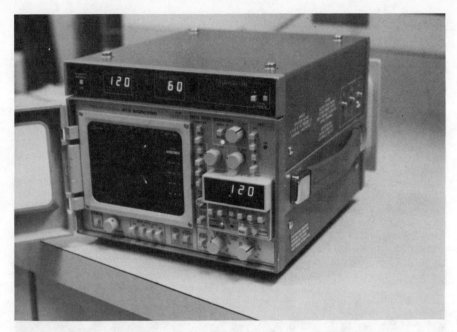

Fig. 12-4. Spacelabs 413 physiologic monitor (Spacelabs, Inc., Redmond, WA).

may hold some interesting possibilities. The use of a liquid crystal display (LCD) in place of the cathode ray tube (CRT) has already been accomplished by one manufacturer and others may follow. The resulting monitor would provide both waveform and digital data on a large flat display. The monitor would be lightweight, have a very low power requirement, and be only about 5 or 6 inches deep.

INTRAVENOUS DELIVERY SYSTEMS

The Travenol Auto Syringe Model AS20A (Travenol Laboratories, Inc., Auto Syringe Division, Hooksett, N.H.) (Fig. 12-5) is the ideal intravenous pump for infant transport. This syringe pump is battery powered, microprocessor controlled, and easy to set up and use. Accurate flows are delivered with a wide variety of syringe sizes, up to and including 50 ml. Because of its small size, it can be placed inside the incubator with the infant (Fig. 12-6). The syringe pump has several advantages over traditional volumetric pumps: (1) there is no tubing external to the incubator that can get caught or snagged, and no open port is required in the incubator hood to admit the tubing; (2) the fluid is warmed inside the incubator, which can be very important during transports in winter; and (3) when multiple infusions are required, up to four of these pumps can be placed inside the incubator.

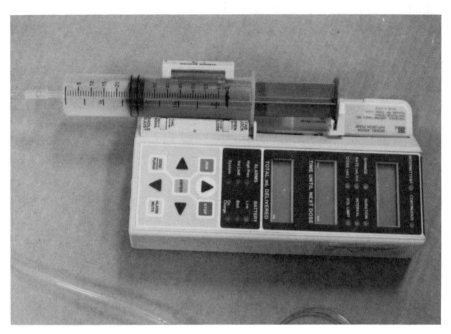

*Fig. 12-5. Travenol Model AS20A IV syringe pump (Travenol Laboratories, Inc., Auto Syringe Division, Hooksett, N.H.).*

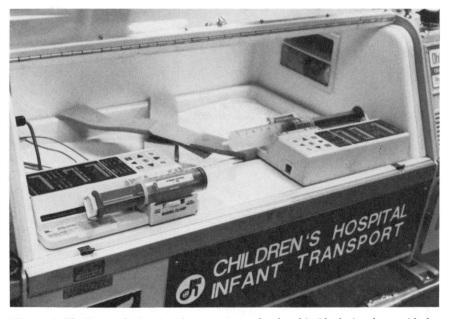

*Fig. 12-6. The Travenol AS20A syringe pumps can be placed inside the incubator with the patient, keeping the IV fluid warm and eliminating dangling external IV tubing.*

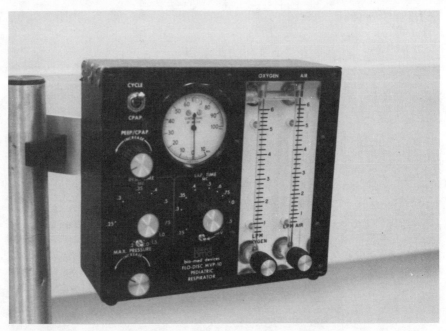

Fig. 12-7. MVP-10 ventilator from Bio-Med Devices (Stamford, CT).

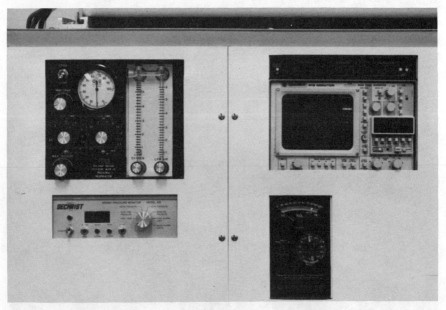

Fig. 12-8. Supplemental ventilatory monitoring includes an airway pressure monitor (lower left) and an in-line oxygen monitor (lower right).

VENTILATOR AND OTHER RESPIRATORY SUPPORT EQUIPMENT

A reliable ventilator is essential for transporting critically ill infants. Although there are a number of ventilators currently used for transport, one of the most popular is the MVP-10 (Bio-Med Devices, Inc., Stamford, Conn.) (Fig. 12-7). This unit is a continuous flow, time-cycled, pressure-limiting ventilator that can also be used to provide continuous positive airway pressure (CPAP). The ventilator logic is powered by a 50 psi oxygen source (consumption is approximately 2−3 liters/minute) eliminating the need for electrical power. Built-in air and oxygen flowmeters provide blended gas mixtures and breathing rates of up to 120 per minute. The physical size (8 × 9 × 3 in.) and weight (5 lb) of the MVP-10 are added assets for transport purposes.

Supplemental ventilatory monitoring can be added as shown in Fig. 12-8. The pressure monitor measures peak, mean, and baseline airway pressures and alarms in the event of any significant pressure change. The oxygen analyzer is placed in the patient circuit to verify the oxygen level delivered to the patient and to provide an alarm when limits are exceeded. Either a Clark electrode or a fuel cell are suitable for this application; however, the Clark electrode will require membrane changes at regular intervals. This changing can be done during routine preventive maintenance (PM) of the system.

The NMICU must carry an ample supply of pressurized air and oxygen, which is usually achieved by on-board E cylinders. However, the compressed air tank may be replaced by an on-board air compressor. The advantage of an air compressor is that it provides an unlimited air supply. The disadvantages are increased electrical power consumption and the added weight of the compressor and power supply.

E cylinders are a logical choice as an on-board source for air and oxygen because they are relatively lightweight, easy to handle, and readily available in most hospitals. Typically, a steel E cylinder is pressurized to 2000 psi and contains about 680 liters of usable gas. Aluminum E cylinders are also available, and Table 12-1 provides a comparison of steel and aluminum tanks. The use of aluminum cylinders makes it possible to reduce the overall weight of the transport system without reducing the on-board gas supply, or to increase the on-board gas supply by about 50 percent without changing the overall weight of the system. Since the on-board gas supply is limited, it is important to know how long it will last in a variety of situations. Figure 12-9 illustrates the time until depletion of an E cylinder, as a function of gas flow. To provide a safety factor, these curves are based on 80 percent of the usable gas volume.

*Table 12-1. Typical E cylinder characteristics*

| Tank material | Weight (lbs) | Maximum tank pressure (psi) | Usable gas volume (liters) |
|---|---|---|---|
| Steel | 17 | 2000 | 680 |
| Aluminum | 7 | 2000 | 680 |
| Aluminum | 14 | 3000 | 1020 |

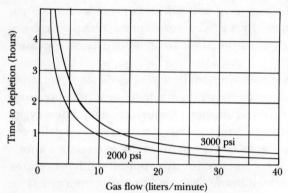

*Fig. 12-9. Time to depletion of an E cylinder as a function of gas flow. Curves are provided for cylinders pressurized to 2000 and 3000 psi. (Curves are based on 80% of usable gas volume.)*

Another important aspect of the transport ventilator system is the ability to provide for alternate gas sources. A simple valve system can be installed in the NMICU to permit switching from the on-board tanks to an external gas supply. Valves can be installed for both air and oxygen, which allows use of the in situ gas supplies when in the hospital, ambulance, or aircraft, while preserving the on-board supply. Thus, the only time that use of the on-board gases is required is in moving the patient between the hospital and vehicle or from vehicle to vehicle. The flexibility of this system is enhanced by the use of adapters. By carrying a series of adapters for medical gas quick connects, it is possible to adapt to almost any medical gas system. Examples of these adapters are shown in Fig. 12-10.

BATTERIES

Rechargeable battery technology has made significant advances over the last several years. There is a wide selection of sealed, maintenance-free batteries that are commercially available, both in nickel-cadmium and lead-acid configurations. Both of these types are suitable for transport applications. They are capable of handling the high current requirements associated with equipment such as incubators and air compressors and can provide several hours of operation in a relatively small package.

Battery performance is expressed in terms of operating voltage, maximum discharge current, maximum charging current, battery capacity, and cycle life. The operating voltage is that voltage that is maintained throughout the discharge cycle of the battery. In the case of most transport instrumentation, the operating voltage is 12 volts. The maximum discharge current is the highest current that can be supplied by the battery without a resulting voltage drop, and the maximum charging current is the highest current that can be used to charge the battery without causing damage to the battery cells. The battery capacity is the total amount of electrical energy available from a fully charged battery and is expressed in ampere-hours (ah). For example, a battery with a 20-ah capacity will run an instrument that uses 10 amperes of current for approximately 2 hours. Finally, the cycle life is an estimate of the number of charges and discharges that a battery can undergo before it begins to deteriorate. A typical cycle life for the nickel-cadmium and lead-acid batteries is between 1000 and 2000 hours.

*Fig. 12-10. Examples of medical quick-connect adapters for Chemetron 50 psi oxygen system. Left column, top to bottom: Oxequip, Shraeder, Puritan-Bennett, Chemetron. Right column, top to bottom: Ohmeda, female DISS, male DISS. Similar adapters can also be made for medical air systems.*

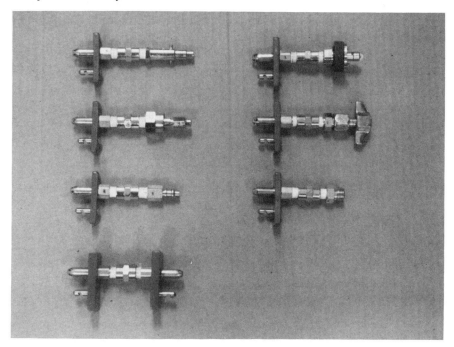

In summary, to choose a suitable battery for a transport system the operating voltage and the current requirements of the instrumentation must first be identified and the maximum time of operation determined. The system can then be matched to a battery with the proper operating voltage, maximum discharge current, and ampere-hour capacity.

Selection of the proper battery charger is also important for overall transport system performance, as well as for extended battery lifetimes. An automatic dual-rate charger can provide a rapid charge for a low battery and will automatically switch to a "float" charge, or trickle charge, once the battery is fully charged. The result is quick recovery of a depleted battery without the risk of overcharging and sustaining permanent battery damage. It is important to realize, however, that a fully depleted battery may require 10 to 16 hours to recover to full charge.

## The Transport System

The objective in designing an NMICU is to provide all of the required monitoring and therapeutic capabilities in the smallest, lightest possible package. In many cases, the medical advantage of including a particular device must be weighed against its impact on the overall size and weight of the resulting system. Typical weights of the routine building blocks are listed in Table 12-2. Depending on the selection of these items, the resulting NMICU may weigh anywhere from 175 to 275 lb and, as additional equipment is added, the system weight will obviously increase.

Integration of each instrument into the system configuration is an important consideration and will result in an NMICU with highly visible displays, easily accessible control panels, and, most importantly, easy access to the patient. When designing the instrument panel, it is important that transport personnel are able to see and have access to it while sitting in the

*Table 12-2. Estimated weights of transport instrumentation\**

| Equipment | Typical weight (lb) |
| --- | --- |
| Incubator | 80–90 |
| Physiological monitor | 18–25 |
| Ventilator | 5–10 |
| Battery | 30–40 |
| E cylinders (pair) | 14–34 |
| IV pump (each) | 1–15 |
| Transport frame | 30–60 |
| Total | 178–274 |

*Approximate system weight

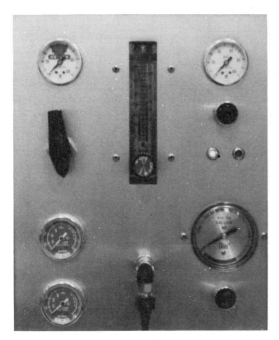

Fig. 12-11. Instrument panel for NMICU gas systems. Left side, top to bottom: oxygen line pressure
gauge, valve to switch between on-board tanks and external oxygen, two content gauges for on-board tanks.
Center: oxygen flowmeter. Right, top to bottom: compressed air line pressure gauge, suction gauge for
medical vacuum.

transport vehicle. For vertical systems (with instrumentation below the incubator (Fig. 12-1), a 10- to 15-degree backward tilt of the panel is helpful
in achieving this goal. For horizontal systems (with instrumentation at either end of the incubator (Fig. 12-2), a slight angle toward the center of the
system may be in order. An integral part of the instrument panel is the information pertaining to the on-board gas supplies. Both cylinder content
gauges and line pressure gauges should be readily visible and accessible to
transport personnel. One such instrument panel is illustrated in Fig. 12-11.

The method of handling patient interfaces (or connections to the patient) is another problem to consider. On a typical transport, connections to
the patient may include an ECG cable, a blood pressure transducer, a temperature probe, a ventilator hose, and one or more intravenous lines. To
eliminate, or at least minimize, the resulting "spaghetti" external to the incubator, a patient bulkhead can be incorporated into the incubator as
shown in Fig. 12-12. This bulkhead provides connections for the physio-

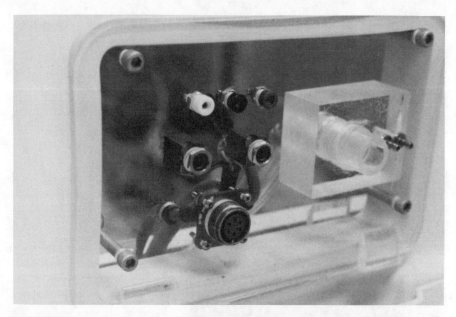

A

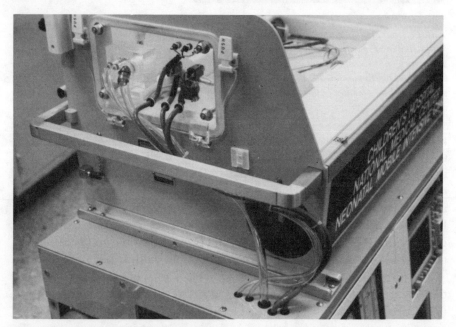

B

*Fig. 12-12. Patient bulkhead for monitoring cables and ventilator lines. A. Inside view shows ECG, temperature, and blood pressure connections on the left and ventilator connections on the right. B. Rear view of patient bulkhead.*

logical monitor and ventilator lines inside the incubator, thus eliminating the possibility of snagging or damaging these lines while mobile. Note that this bulkhead is inserted into an existing access port in the incubator wall and, therefore, does not require any modifications to the incubator body.

The way that the NMICU is used is just as important as the physical configuration and in many cases will have a direct impact on the physical design. For example, by providing sufficient medical gas (oxygen, air, and vacuum) and electrical capability in the transport vehicle, the on-board resources of the NMICU can be preserved.

In summary, designing an NMICU is equivalent to solving a three-dimensional jigsaw puzzle. All instrumentation should be located within view and reach of transport personnel without impeding access to the patient. Efforts should be made to minimize the number of patient-monitoring and intravenous or intraarterial lines drooped outside the incubator, and provisions should be made to adapt to the gas and electrical resources of the referring hospitals and transport vehicles.

### Transport Vehicles

Ground transport is usually accomplished by motor ambulance whereas air transport may involve helicopter or fixed-wing aircraft. There are several requirements, however, that are common to all vehicles.

Adequate supplies of oxygen and compressed air are imperative. These gases are usually supplied in M cylinders, which contain approximately 3400 liters of usable gas pressurized to approximately 2500 psi. These tank pressures must be regulated down to 50 psi for use with medical equipment. The bulkhead connections should use one of the medical gas safety-indexed connectors to eliminate the possibility of cross connecting oxygen to air or vice versa. The compressed air cylinder may be replaced by an air compressor.

Medical suction should also be provided, which can be accomplished with a portable suction system or with a vacuum pump installed in the vehicle. If a bulkhead connector is provided, it must also be safety indexed. A suction regulator and a fluid trap must be connected between the vacuum pump and the patient.

Electrical power should be provided in the form of 120 volts AC, with the standard hospital grade "three-prong"–grounded AC wall receptacles. In this way, the NMICU can be plugged into an AC power source during most of the transport, not only conserving the on-board battery but also charging it. The 120 volts AC is provided by an inverter, a device that converts the vehicle's direct current to alternating current at 120 volts. Proper sizing of the inverter is important in meeting the AC current requirements of the NMICU (e.g., a 1200-volt ampere inverter can deliver approximately 10 amperes at 120 volts AC). Most transport systems will draw between 4 to 8 amperes at 120 volts. This load could be handled by a 1000-volt ampere inverter.

Another important feature of the transport vehicle is the mounting system for the NMICU. Contrary to popular belief, there is no such thing as a "standard stretcher mount." As an example, one supplier of ambulance cots provides three or four different mounting protocols. It is therefore up to the transport program administrators to standardize within their program. Difficulty may still arise during air transports because the ambulances that convey patients to the landing area may not be equipped with compatible mounting gear. Improvisation and the use of heavy-duty securing straps will usually solve this problem.

GROUND AMBULANCE

When one designs an NMICU only for land-based transport, weight and size are relatively less important criteria. Although weight is still a significant factor when loading and unloading the NMICU, a powered lift can be installed in the ambulance to assist the staff with this maneuver (Fig. 12-13).

*Fig. 12-13. A power lift is used to load a transport incubator onto an ambulance. (© 1987, David W. Wooddell. Reproduced with permission.)*

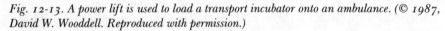
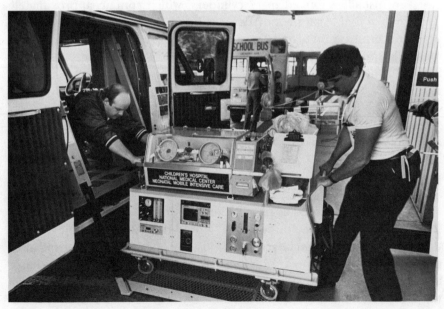

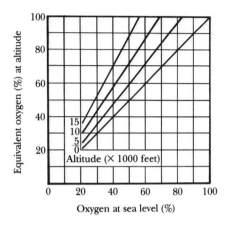

Fig. 12-14. Effect of altitude on patient oxygen requirements.

## HELICOPTER

Helicopter transport is very effective within a 150-mile radius. However, the helicopter creates the most difficult transport environment in which to work. The medical instrumentation is subjected to intense vibration, and the transport staff is placed in a noisy environment in which it is often impossible to hear an audible alarm. It is, therefore, important that all alarms have a visual component and that indicators can be easily observed and identified by the transport staff.

## FIXED-WING AIRCRAFT

The most stringent NMICU design criteria are imposed by the "executive-size" airplane. Whether a jet or a turbojet, loading the NMICU requires a 90-degree turn through a small doorway at some distance above the ground. Therefore, the weight, length, and width of the NMICU become very important.

When flying at high altitude, it is important to realize that the partial pressure of oxygen ($PO_2$) will decrease as altitude increases (see also Chaps. 11 and 13). For example, as illustrated in Fig. 12-14, a patient receiving 60 percent oxygen at sea level will require 87 percent oxygen at 10,000 ft to achieve the equivalent $PO_2$. If the patient requires 100 percent oxygen at sea level, then the aircraft must fly at an altitude where it can maintain cabin pressure at sea level. This altitude is typically approximately 20,000 ft for an executive-size jet.

## Maintenance

Preventive maintenance (PM) is an important aspect of any infant transport program. During normal use, the NMICU is continuously subjected to bumps, bounces, and vibration. This type of physical wear and tear can easily result in decreased instrument performance or outright equipment failure. Although an electronic instrument failure can occur at any time, a PM program is designed to decrease the probability of equipment failure and to identify and correct minor deficiencies before they develop into major problems. PM intervals of 3 months or less should be considered for most transport instrumentation. Individual transport programs may require shorter PM intervals if equipment histories indicate a significant number of preventable failures.

The NMICU is a complex piece of equipment consisting of a series of individual medical instruments and systems. During PM, the performance of each instrument and system must be checked, verified, and corrected if necessary. A sample checklist of medical instrument functions that require performance verification during routine PM consists of the following:

1. Incubator
   a. Temperature control system
   b. High-temperature safety thermostat
   c. High- and low-temperature alarms
      (1) Audible
      (2) Visible
2. Physiological monitor
   a. Digital display
      (1) Heart rate
      (2) Respiration rate
      (3) Blood pressure
      (4) Temperature
   b. Waveform display
      (1) ECG
      (2) Respiration
      (3) Blood pressure
   c. High and low alarms for all physiological parameters
      (1) Audible
      (2) Visible
3. Ventilator system
   a. High-pressure relief valve
   b. Controls
      (1) Breath rate
      (2) Maximum pressure
      (3) Minimum pressure
      (4) Airflow and volume
      (5) Oxygen-air blending

   c. High- and low-pressure alarms
     (1) Audible
     (2) Visible
   d. High- and low-oxygen alarms
     (1) Audible
     (2) Visible
   e. Integrity of gas delivery circuit
     (1) Absence of leaks
     (2) Absence of kinks
4. Infusion pumps
   a. Fluid delivery
     (1) Volume accuracy
     (2) Flow accuracy
   b. Occlusion pressure alarm
     (1) Audible
     (2) Visible
5. Medical gas systems (air, oxygen, vacuum)
   a. Integrity of all high-pressure gas lines and connections
   b. Accuracy of content gauges and line pressure gauges
   c. Operation and proper setting of regulators
   d. Operation of air compressor and vacuum pump if applicable
6. Electrical system
   a. Automatic switching between AC and DC operation
   b. Integrity of all wiring and connections including ground connections
   c. Battery system
     (1) Battery charger
     (2) Battery capacity
7. Transport frame
   a. Structural integrity
     (1) Frame
     (2) Wheels and casters
   b. Stress points
   c. Structural cracks
   d. Cosmetic damage

This list, although not necessarily complete, gives an indication of the complexity of PM procedures. In addition each instrument is tested for ground integrity and electrical leakage, both individually and as part of the total system.

The NMICU can be designed for ease of maintenance and repair. For example, the instrument layout in Fig. 12-15 uses a rack-mount design.

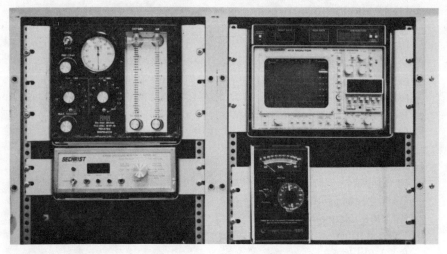

*Fig. 12-15. Rack-mount design for easy installation and removal of equipment.*

Each instrument sits in its own mount, which, in turn, is attached to the side rails. With this type of approach, each instrument can be easily removed and replaced if necessary. The front panels (not shown) are also easily removed because each panel is secured with four quarter-turn fasteners. Each instrument should be easily accessible, removable, and replaceable without dismantling the system. Any modifications that are made to the system should be designed to facilitate the swapping of equipment when repairs are needed. The design of the patient bulkhead in Fig. 12-12 is a good example. By removing the bulkhead from the access port, the incubator can then be easily replaced by another "stock" unit.

Whenever possible, backup instruments should be kept available at the base hospital. Swapping these for a defective instrument in the NMICU results in fast turnaround times and allows the NMICU to remain in service while the malfunctioning item is repaired.

The NMICU is subjected to the harshest medical environment. Consistent satisfactory performance of the system is highly dependent on the availability of competent biomedical engineering support with a strong PM and repair program.

### Future Considerations
New monitoring and therapeutic technologies are constantly being developed and refined. Currently, transcutaneous oxygen and carbon dioxide levels are routinely monitored during many patient transports. Pulse oximetry and noninvasive blood pressure instrumentation are also available

in portable configurations. When determining whether to add a new technology to the NMICU, several questions must be addressed. Will it improve the management of the patient? Is there an alternative way of accomplishing the same result? Does the improvement in patient management override the consideration of added weight and increased size of the transport system? Can the new instrument be easily added to or integrated into the system configuration? Most important, will the new technology work properly in the transport environment? Automatic noninvasive blood pressure units, for example, because of the nature of the measurement, may not function properly in a moving vehicle.

As new technology is developed and additional portable monitoring capabilities become available, decisions will have to be made regarding the information that is most useful for patient management during transport. The NMICU has very identifiable size limitations that cannot be exceeded.

The use of lighter, stronger materials should be considered for frame construction. Materials such as titanium or fiberglass compounds could provide added strength while reducing the overall weight of the system.

Technological advances can be separated into two distinct categories:

1. Development of new sensor technologies to measure or monitor physiological parameters
2. Refinement of proved technologies into smaller packages with lower power requirements

In either case, advances in technology will have a significant impact on the future configuration of the NMICU.

The use of new technology is not the goal of a transport program. The goal is to improve patient care, and new technology, if used appropriately, can be a means of achieving that goal.

## References
1. LeBlanc, M. H. The physics of thermal exchange between infants and their environment. *Med. Instrum.* 21:11, 1987.
2. Marks, K. H. Incubators. *Med. Instrum.* 21:29, 1987.

## Bibliography
Bell, E. F. Infant incubators and radiant warmers. *Early Hum. Dev.* 8:351, 1983.
Darnall, A. The thermophysiology of the newborn infant. *Med. Instrum.* 21:16, 1987.
Perlstein, P. H. Future directions for device design and infant management. *Med. Instrum.* 21:36, 1987.
Scopes, J. W. Thermoregulation in the Newborn. In G. B. Avery (ed.), *Neonatology-Pathophysiology and Management of the Newborn* (2nd ed.). Philadelphia: J. B. Lippincott, 1981.

# 13 Ensuring Safety During Air Transport

Don Wright
Tom Einhorn
Robert A. Margulies

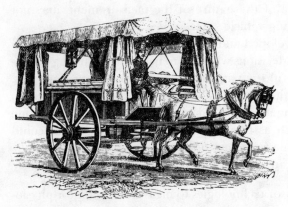

13A. *A class 4 sick transport conveyance (conveyance drawn by animals). "Ten of these carts have round tops or covers, ten have flat ones . . . the ten flat-topped carts carry two stretchers on vulcanized springs and rollers on the floor of the cart, and nine persons before and behind, in all eleven, while a twelfth may be added on a stretcher slung to the roof." (Reproduced from* Longmore, T. A Treatise on the Transport of Sick and Wounded Troops. *London: Her Majesty's Stationery Office, 1869.)*

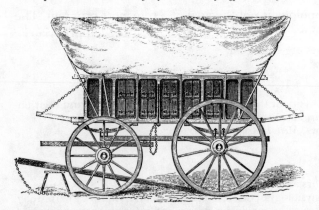

13B. *A class 4 sick transport conveyance (conveyance drawn by animals). (Reproduced from* Longmore, T. A Treatise on the Transport of Sick and Wounded Troops. *London: Her Majesty's Stationery Office, 1869.)*

The air transportation of patients is a rapidly expanding component of modern health care networks. The aircraft has provided a significant benefit in linking the patient with appropriate and timely medical care. Although it was inaugurated with a certain degree of skepticism, the benefits of civilian use of this military concept have been proved repeatedly. Most major trauma centers in the United States either operate their own aeromedical program or have direct access to air transportation.

The air transportation industry is experiencing phenomenal growing pains and ever-increasing competitiveness [6]. Compromises in safety must not enter the bargaining arena. A recent study at Johns Hopkins School of Public Health [20] demonstrated the dire need to address specific safety issues associated with emergency helicopter transports. Data indicate that the risk of death or injury in an emergency medical helicopter is 30 times greater than in an emergency ground transportation vehicle, 100 times greater than in private planes, and 5 times greater than in helicopters in general use (see Chap. Appendix I for accident data).

Unfortunately, the deficiencies that have led to this dismal state in the aeromedical industry have been primarily caused by misguided attempts to cut costs. In the short term, safety is costly in time and money. In the long term, however, safety saves money. Good safety practices prevent accidents and injuries, save lives, protect equipment, eliminate unnecessary law suits, and keep insurance rates at an affordable level.

No other aspect of an aeromedical service should overshadow the need to provide safe and efficient transportation for medical personnel and patients. Safety elements encompass a broad spectrum, including utilization, aircraft, equipment, mission, operations, weather, crew members, medical personnel, and patients. Each element must be evaluated as it relates to and impacts on all others. "Most harmful events are occasioned by known, identifiable and controllable causes" [11].

## Use

The efficacy of air transportation has come under scrutiny by several groups and individuals [4]. Beyond the potential for misuse of service lies the unnecessary exposure of crew and patients to a number of hazards. The determination of when and where to use air transport is initially a medical decision. At accident sites, the decision to request an air ambulance for evaluation is made by first responders, usually paramedics. In rare cases, police or other agencies may request air transport services to act as first responders on notification of a mishap or disaster. For hospital transfers, the referring and receiving physicians consult and decide whether air transport is necessary. The criteria used in making this determination should include the seriousness and nature of the illness or injury, necessity to reduce time in transport, necessity to deliver needed medical expertise in a timely fashion, necessity to deliver specific medical equipment in a timely fashion, and the avoidance of taking limited ground ambulance services away from the local area for an extended period of time.

The legitimate use of air transport services must be based on sound and specific guidelines. Otherwise, abuses of the system will produce additional safety risks and increase the potential for complacency among flight crews and medical personnel.

## *Aircraft*
Not all aircraft are suitable or adaptable for air transports. Basically two types or categories of aircraft exist. Fixed-wing aircraft (airplanes) are used for long flights between airports; rotary-wing aircraft (helicopters) are used for shorter flights and allow for more direct routing and shorter response times.

Fixed-wing aircraft are essentially stable platforms that do not require constant pilot control for operation. Compared with rotocraft (depending on the model), they are generally faster, are more efficient, require less maintenance, are quieter, provide more interior room, and may provide pressurization.

Helicopters, however, are unstable vehicles and usually require constant pilot control. This latter aspect accounts for the helicopter pilot workload being approximately 8 times greater than that of an airplane pilot [12]. Helicopters are somewhat slower in speed than airplanes and are less efficient. Their range of operation is smaller, and they cost more to operate. They also have less available working space, and pressurization is not currently available.

An aircraft used for patient transport must provide for ease of loading of a transport module or a patient on a stretcher, stretcher-securing devices, patient restraints, adequate room to prevent the patient from interfering with the pilot or controls, sufficient room to allow medical personnel maximum body access to administer advanced cardiac life support, adequate lighting for patient monitoring without interfering with the flight crew, inflight access to necessary medical supplies and equipment, and sufficient radios or intercom systems to provide for internal and air-to-ground communication (see also Chap. 11).

### SELECTING AN AIRCRAFT FOR PATIENT TRANSPORT
Each type of aircraft has its own assets and liabilities, depending on the mission. For transports covering distances of greater than approximately 300

miles or requiring significant altitude changes, or both, fixed-wing aircraft provide for greater speed and comfort. However, the advantage of greater speed is offset by the airplane's requirement to land and take off from air fields. Thus, two additional transports of the patient are required, between the hospital and airfield.

Helicopters can land close to the hospital and at or near accident sites (scene flights). Scene flights use all the advantages of the helicopter, which can land in areas as small as 60 × 60 ft. Medical personnel and equipment can be delivered immediately to the patient, and the patient can be flown directly to the receiving facility.

The choice of a suitable aircraft type will depend on several patient-related factors, which include

Seriousness of illness or injury
Altitude and pressurization considerations
Distance to be transported
Specialized treatment or equipment needed
Type of illness or injury
Medical personnel needed

Other specific considerations include

Speed and range of vehicle
Service ceiling (altitude capability)
Instrument certification (adverse weather capability)
Interior space available and configuration
Equipment (e.g., oxygen, suction, or electrical power source)
Useful load (amount of weight that can be carried)
Single versus multiengine
Pressurization capabilities
Communication capabilities
Environmental control capabilities
Patient/stretcher loading and securing system
Noise and vibration levels
Interior lighting

It is likely that a compromise will be necessary when selecting the type of aircraft for patient transport (Table 13-1 and Book Appendix 8). Personnel and equipment to accompany patients will be limited because of weight and size restrictions and the center of gravity limits of an aircraft. Any unusual equipment or specialized handling required for a patient should be reported to the flight crew prior to making arrangements for transport. If a

Table 13-1. Important Basic Considerations Before
Starting a Medical Air Transport Program*

1. Be informed. Review available literature on suitable aircraft models and the administrative and safety aspects of aeromedical services.
2. Make an area analysis for operating altitudes, temperature ranges, hospital pad location and size, fuel availability, and possible noise problems.
3. Consult commercial operators and pilots in the area about aircraft performance, reliability, and operating costs.
4. Consult more than one operator.
5. Prepare a list of specifications before contacting local operators. This list should include both general aircraft specifications and specific requirements for the patient care area.
6. Select an authorized and certified operator who is willing to meet your specifications as long as they are compatible with safety requirements.
7. Develop a contract that definitively describes the responsibilities, liabilities, and compensation of the involved parties. (In a lease agreement the operator is obligated to ensure that the aircraft are airworthy and properly maintained and that the pilots are qualified.)
8. Be aware that the hospital must supply adequate administrative support for their component of the transport service and be committed to work closely with the air service to develop an optimal program.
9. Know all the costs involved in optional equipment and medical equipment installations before buying an aircraft.
10. Remember (if buying an aircraft) that insurance costs are significantly higher for new operators, and that a backup vehicle is required when the primary vehicle is out of service for repairs or other reasons.
11. Include the vehicle and usage costs in your calculations. The cost of operation includes pilot salaries, insurance, fuel, maintenance, and a replacement part reserve. Most manufacturers will supply projected usage costs tailored to your specific program. However, their figures generally tend to be lower than actual costs.
12. Remember that new aircraft sometimes require costly modifications mandated by the FAA (or equivalent national body) at the owner's expense. Older models and out-of-production aircraft are harder to find parts for.
13. Ensure that the interface between the medical dispatch system and the vehicle dispatch system is well planned.

*Refer to Book Appendix 8 for a detailed list.

particular aircraft is unsuitable for the mission, the flight crew can either provide or recommend the most suitable alternative without compromising the safety of the mission. Each mission should be evaluated on a case-by-case basis, with nothing being taken for granted [9].

## Medical Equipment
The limits of weight and space, which are so critical on an aircraft, will dictate how much medical equipment and the number of personnel that may

be carried. Essential items, based on patient needs, of course assume priority. Nonessential items may occupy precious space and infringe on aircraft performance; thus, medical personnel must prioritize their needs while allowing for unforseen emergencies.

Since specific medical needs cannot always be predetermined, especially on emergency flights, prepared kits offer flexibility. Kits designed for trauma, adult medical, pediatric, obstetric, and neonatal care can be quickly loaded on or off aircraft as needed. Although medical supplies and equipment may, in some cases, be obtained from the referring facility, this source should not be depended on. The more thought that goes into the premission planning for equipment needs, the better prepared the medical personnel will be (see Chaps. 11 and 12).

Each piece of medical equipment should be evaluated by a biomedical engineer prior to use for air transport. Some equipment may function improperly or have limited use aboard an aircraft. Helicopters may produce enough vibration to damage or severely limit the capabilities of sensitive medical gear, and airplanes may expose equipment to sudden changes in barometric pressure. Sealed containers and gases are especially prone to the effects of altitude. Some items, such as medical antishock trousers, must be closely monitored during pressure changes.

When aircraft are not equipped with systems capable of providing an adequate electrical source for medical equipment, portable equipment powered by batteries must be used. Dependence on batteries adds problems associated with battery weight, volume, and endurance and the possibility of corrosive liquid spills. Any electrically- or battery-operated equipment that produces electromagnetic interference may cause the aircraft navigation systems to malfunction.

Certain equipment may require special consideration in relation to the fuel and oil systems in the aircraft. Oxygen tanks must be appropriately located and the related delivery system well designed and routed. To avoid the possibility of an on-board fire, all oxygen lines must avoid areas that could become saturated in the event of an oil leak.

Equipment must be stored and secured properly. Certain parts or components on an aircraft are fragile and susceptible to damage from unsecured equipment. In the event of turbulence or sudden stops, any loose objects could become dangerous missiles.

### Operations
Operational safety begins with the management of the aviation assets (see Book Appendix 10). Although the pilot in command is the final authority as to the safe operation of an aircraft, operational issues are dictated

and controlled by management personnel (including the hospital administrator). It is the responsibility of management [11] to provide the necessary support, supervision, and direction to ensure that all aspects of an air
transport service function properly. Key areas requiring review include
personnel, training, equipment, and procedures.

PERSONNEL
The first line of safety in any program begins with the individuals involved.
Since 90 percent of emergency medical service (EMS) aviation accidents are
attributable to human factors [5], the choice of personnel requires meticulous scrutiny. In the case of both aviation and medical personnel, more
than the minimum requirements are necessary to ensure safe and efficient
air transport operations. A solid experience base relative to the demands of
the mission is crucial for optimal team performance.

TRAINING
"The best safety device in any aircraft is a well-trained pilot," according to
Flight Safety International, the largest civilian flight training facility in the
nation. Continuing education and application of training are necessary for
maintenance of operational skills. Safety training addresses not only operational safety but also emergency procedures that one hopes will only be
used in the training environment. Regular, ongoing refresher training can
reinforce proper safety procedures, identify unsafe or problem areas, and
allow personnel to practice procedures that are used infrequently.

EQUIPMENT
Equipment used for air transport should always be evaluated from the
safety perspective. Equipment carried on the aircraft must be compatible
with the aviation environment. Equipment used around the aircraft must
be considered for suitability and potential damage to or from the aircraft.
Personal safety equipment must be evaluated as to need and type. This may
include headsets, helmets, fire resistant clothing, foot gear, and eye and ear
protection (see also Crash Survival). The aircraft itself must be considered
for the element of safety it provides for crew members, medical personnel,
and patients. Many aircraft are designed with a single specific use in mind.
Thus, an aircraft may be safe and efficient in one role but unsuitable and
unsafe in another.

PROCEDURES
The safety procedures used by any organization must be well developed
and properly implemented to ensure satisfactory results. In the same way
that sound medical practices are used (whenever possible) regardless of the

situation, no compromises to safety procedures should be dictated or tolerated, regardless of the urgency of the mission.

A wealth of tried-and-true aviation safety principles are available for review [1]. These principles should be applied with the same vigor by aeromedical services as in any other area of aviation. Their application necessitates a thorough understanding of risk management [14]. Risk factors must be identified, accepted, and understood before appropriate decisions can be made. Once the risk-management decisions are made, air transport and hospital management personnel must uniformly support and implement them.

An active safety program is a necessary element of any flight program. Safety programs provide methods of identifying safety concerns, bring these concerns to the attention of the management, and require that they be addressed. Safety committees provide a forum for issues to be discussed and ensure that safety maintains a proper priority in the overall scope of air transport programs. A written statement by management personnel, emphasizing their support for safety, contributes significantly to the commitment of all participants in an aeromedical service. Any detectable hesitation in this commitment will eventually be reflected in the day-to-day activities of the program. It is recommended that every program have an annual safety audit. The purpose of a safety audit is to obtain a comprehensive review by a qualified outside source. This provides an unbiased, objective critique to promote positive change and reinforce existing safety practices.

## SCENE WORK

Fixed-wing aircraft generally present no additional safety considerations for ground personnel when landing and taking off. Commercial and military airports usually provide at least minimum safety procedures, equipment, and facilities to prevent injury to waiting medical crews and patients.

Helicopters, however, may land and take off directly from the scene of an accident at an unimproved site. Their unique capabilities also create additional safety considerations for those on the aircraft, the patient, and ground personnel.

A selected landing site must, first of all, be large enough to accommodate the particular type of helicopter being used (see Book Appendix 11). The required area ranges from as little as 60 × 60 ft for smaller helicopters to as large as 120 × 120 ft for larger helicopters. For night landing this area must be increased.

The area selected must be free of wires, obstacles, debris, or other matter that could restrict the pilot's vision or be ingested by the helicopter engines.

The helipad should be regularly inspected (at least weekly), and protocols should include the procedure for closing down the pad (e.g., whom to notify) should safety hazards be detected.

All involved ground personnel should undergo special training that includes an emphasis on safety aspects. This training should be regularly updated. Ground personnel should be at least 200 ft from the landing area, and they should ensure that all loose equipment and clothing are secured. The wind generated by a helicopter in a landing configuration can be very strong, turning debris and equipment into potentially dangerous missiles. The dangers associated with wet or slippery surfaces are compounded by the high winds produced by the helicopter.

For night landings, the area must be marked at each corner with a light or flare. If flares are used, they must be closely managed. No lights should be pointed at the aircraft itself. White lights cause pilots to lose their night vision and may temporarily blind them. Lights pointed toward the landing surface help the pilot determine the exact touchdown area.

After landing, the most serious threat to safety is the rotor blades. The blades of a helicopter turn at sufficient speed and force to cut through small trees and poles. Any contact with the main (overhead) rotor or tail (rear) rotor can be catastrophic. Therefore, the landing site must be provided with specially trained security personnel who are designated to keep spectators away.

Extreme caution must be exercised when personnel are moving around an operational helicopter. Unloading the patient with the rotors running ("hot" unloading) should be done only when the few minutes saved might make a difference in the outcome for the patient. The aircraft may only be approached from the front with permission from the pilot. The tail of the helicopter is extremely dangerous because of the high-speed tail rotor and its proximity to the ground. Running is prohibited in the vicinity of the aircraft. Nothing, including intravenous lines, should be raised above one's head. Because the rotors on some helicopters dip quite low, a crouched approach is always recommended (Fig. 13-1).

The same precautions taken during landing are used for takeoff. Trained personnel who are available to assist the flight team are essential, since the pilot has the responsibilities of conducting a ground reconnaissance and preparing for takeoff (Fig. 13-2).

No one should approach the aircraft unless instructed to do so by the pilot. Cabin and compartment doors should be operated only by those trained to do so. The aircraft has many fragile components that, if misused, may break and render it unsuitable for flight. Equipment on the aircraft

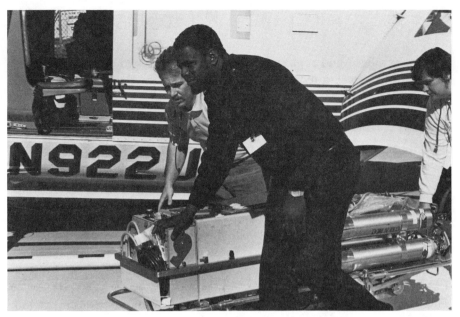

Fig. 13-1. "Hot" unloading. A crouched position is adopted. Neither the stretcher bearing, the incubator, nor the IV lines are raised until well clear of the rotor blades. For optimal safety, eye and ear protection are recommended (not shown) whenever personnel are engaged in "hot" loading or unloading. (Copyright © 1987, David W. Wooddell. Reproduced with permission.)

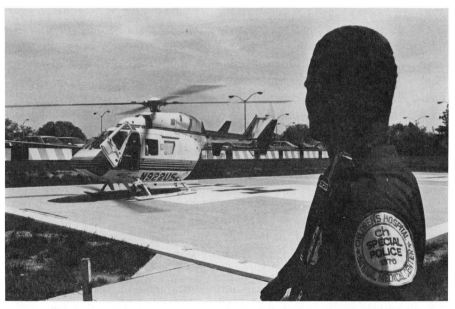

Fig. 13-2. Preparing for takeoff. Security coordination is necessary for safe transport operations. The incorporation of the communications equipment (microphone shown on shoulder epaulet) into a helmet that also provides hearing and vision protection would be optimal. (Copyright © 1987, David W. Wooddell. Reproduced with permission.)

must be removed and replaced by the flight team. Serious injury or death can result from well-intentioned "help" from untrained ground personnel.

### Weather

The decision regarding the acceptability of weather conditions for flying a patient transport mission must be made by the pilot (see Book Appendix 10 for weather minimums). Medical staff should never inform the pilot of details of the condition of the patient or use other tactics intended to pressure him or her into flying in adverse conditions. Flight crew members must obtain regular weather updates between missions.

### Flight Crewmembers

Flight crewmembers are governed by the Federal Aviation Administration according to the specific type of operation in which they fly [8], type of aircraft being flown, and type of mission being performed (see Book Appendix 9). Pilots are federally licensed and must undergo annual physical and performance checks. Aeromedical flights demand that the flight crewmember obtain additional training specific to emergency medical service missions.

The need for additional specialized training is mandated by the unique operations associated with a full-time 24-hour air ambulance program. The urgency and intensity of time commitment that is associated with most patient transports places some unusual demands on both personnel and equipment. Flight crews must contend with the stress and emotion of short response times while transporting the critically ill and injured. Premission planning is severely restricted in many cases. Therefore, crews must maintain the aircraft in a constant state of readiness. For some flight personnel, the nature of an aeromedical mission can have an emotional and psychological impact that may adversely affect their performance capabilities.

Just as equipment must be maintained in a ready state, so must flight crews. Adequate rest, exercise, and nutrition become even more important because of the demands of the mission. The anxiety that results from maintaining a constant state of anticipation can be more stressful than the actual mission.

The responsibility of the pilot in aeromedical missions is significant and the consequences of making a mistake can be devastating. In most cases, the safety of the medical flight personnel, patients, and the aircraft rests in the hands of a single individual. It is imperative that nothing will interfere with the pilot's judgment and decision-making capabilities [1]. *Medical per-*

*sonnel should accept the pilot's decision regarding aviation matters without question.* After the immediate crisis has passed, explanations can be obtained with respect to the specifics of any aviation decisions made.

## Medical Flight Personnel

Medical flight personnel are unique in the health care industry. Combinations of physicians, nurses, and paramedics generally compose medical teams to accompany patients during air transport. The demands of patient care in this type of environment can be tremendous [15]. Some procedures are more difficult or impossible to do while in flight.

By necessity, medical flight personnel must be experienced, strong-willed, quick to perform assessments, independent, and confident in their abilities. Because most patients who need air transport are in critical condition, a strong background in emergency medicine and critical care is essential. Certified expertise in basic cardiac life support (BCLS), advanced cardiac life support (ACLS), and advanced trauma life support (ATLS) is recommended [17].

More than clinical skill is required. Medical flight personnel may have to perform in stressful situations and under adverse conditions. The ability to maintain composure and perform necessary duties in the midst of chaos may at times stretch the limits of even the most competent practitioner.

Medical flight personnel must also receive specialized training for air transportation. Not only are greater demands placed on medical crews but also additional medical considerations must be evaluated [15]. Fitness for flight duties should be a primary consideration for medical personnel. Not everyone adapts to the sensations of flight, and some individuals may become quite ill. Motion sickness may severely impair the ability to treat patients. Other physical considerations include height and weight limitations and muscular strength necessary to load and unload patients in confined spaces. Aeromedical personnel should also receive training in altitude physiology and aerospace medicine.

Without appropriate specialized knowledge, otherwise competent and qualified medical crews can unnecessarily compromise patient care, damage equipment, or inadvertently create or contribute to an unsafe condition on board the aircraft. Initial and continuing education is necessary to keep abreast of new procedures and new equipment designs, especially for air transports. Retraining also provides a method of evaluation and contributes to the prevention of complacency. Safety training is an ongoing process and requires the cooperation of everyone working on or around the aircraft.

## Patients

The responsibility for patient safety rests with the medical personnel and flight crew. Patients who require air transport are generally in no condition to assume even minimal safety precautions for themselves. Therefore, reasonable and appropriate safety measures must be provided by those assigned duties during flight time. If the patient is conscious, it is important that he or she realize the method and need for air transport, if possible. This information can increase cooperation and may also allay any anxiety the patient may have about flying [21].

In most cases, loading a patient on a stretcher onto an aircraft is no simple task. Whereas some aircraft have mechanical features for ease of loading, the majority have either no loading system or one that is inadequate for patient loading. The flight and medical crew must combine efforts to protect the patient and the aircraft during loading and unloading operations. Negotiating narrow cabin doors and confined quarters requires careful maneuvering of the patient. Oxygen tubing, intravenous lines, or any other tubes that are accidently dislodged during loading could delay the transport and jeopardize the patient.

Once inside the aircraft patients must be properly secured in the transport module or to the stretcher, and the stretcher properly secured to the aircraft. In the case of neonatal transports, the transport module is secured to a stretcher or directly to the aircraft (Fig. 13-3). Proper restraints ensure the safety of the patient as well as the flight crew, in case an adult patient becomes combative. Ear protection for the patient is also recommended, especially for helicopter transports (see Chap. 11).

During transport the patient must be constantly monitored, not only from the medical perspective but also to ensure that restraints and other safety equipment remain in place. The medical condition of the patient should be closely observed throughout the flight. The flight crew should be advised of the patient's condition only if it becomes necessary for the pilot to deviate from the flight path, descend, or take other action necessary for patient care. It must also be understood that the safety of the mission takes precedence over patient care.

Once the patient has been delivered to the receiving facility, the same safety precautions must be used when unloading. Assistance during these procedures should come only from those who are adequately trained and are familiar with aircraft operations (Fig. 13-4). The patient must be made ready to unload before anyone moves the stretcher. All intravenous lines and tubing must be free of the aircraft, and other ancillary equipment should be removed or disconnected. After the patient has left the area, a

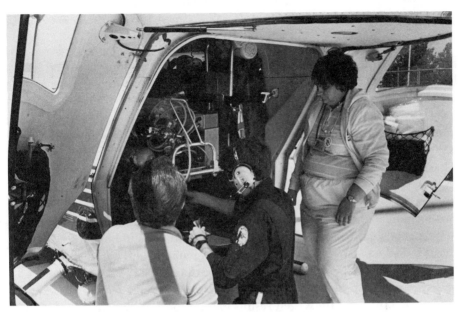

Fig. 13-3. Preparation for air transport. A flight nurse secures the transport incubator inside the helicopter. Questions raised by this picture are (1) Should all personnel be wearing protective eye and ear coverings? (2) Should all three be wearing one-piece flame retardant flight suits? (Copyright © 1987, David W. Wooddell. Reproduced with permission.)

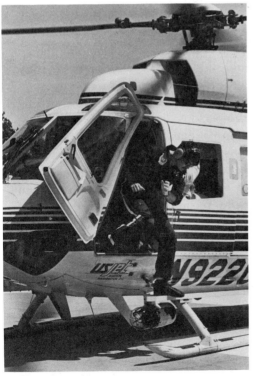

Fig. 13-4. Immediately after landing, a flight nurse leaves the helicopter to help with unloading the patient. The pilot never leaves the helicopter while the rotors are turning. Questions raised by this picture are (1) Is the flight suit made of flame retardant material? (2) Does the suit cover as much of the body as possible? (3) Is the nurse wearing protective eyewear, and do his shoes have crush-resistant steel tips? (Copyright © 1987, David W. Wooddell. Reproduced with permission.)

final search of the aircraft is needed to ensure that nothing has been left behind, such as medical records or radiographs.

## Other Important Safety Considerations
### EFFECTS OF ALTITUDE ON HUMAN PHYSIOLOGY
There are many aspects of the aviation environment that may affect the ability to function of the flight crew and medical flight personnel. The effects on each individual will, to a greater or lesser degree, depend on several factors that include adaptability, general health, and self-imposed limitations [22].

When considering the effects of altitude on the human body (see Chap. 11), two distinct areas must be evaluated: oxygenation and barometric pressure. With an increase in altitude, there is a reduction of the partial pressure of oxygen. At a certain altitude, which varies between individuals, lowered partial pressure of oxygen results in symptomatic hypoxia. There is a marked individual variability in the susceptibility and reaction to hypoxia, and both patients and crew are at risk. Those who smoke or are in less than ideal physical condition are more likely to be affected early by hypoxia. Depending on the amount of oxygen that is available and the duration of exposure, a variety of symptoms may develop. These include drowsiness, nausea, headache, euphoria, blurred or tunnel vision, mental impairment, psychomotor function deterioration, hyperventilation, and cyanosis. A significant deterioration of night vision can occur at an altitude of only 4000 ft [22]. At 25,000 ft, if an aircraft should suddenly lose cabin pressure, complete incapacitation can occur in as little as 2 minutes [22].

The contraction and expansion of some gases may affect certain medical equipment and supplies as well as the persons on board the aircraft. (See also Chap. 11 for effects of altitude on patients.) Changes in gases found throughout the body can cause serious problems when there is a decrease in barometric pressure with an increase in altitude. Trapped gases in the gastrointestinal tract, middle ear, or sinuses can cause excruciating pain during altitude changes. It is, therefore, recommended that personnel do not fly when they have a cold, congestion, respiratory infection, or sinusitis. Sometimes a sinus block can be prevented by frequent use of the Valsalva maneuver during descent. If this technique is unsuccessful, an ascent may ventilate the sinus, and a slower descent may prevent return of symptoms.

Evolved gas disorders are another area of concern in pressurized aircraft. These may develop with rapid decompression when nitrogen supersaturation of the body occurs because of a decrease in barometric pressure, and the body is unable to reestablish an equilibrium (degas). Nitrogen bubbles may form in the tissues and in the blood. Rapid decompression can result in the bends, chokes, paresthesia, or central nervous system disorders. If any of these problems develop, the use of 100 percent oxygen, increased cabin pressurization (if possible), or descent in altitude, or a combination of these will help alleviate some of the problems. It is also recommended that the patient be immobilized to reduce further circulation of the nitrogen bubbles. Because the risk of decompression sickness is increased, no crewmember who has engaged in any type of diving using compressed gas should fly within 48 hours of doing so.

Acceleration and deceleration forces are also factors associated with air transportation [15]. Although sudden and drastic flight maneuvers are avoided if possible by conscientious pilots, turbulence or certain emergency operations may induce a variety of gravitational forces acting on the body. Fixed-wing aircraft operations are more prone to generate such forces, especially during takeoff and landing. The effects of these forces on the patient are probably the most important concern because of their effects on the cardiovascular system. Acceleration and deceleration forces tend to push or pull on internal organs and pool blood in the direction of the inertial force. A loss of blood and blood pressure will occur in the opposite end of the body, in the direction of acceleration. Specific injuries, such as those affecting the head, may require special consideration when one decides where to position the patient in the aircraft.

STRESS
Stress in the aviation environment is of particular importance because of its effect on the flight crew [22]. Any interference with the decision-making capability of the pilot can jeopardize the safety of the entire mission. Stress, as it affects the medical flight personnel, can jeopardize patient care, and stress imposed on the patient can jeopardize his or her welfare.

Stress occurs in two forms: acute and chronic. Acute stress is the more serious of the two and is associated with very short and intense fear, demands, or pressure. Chronic stress is not as severe and generally persists for months or years. Stresses involved in air transport include the nature of the mission, short response times, limited time for premission planning, altitude factors, aircraft environment, weather, duty schedules, and the patient's clinical status.

Some types of stress are self-imposed and, therefore, can and should be controlled. Drugs, alcohol, tobacco, and caffeine all have an effect on performance and may increase stress levels.

The effect of increased anxiety and stress on patients with conditions such as acute myocardial infarction should also be considered when electing to transport by air.

FATIGUE

The effects of fatigue are extremely important to the flight crew [22]. Fatigue is a decrease in performance brought on by the effects of stress [1]. Fatigue can also be categorized as acute or chronic. In the case of air transport chronic fatigue has more serious consequences. Acute or short-term fatigue is the physical tiredness one normally experiences after a long day's work. This type of fatigue can cause coordination as well as awareness problems. The flight environment can contribute to acute fatigue. For instance, night flying is 40 percent more demanding than day flying when all other factors are equal [22]. Proper rest and sleep will overcome the effects of acute fatigue.

Chronic or long-term fatigue will significantly affect pilot judgment and decision making [1]. The *Airman's Information Manual* states, "Fatigue continues to be the most treacherous hazard to flight safety" [1]. The effects of fatigue are insidious and may not be recognized until serious errors are made.

Helicopter operations, in particular, have come under scrutiny recently because of their relatively high accident rate. Many groups, individuals, and government agencies are beginning to examine this problem and offer solutions. The most comprehensive and determined efforts offered in this area have come from the pilots in aeromedical transport themselves [7, 12]. A recent decline in the aeromedical accident rate supports the fact that the essential components of accident prevention are well known and, if they are used, a high accident rate is not an essential part of flight operations [24].

The National EMS Pilots Association (NEMSPA) was formed for the specific purpose of addressing safety issues as they relate to air ambulance services and to educate the medical community as to their own responsibility in this area. NEMSPA has identified working during fatigue as the most serious violation of safety practice in the aeromedical industry [16]. In the past, most aeromedical pilots were on duty 240 to 360 hours per month. The number of hours on duty, combined with rotating shifts, stress, and fatigue created a very undesirable set of conditions. The type of mission being flown, along with the hours of operation, demand that pilots be at their peak of performance every time the aircraft leaves the ground.

Proper diet, rest, and physical fitness all contribute to preventing fatigue and helping to ensure the flight crew's capability to properly prepare for and fly a mission.

NOISE

Noise has been defined as sound that is loud, unpleasant, or unwanted [22]. Noise, in addition to causing stress, can interfere with concentration and communication. In certain cases, noise can result in hearing loss. Noise levels and time of exposure determine the amount of damage suffered. The greater the intensity of the noise, the less time one should be exposed (see Chap. 11).

VIBRATION

Vibrations, like noise, can contribute to fatigue [13]. In a helicopter, vibrations can be quite significant. Certain procedures, such as starting intravenous fluid lines, may be impossible. Certain injuries may be aggravated by vibrations and cause discomfort for patients.

The combination of noise and vibration has been shown to affect performance and may have adverse effects on cardiovascular status. A study has shown a significant increase in the mean duration and amplitude of fetal heart rate acceleration caused by sound and vibration [10].

TOXIC HAZARDS

There are many chemical hazards associated with the operation of aircraft. These chemicals may enter the system either through the skin by direct contact or by inhalation. Any unusual odors or fluids inside the aircraft should be brought to the attention of the flight crew. Substances of concern include exhaust fumes, carbon monoxide, aviation fuels, hydraulic fluids, oil and lubricants, coolants, and fire extinguishers. In addition, any inflight fire will cause release of toxic substances. The effects of any of these chemicals can range from mild irritation to death. They can all decrease performance, create complications for the patient, and affect the safety of the mission.

SPATIAL DISORIENTATION

Spatial disorientation is a phenomenon associated with an inaccurate perception of position, attitude, and motion. False information provided by body senses is so overpowering that the pilot is rendered incapable of perceiving and interpreting accurate and reliable information available through the flight instruments. Experience is not protection against this illusion [18].

When a pilot is at the controls, spatial disorientation is an emergency situation. The false information will invariably cause the pilot to make the wrong adjustments to the controls. All too often the results of spatial disorientation, especially at lower altitudes, are disastrous.

Prevention of this phenomenon includes maintaining visual ground references, believing the aircraft instruments, avoiding staring at lights at night, developing night vision rather than going directly from a well-lit area to the aircraft, and maintaining good health and nutrition.

Once spatial disorientation has occurred, a pilot must immediately refer to the aircraft instruments and believe they are accurate. If one tries to maintain visual reference the problem will only be compounded. Perhaps the hardest part is ignoring body sensations. Instrument training for pilots is the greatest safety measure implemented to avoid spatial disorientation accidents. It has been shown that qualified instrument pilots required as long as 35 seconds to regain control of an aircraft once visual references were lost, while noninstrument-rated pilots were not able to maintain control at all [18].

Medical attendants are also susceptible to spatial disorientation and may contribute to the problem by distracting the pilot when concentration is needed most.

CRASH SURVIVAL

It is everyone's intent to avoid accidents; however, it must be accepted that some will occur. Not all aircraft accidents are immediately fatal, and not all occur in accessible areas where rescue services are readily available. Thus, the flight crew must be prepared for the necessity of attempting to survive, summoning help, and providing localizing information for rescue crews. Although weight and volume restrictions are of prime importance, and medical equipment and space for the care of the patient are major priorities in the minds of the medical air crew, the survival of all aboard should concern and involve the entire crew.

The importance of wearing suitable clothing for the weather conditions cannot be overemphasized. Even accidents that occur close to well-populated areas can be unobserved, and rescue may be significantly delayed when personnel are immobilized by serious injury or trapped in or under the aircraft. In such circumstances, adequate clothing can significantly contribute to survival.

All personnel involved in routine flight operations should wear garments made of Nomex or similar fire retardant materials. These garments should be worn over cotton, wool, or wool-cotton mixtures. Polyester synthetics are extraordinarily dangerous in flight operations because of their physical properties, which lead to melting and severe skin burns if exposed to flame or high heat. Since Nomex garments are fire retardant but not fireproof they will burn if a flame is kept in direct contact with them. Thus, overgarments that will ignite and burn are not suitable for cold weather protection in aircraft. The fire retardant shell must be the outermost garment, or a *fire retardant* coat or jacket can be worn over the flight suit. Whenever possible, flight personnel should wear long sleeves and fire retardant gloves (regardless of weather conditions), except when doing so will interfere with the provision of optimal patient care. These precautions may appear extreme to the uninitiated until they consider the possibility of surviving an aircraft accident only to be killed or permanently disabled as a result of burns. Patients should also be protected. Flight crews should carry fire retardant blankets and sheets with them, including some suitable for use in isolettes. The infant receiving oxygen is in a particularly high-risk situation.

Although weight and volume constraints are paramount, it is in everyone's best interest to have specific items permanently stowed in the aircraft. These items will require preventive maintenance checks and rotation in accordance with the manufacturer's shelf life recommendations. Such items include

1. Drinking water and food, amount and type dependent on the size and geographical conditions of the area over which the mission is flown.
2. Battery-powered survival-type radios are readily available commercially and should be included in the weight/volume allowance for the aircraft. The functional status of the batteries and the radios must be frequently and routinely checked. The radios should be preset to search and rescue (SAR) frequencies used in the local area.
3. Flares, smokes, and signal mirrors should be available for night and day signaling purposes.
4. Self-inflating rescue rafts, preferably incorporating self-deploying automatically activated transponders (locator devices), should be carried on flights over water.

All personnel must be trained and proficient in the use of all survival items and communication equipment, in case only one individual retains functional capabilities.

Other items that could be considered will depend on the area of flight, the duration of flight, and the time of year and expected weather conditions. What might be routine for parts of Alaska (e.g., firearms) might be excessive in major metropolitan areas. Each aircrew must determine what survival equipment is required. However, being based in a major metropolitan area does not preclude the possibility of extended flight over relatively unpopulated territory.

Medical personnel should also undergo careful annual evaluation of their individual medical status and physical condition in the context of their potential to survive an aircraft accident.

## Safety Is a Shared Responsibility

In the final analysis, it is apparent that everyone involved contributes to the safety of an air transport.

Mechanics are responsible for the mechanical condition and maintenance of the machine. They constantly perform inspections on practically every facet of the aircraft. Mechanics provide expertise in aircraft analysis and incorporate troubleshooting procedures to isolate problem areas. Once problems have been identified, they are corrected and components are replaced or rebuilt.

Pilots are responsible for the safe operation of the aircraft. Medical personnel are responsible for their patients and for their own actions relative to safety procedures.

A cooperative effort between the medical and aviation contingent contributes greatly to the level of safety attained. Open communication is necessary to allow appropriate risk-management evaluation of each mission.

Although everyone may contribute to safety, the overall responsibility remains with the hospital and aviation service management personnel. Their operational policies, involvement in day-to-day operations, and support of safety practices will determine whether or not a transport program is safe.

Air transportation has contributed significantly to saving many lives. It may be years before an accurate evaluation can determine the number of patients who have benefited from aeromedical transports. It has been estimated that of approximately 350,000 patients transported, as many as 20 percent [19] owe their lives directly to the availability of aircraft. However, such glowing statistics are readily tarnished by misuse of aeromedical transport and insufficient attention to safety issues.

## References

1. *Airman's Information Manual.* Seattle: A.S.A. Publications, 1967.
2. American College of Surgeons. *Guidelines for the Operation of a Critical Care Air Ambulance Service,* 1986. Appendix 2.
3. American Society for Testing and Materials. F 30.01.02 Philadelphia: 1986. Pp. 34–40.
4. Burney, R. E., and MacKenzie, J. R. Proving the efficacy of hospital-based HEMS. *Ann. Emerg. Med.* 14:9, 1985.
5. Collett, H. M. An Editorial Opinion, By Pilots, For Pilots, *Hospital Aviation,* August 1985. P. 2.
6. Collett, H. M. Competing Aeromedical Services: More to Come, *Hospital Aviation,* October 1987. P. 8.
7. Crockett, D. Accident Epidemic—Aeromedical Helicopter Operations. *Business Aviation Safety* 3:116–119, 1987.
8. *Federal Aviation Regulations.* Part 91, 135, 121. Seattle: A.S.A. Publications, 1987.
9. Fedorowicz, R. J. REARM: Risk Evaluation and Aviation Resource Management. *AirNet* 2(11):1–3, 1987.

10. Gagnon, R., Patrick, J., Foreman, J., et al. Stimulation of human fetuses with sound and vibration. *Am. J. Obstet. Gynecol.* 155(4):848–851, 1986.
11. Grimaldi, J. V. Safety and Safety Management. In W. M. Rom (ed.), *Environmental and Occupational Medicine.* Boston: Little, Brown, 1983.
12. Harvey, D. Do the Pilots Have the Answers to EMS Safety? *Rotor and Wing International* December 1986. P. 15.
13. Landstrom, U., and Lofstedt, P. Noise, Vibration and Changes in Wakefulness During Helicopter Flight. *Aviation, Space and Environmental Medicine* February 1987. Pp. 109–118.
14. McLean, D. *AirNet,* October 1987. P. 1.
15. McNeil, L. *Airborne Care of the Ill and Injured.* New York: Springer-Verlag, 1983. Pp. 9–13.
16. National EMS Pilots Association. *Safety Guidelines for Pilots, Aircraft and Operations* EMS Helicopters, 1987.
17. National Flight Nurses Association. *Practice Standards for Flight Nursing,* 1986.
18. Negrette, A. J. P. Spatial disorientation: It plays no favorites. *Rotor and Wing International* December 1986. P. 21.
19. Popkey, D. Medical Flights Catch Flak Over Safety. *The Idaho Statesman,* 352, July 12, 1987. P. 1.
20. Staff. Report Finds High Risks with Medical Helicopters. *Wall Street Journal,* October 21, 1987. P. 14.
21. Topal, E. J., Fung, A. Y., Kline, E., et al. Safety of helicopter transport and out-of-hospital intravenous fibrinolytic therapy in patients with evolving myocardial infarction. *Cathet. Cardiovasc. Diagno.* 12:151–155, 1986.
22. U.S. Army, Altitude Physiology, *Aeromedical Training for Flight Personnel.* FM 1-301, 1983. Pp. 2.1–2.30.
23. U.S. Army Safety Center. *Flightfax.* Ft. Rucker, AL: U.S. Army Safety Center. Jan–Feb, 1983. P. 2.
24. Ver Berkmoes, R. Aeromedical Accident Rate Shows Decline. *American Medical News,* January 15, 1988. P. 5.

## Bibliography

*Airman's Information Manual.* Seattle: A.S.A. Publications, 1987.
*Federal Aviation Regulations.* Seattle: A.S.A. Publications, 1987.
Helicopter Association International. *Safety Manual: A Safety Management Guide for Helicopter Operators,* 1984.
McNeil, E. L. *Airborne Care of the Ill and Injured.* New York: Springer-Verlag, 1983.
U.S. Army, *Aeromedical Training for Flight Personnel.* FM 1-301, 1983.

## Chapter Appendix I: Accident Rates for Commercial EMS Helicopters and 14 CFR Part 135 Non-Scheduled Helicopter Air Taxis

Accident rates for commercial EMS helicopters and CFR Part 135 non-scheduled helicopter air taxis are shown in Fig. A-1. Although the information provided from the National Transportation Safety Board (NTSB) safety study portrays a dismal picture for EMS helicopters, the reality is perhaps much worse because of the limitations imposed by the methodology used to determine the number of accidents. The study includes only accidents that met the following conditions: (1) the helicopter used was dedicated primarily to the EMS mission, it was configured with at least a patient stretcher, and it had the equipment on board to provide basic life support; (2) the helicopter, when used for EMS missions, had trained medical personnel on board to care for the patient; and (3) the pilots were employed primarily to fly the dedicated helicopter on EMS missions, although other duties such as public relation flights or personnel transfers may also be required of them at times.

Furthermore, neither public-use EMS helicopter accidents nor known accidents that were not reported to the NTSB were included. The criteria used by the NTSB to determine EMS helicopter accidents reduced a total of 92 industry-reported accidents to only 47. Thus, the accident rates shown may represent a significant underestimate.

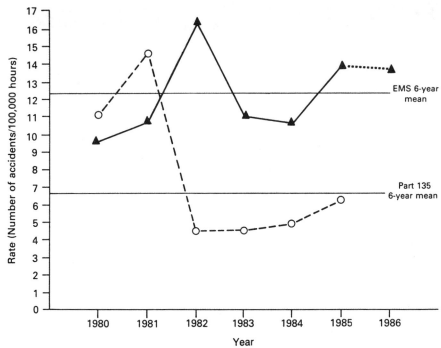

*Fig. A-1. Commercial EMS helicopter and 14 CFR Part 135 non-scheduled helicopter air taxi accident rates. EMS helicopter data are based on accidents that involved patient transportation. Air taxi data include the data for EMS helicopters.* ▲—— = *EMS helicopters;* ○---- = *Part 135 non-scheduled helicopter air taxis. (Data is derived from the National Transportation Safety Board Safety Study: Commercial Emergency Medical Service Helicopter Operations. Report no. NTSB/SS-88/01. Washington, D.C.)*

# V  *Transport of the Pregnant Woman*

# 14

# Indications for Maternal Transport

Jean C. Bolan

*14A. Perspective view of Director-General Smith's sick transport wagon showing compartments for recumbent patients and the plan for forming an operation table in the rear of the vehicle. A class 4 sick transport conveyance (conveyance drawn by animals).* (Reproduced from Longmore, T. A Treatise on the Transport of Sick and Wounded Troops. *London: Her Majesty's Stationary Office, 1869.*)

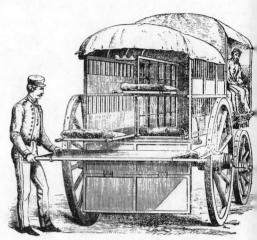

*The compartments were made narrow designedly. The Director-General, Dr. Smith, stated that his object in not having them made wider was, because if a man severely wounded be put in a position in which he can roll about, he would be much hurt. But it did not appear that it was so much the narrowness which was found objectionable by those who were carried in them, as the confined limits and restricted power of movement in consequence in all directions. It was this feeling of imprisonment which caused some persons to liken them to "cells" and even to "coffins."*

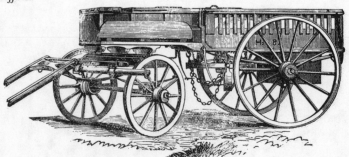

*14B. Side view of Director-General Smith's sick transport wagon altered for use as a store-transport wagon. A class 4 sick transport conveyance (conveyance drawn by animals).* (Reproduced from Longmore, T. A Treatise on the Transport of Sick and Wounded Troops. *London: Her Majesty's Stationary Office, 1869.*)

A smoothly functioning maternal transport system is an integral component of regionalized perinatal services. Perinatal services can be regionalized because the majority of patients, both obstetrical and newborn, do not require the sophisticated care that may be desperately needed by a few patients. In the United States, because neonatal intensive care was one of the first services to be regionalized, organized transport of the neonate has preceded development of obstetrical transport programs. Systems for the transport of the pregnant woman have evolved primarily as a result of data suggesting that premature newborns do not tolerate the stresses of transport in the immediate neonatal period well.

## Advantages of Maternal Transport

Numerous studies have shown decreased neonatal mortality rates following maternal transport, as compared with those following neonatal transport. Harris et al. studied the results of a maternal transport system in Arizona [9]. During 1974 to 1976, they compared 239 infants born after maternal transport with 642 infants transported in the neonatal period. After excluding those babies who died of congenital anomalies incompatible with life, they found an overall mortality of 9.6 percent for the babies born after maternal transport versus a mortality of 12.5 percent following neonatal transport. In addition, the mean birth weight of babies dying in the neonatal period after transport in utero was 1407 g versus 1866 g for deaths after neonatal transport.

Levy et al. investigated the impact of the maternal transport system established in Louisiana in 1978 and they found that (1) in the group of infants weighing greater than 2000 g at birth, survival was better for babies following maternal transport than it was after neonatal transport, and (2) the overall survival of in-born babies was 98 percent versus 82 percent after neonatal transport [14]. Similarly, in a study from Alabama during 1975 to 1977, the survival of infants after maternal transport was 90.5 percent versus 76 percent for infants after neonatal transport [8]. In addition, the length of hospital stay was 20 days for babies transported postnatally versus 13 days for those who were transported in utero.

Lamont et al., reviewing data from Hammersmith Hospital in London, found an 83 percent survival after in utero transport versus 70 percent after neonatal transport [13]. Their population consisted of 206 obstetrical patients who were transported to Hammersmith Hospital and who delivered 212 infants of less than 34-weeks' gestation. These were compared with 166 transported infants of gestational ages of 26 to 34 weeks. The mean birth weights were the same in both groups (Table 14-1).

*Table 14-1. Survival rates by birth weight and gestational age in
infants of less than 34-weeks' gestation at Hammersmith Hospital, London*

|  | Neonatal transfer [no. (%)] | In-Utero transfer [no. (%)] | Significance |
|---|---|---|---|
| **BIRTH WEIGHT** | | | |
| Mean ± 1 SD | 1398 ± 436 | 1391 ± 415 | NS |
| < 1000 g | 48 (29) | 47 (38) | NS |
| 1000–1499 g | 69 (77) | 86 (92) | < 0.01 |
| 1500–1999 g | 81 (42) | 95 (66) | < 0.02 |
| > 2000 g | 94 (18) | 100 (16) | NS |
| Total | 70 (166) | 83 (212) | < 0.01 |
| < 1500 g | 63 (106) | 75 (130) | < 0.1 |
| ≥ 1500 g | 85 (60) | 96 (82) | < 0.02 |
| Total | 70 (166) | 83 (212) | < 0.01 |
| **GESTATIONAL AGE (WEEKS)** | | | |
| Mean ± 1 SD | 29.9 ± 2.2 | 29.9 ± 2.1 | NS |
| 26 and 27 | 46 (28) | 39 (23) | NS |
| 28 and 29 | 49 (47) | 71 (58) | < 0.05 |
| 30 and 31 | 92 (38) | 94 (63) | NS |
| 32 and 33 | 89 (53) | 99 (68) | < 0.05 |
| Total | 70 (166) | 83 (212) | < 0.01 |
| 26–29 | 48 (75) | 62 (81) | < 0.001 |
| 30–33 | 90 (91) | 96 (131) | < 0.1 |
| Total | 70 (166) | 83 (212) | < 0.01 |

NS = no significance; SD = standard deviation. From Lamont, R. F., et al. Comparative mortality and morbidity of infants transferred in utero or postnatally. *J. Perinat. Med.* 11:200, 1983. With permission.

The results of regionalization in north Georgia were reported by Kanto et al. in 1980 [11]. The survival for infants with birth weights greater than 1500 g who were transported in utero exceeded that for transported neonates of similar birth weights (Table 14-2). Kanto stresses that there may be some intrinsic selection bias, particularly in the smaller weight categories, in that many of the sicker infants with birth weights less than 750 g probably did not survive long enough to be transported. In addition, five infants with severe congenital anomalies who were born after maternal transport might not have been transported as neonates from their referring hospitals. If the group weighing 750 to 1000 g was considered separately (excluding those infants born weighing <750 g), the survival rate following maternal transport would increase from 39 to 58 percent. A bias in the opposite direction may be operative at the high end of the birth weight spec-

Table 14-2. Survival of infants transferred in
utero versus those transferred as neonates in 1980

| Birth weight (g) | In utero transport | | | Neonatal transport | | |
|---|---|---|---|---|---|---|
| | Number | Survived | % | Number | Survived | % |
| < 1000 | 28 | 11 | 39 | 33 | 17 | 52 |
| 1001–1500 | 38 | 31 | 82 | 68 | 57 | 84 |
| 1501–2500 | 69 | 68 | 99 | 133 | 124 | 93 |
| > 2500 | 18 | 18 | 100 | 131 | 115 | 88 |
| Total | 153 | 128 | 84 | 365 | 313 | 86 |

From Kanto, W. P., et al. Impact of a maternal transport program on a newborn service. *South. Med. J* 76(7): 834, 1983. With permission.

trum. There was 100 percent survival of infants transferred in utero who had birth weights greater than 2500 g versus an 88 percent survival of transported neonates with birth weights in the same category. Kanto points out that the transported neonates in this high birth weight group were presumably transported because of demonstrated problems, as opposed to those transported in utero because of the potential for problems that may not have materialized.

Because of these biases, Miller et al. stress that data on the outcome of patients transported in utero should be compared with data on the entire population of women delivering in that region, which they call the "perinatal denominator" [15]. Miller's group studied all mothers delivering liveborn infants in 1979, with birth weights between 1000 and 1500 g, in the north central Illinois catchment area. Cases were grouped into (1) in-born—those who received all prenatal and intrapartum care at a Level III facility, (2) maternal transports—those who were delivered at a Level III facility after prenatal care elsewhere, and (3) out-born—mothers in the region who delivered infants who died, required prolonged hospitalization, or required transfer to a Level III intensive care nursery. The overall neonatal survival for all three groups in this region was 78 percent. Survival of infants born at the perinatal center (groups 1 and 2) was 91 percent and that of the out-born infants (group 3) was 67 percent. Miller views this data as confirming other studies that have shown a significant improvement in survival for infants born following maternal transport to a Level III facility.

## Disadvantages of Maternal Transport
There are few disadvantages to a maternal transport program (see also Chap. 2). However, several theoretical reasons why opposition might be

raised were pointed out by Levy et al. who emphasized that regionalization is viewed by some as demonstrating excessive governmental intervention into medical care, or a step toward socialized medicine [14].

A maternal transport system depends on the ability of the doctor at the referring hospital to make an accurate, timely evaluation of the degree of risk to the mother and to the fetus, and to be willing to act on that risk assessment. In most cases, transport means that he or she must give up the patient to the care of another group of physicians at the receiving facility.

Psychological stress for the patient is also a disadvantage of maternal transport: The patient must be taken either by ambulance or by helicopter to a different hospital that is often located many miles from her home and is inconvenient for her husband and family to visit. This experience can add to the trauma of a very painful and frightening situation, such as premature labor. Losing contact with her own obstetrician may add to the stress for the mother being transported. However, most patients are willing to undergo the inconvenience and psychological trauma of transport for the expectation of a better prognosis for their premature infants.

In some areas, the private obstetrician may be granted temporary privileges at the Level III facility to which the patient is transported. In Washington, D.C., the private doctor seldom chooses this option. Reasons for this choice include unfamiliarity with the Level III hospital and his or her responsibility to other patients. In addition, some hospitals are becoming unwilling to grant temporary privileges because of the threat of legal liability.

### Indications for Maternal Transport

The most common indication for maternal transport is the potential delivery of an infant who is too premature to be cared for properly at the referring hospital. Although many indications exist for transfer of the mother because of maternal medical problems during the pregnancy, the bulk of maternal transports are still for neonatal care. Obviously, referring hospitals vary greatly in their capability to handle infants of low gestational age. Many of the hospitals in the District of Columbia area now have full-time neonatologists and have the capability for assessment and stabilization of the premature newborn on delivery. Most hospitals do not transfer the mother if the gestational age at delivery is estimated to be greater than 34 weeks.

In a study of 124 pregnant patients transferred to the Washington Hospital Center (WHC) between January 1, 1983 and December 31, 1985, we found that 80 percent of these patients were transferred for premature la-

*Table 14-3. Indications for maternal transport*

| Study | Total number of pa- tients | Premature labor | | Premature rupture of membranes | | Hyper- tensive disorder | | Bleeding | |
|---|---|---|---|---|---|---|---|---|---|
| | | No. | % | No. | % | No. | % | No. | % |
| Elliott [6] | 100 | 56 | 56 | 14 | 14 | 12 | 12 | 12 | 12 |
| Anderson* [1] | 85 | 32 | 40 | 25 | 31 | 16 | 20 | 19 | 24 |
| Lamont [13] | 212 | 155 | 75 | NR | NR | 52 | 25 | 5 | 3 |
| Cho [4] | 201 | 74 | 37 | 50 | 25 | 16 | 8 | 13 | 6 |
| Kanto* [11] | 150 | 55 | 37 | 60 | 40 | 29 | 19 | 13 | 9 |
| Knox [12] | 100 | 53 | 53 | 29 | 29 | NR | NR | 9 | 9 |
| WHC | 124 | 48 | 39 | 43 | 35 | 12 | 10 | 7 | 6 |

*Some patients had more than one indication for transport. NR = Data not reported.

bor (48 patients—39 percent), premature rupture of membranes (43 patients—35 percent), or both (Table 14-3). A number of other studies have shown similar findings. In the report by Elliot and coworkers on patients transferred by helicopter in the Long Beach, CA area in 1978, premature labor was the indication for transport for 56 of their first 100 patients [5]. Fourteen patients had premature rupture of membranes and 18 patients had both factors. Knox et al. reported their experience in the Minneapolis area from July to December of 1982 [12] (Table 14-3). They found that 90 percent of their patients were transferred because of possible premature delivery. Of those, 78 percent were in premature labor before or during the transport.

Maternal transfer does not always mean that the patient will be at the referral hospital until delivery. Nineteen of the 124 (15%) mothers transported to the Washington Hospital Center (the majority with the diagnosis of premature labor or vaginal bleeding) were discharged undelivered. Many of these mothers delivered at term at their original referring hospital. Ten patients (8%) were hospitalized for 7 days or more prior to delivery, thus gaining a significant period of time for additional fetal maturation. Knox reports that 46 percent of his patients admitted with diagnoses of premature labor, premature rupture of membranes, placental abruption, and other conditions, underwent successful tocolysis as defined by a delay in delivery of greater than 48 hours from admission, or until documented pulmonary maturity [12]. Gestational age, diagnosis, cervical dilation, and distance transported were not significant factors in determining which patients underwent successful tocolysis. Elliott and coworkers found that in 6 percent of their patients delivery was delayed for more than 7 days from the time of transport, thus allowing for increased fetal maturity [6].

All of the fetuses who had a time interval of more than 72 hours from admission to delivery survived the perinatal period. He strongly recommends immediate transfer of the fetus of less than 34-weeks' gestation with premature ruptured membranes, rather than awaiting labor at the referring hospital. He found that the chances of delaying delivery for more than 48 hours were significantly reduced if the patient arrived at the tertiary care center already in labor ($P < 0.004$).

The question of the minimum gestational age at which maternal transport is indicated is frequently debated among obstetricians. At Washington Hospital Center, we have taken the position that maternal transport should not be refused, even if the gestational age reported to us is not associated with a significant likelihood of fetal survival. The rationale is based on the data presented above: In many patients the time from admission to delivery may be prolonged (up to 9 weeks in one patient originally transported to us for bleeding secondary to placenta previa), so that the infant may be viable by the time it is delivered. It is also possible that therapeutic measures taken at the tertiary care hospital, such as aggressive tocolysis or use of corticosteroids, may significantly increase the chance of fetal survival. The gestational age assigned, after reassessment with ultrasound, at the Level III center is frequently significantly different from the gestational age estimation made at the referring hospital based on the patient's dates or uterine size, or both. At birth, the baby may be significantly larger or older than predicted by any prenatal data. Several mothers who have been transferred to us at estimated gestational ages of 22 to 24 weeks have delivered infants that appeared to be 26 or more weeks' gestation by neonatal assessment. However, mothers transferred at gestations of questionably less than 26 weeks should be counseled prior to transport regarding the possibility that their fetus may not be a candidate for heroic medical measures.

Pregnancy-induced hypertension is the most common maternal medical problem for which transport is indicated. Twelve (10%) of the patients transferred to the Washington Hospital Center between January 1, 1983 and December 31, 1985 had hypertension as their primary indication for transfer. Most other studies report similar numbers (Table 14-3). In general, any maternal medical condition that is either severe enough to indicate intensive care or is associated with an increased risk of delivery prior to 34-weeks' gestation is an indication for transport. Other medical problems for which patients have been transported to the Washington Hospital Center include maternal diabetes with ketoacidosis and systemic lupus erythematosus. Levy reports that toxemia and diabetes were the second and third most common indications for transport in his series [14]. Rehm [17] found that maternal indications for transport to the Salt Lake City perinatal center included infection (likely to be associated with premature delivery), cardiac disease, renal disease, and drug overdose. Maternal transport may also be indicated for surgical complications. The most commonly occurring of these is maternal trauma requiring either intensive care or surgical correction. Other surgical indications include an acute abdominal emergency at less than 34-weeks' gestation or a thoracic surgical problem requiring intensive care. In the Washington Hospital Center surgical problems have been rare indications for maternal transport.

## Risk Assessment

It is desirable, although not always possible, to determine prior to labor which patients are sufficiently high risk to require referral. A variety of pregnancy-risk scoring systems have been designed [7,10,16]. The system used by Hobel et al. is one of the most popular: Scores are assigned to the patient at her initial antenatal visit and again at 30-, 35-, and 39-weeks' gestation [10]. The prenatal factors that Hobel uses are shown in Table 14-4. A score of 10 places the patient in the "high-risk" group. Patients are scored again in labor, using a different set of factors (Table 14-5). A score of 10 is again used to classify the patient as "at risk" [10]. Many of the factors on these scoring charts are not automatic indications for maternal transport. Some factors, such as fetal distress or precipitous labor, would be recognized too late in labor for maternal transport to be possible. However, an appropriately modified scoring system could be designed to predetermine the factors that might indicate referral of the mother to a Level III hospital. Use of a scoring system for this purpose was attempted at a small hospital in rural Newfoundland (Table 14-6) [3]. The physicians there found that they were requesting more consultations and transferring more patients, after using the strict guidelines, than had been the practice before the guidelines were instituted. They were unable to reliably predict the rate of nonelective intervention during labor and delivery, such as augmentation of labor, instrumental delivery, cesarean section during labor, and neonatal resuscitation; however, their overall conclusion was that use of the guidelines was helpful in matching the hospital of delivery to the patient's risk category.

## Method of Transport

Selection of the appropriate vehicle for transport and appropriate personnel to accompany the patient during transport is dependent on a host of factors but relates primarily to the patient's overall cardiovascular stability

*Table 14-4. Prenatal factors in risk assessment*

| Factors | Score |
|---|---|
| CARDIOVASCULAR AND RENAL | |
| Moderate-to-severe toxemia | 10 |
| Chronic hypertension | 10 |
| Moderate-to-severe renal disease | 10 |
| Severe heart disease, class II–IV | 10 |
| History of eclampsia | 5 |
| History of pyelitis | 5 |
| Class I heart disease | 5 |
| Mild toxemia | 5 |
| Acute pyelonephritis | 5 |
| History of cystitis | 1 |
| Acute cystitis | 1 |
| History of toxemia | 1 |
| METABOLIC | |
| Diabetes ≥ class A-II | 10 |
| Previous endocrine ablation | 10 |
| Thyroid disease | 5 |
| Prediabetes class A-I | 5 |
| Family history of diabetes | 1 |
| PREVIOUS HISTORIES | |
| Previous fetal exchange transfusion for Rh | 10 |
| Previous stillbirth | 10 |
| Postterm > 42 weeks | 10 |
| Previous premature infant | 10 |
| Previous neonatal death | 10 |
| Previous cesarean section | 5 |
| Habitual abortion | 5 |
| Infant > 10 lb. | 5 |
| Multiparity > 5 | 5 |

and to the likelihood of her imminent delivery. This decision must be made jointly by the physician at the referring hospital and the physician at the receiving hospital. In general, it is preferable to have these decisions made by the most senior person who can be readily obtained at each institution, that is, by the attending obstetrician at the referring hospital and by the attending perinatologist at the receiving hospital. The options for transport vehicle are as follows:

1. Private automobile is for extremely low-risk patients requiring transport of a short distance. In general, if the patient's condition is such that maternal transport is required, this method of transport is not advisable. It

*Table 14-4. (continued)*

| Factors | Score |
|---------|-------|
| Epilepsy | 5 |
| Fetal anomalies | 1 |
| ANATOMICAL ABNORMALITIES | |
| Uterine malformation | 10 |
| Incompetent cervix | 10 |
| Abnormal fetal position | 10 |
| Polyhydraminios | 10 |
| Small pelvis | 5 |
| MISCELLANEOUS | |
| Abnormal cervical cytology | 10 |
| Multiple pregnancy | 10 |
| Sickle cell disease | 10 |
| Age ≥ 35 or ≤ 15 | 5 |
| Viral disease | 5 |
| Rh sensitization only | 5 |
| Positive serology | 5 |
| Severe anemia (< 9 g/dl Hgb) | 5 |
| Excessive use of drugs | 5 |
| History of TB or PPD ≥ 10 mm | 5 |
| Weight < 100 or > 200 lb | 5 |
| Pulmonary disease | 5 |
| Flu syndrome (severe) | 5 |
| Vaginal spotting | 5 |
| Mild anemia (9.0–10.9 g Hgb) | 1 |
| Smoking ≥ 1 pack/day | 1 |
| Alcohol (moderate) | 1 |
| Emotional problem | 1 |

From Hobel, C. J., et al. Prenatal and intrapartum high-risk screening. *Am. J. Obstet. Gynecol.* 117(1): 1, 1973. With permission.

might, on occasion, be used for transfer from the private doctor's office directly to the Level III hospital.

2. Ground ambulance transport is most commonly used for patients with conditions of medium risk, such as premature rupture of membranes prior to labor or early premature labor with cervical dilation less than 4 cm. Preeclamptics requiring magnesium sulfate, but with reasonably stable blood pressure, would fall into this category, as would patients transferred because of vaginal bleeding who are in a stable condition. Ambulance transport may also be the method of choice in conditions of higher risk, such as more advanced cervical dilation of 4 to 8 cm, if the distances

*Table 14-5. Intrapartum factors in risk assessment*

| Factors | Score |
|---|---|
| **MATERNAL** | |
| Moderate-to-severe toxemia | 10 |
| Hydramnios or oligohydramnios | 10 |
| Amnionitis | 10 |
| Uterine rupture | 10 |
| Mild toxemia | 5 |
| Premature rupture of membranes > 12 hours | 5 |
| Primary dysfunctional labor | 5 |
| Secondary arrest of dilation | 5 |
| Demerol > 300 mg | 5 |
| $MgSO_4$ > 25 g | 5 |
| Labor > 20 hours | 5 |
| Second stage > 2.5 hours | 5 |
| Clinical small pelvis | 5 |
| Medical induction | 5 |
| Precipitous labor < 3 hours | 5 |
| Primary cesarean section | 5 |
| Repeat cesarean section | 5 |
| Elective induction | 1 |
| Prolonged latent phase | 1 |
| Uterine tetany | 1 |
| Pitocin augmentation | 1 |
| **PLACENTAL** | |
| Placenta previa | 10 |
| Abruptio placentae | 10 |
| Postterm > 42 weeks | 10 |
| Meconium-stained amniotic fluid (dark) | 10 |
| Meconium-stained amniotic fluid (light) | 5 |
| Marginal separation | 1 |
| **FETAL** | |
| Abnormal presentation | 10 |
| Multiple pregnancy | 10 |
| Fetal bradycardia > 30 minutes | 10 |
| Breech delivery total extraction | 10 |
| Prolapsed cord | 10 |
| Fetal weight < 2500 g | 10 |
| Fetal acidosis pH ≤ 7.25 (stage I) | 10 |
| Fetal tachycardia > 30 minutes | 10 |
| Operative forceps or vacuum extraction | 5 |
| Breech delivery spontaneous or assisted | 5 |
| General anesthesia | 5 |
| Outlet forceps | 1 |
| Shoulder dystocia | 1 |

From Hobel, C. J., Hyvarinen, M. A. Okada, D. M. et al. Prenatal and intrapartum high-risk screening. *Am. J. Obstet. Gynecol.* 117(1): 1, 1973. With permission.

*Table 14-6. Prenatal risk factors according to grade of risk, and recommendations for management outlined in the Newfoundland and Laborador Prenatal Record*

| Grade of Risk and Risk Factor[a] | Number of patients[b] |
|---|---|
| A: No predictable risk | NA[c] |
| B: At risk | |
|     Maternal obesity (75 kg or greater at first visit) | 38 |
|     Pregnant for 42 weeks or more | 34 |
|     Hypertension | 29 |
|         Mild Preeclampsia | 19 |
|         Hypertension alone | 10 |
|     Previous cesarean section | 25 |
|     Significant tobacco intake (20 or more cigarettes a day) | 23 |
|     Breech or malpresentation | 14 |
|     Antepartum hemorrhage, ceased | 13 |
|     Weight gain of $< 4.5$ kg by 30-weeks' gestation | 13 |
|     History of premature labor, stillbirth, neonatal death, or intra-uterine growth retardation | 8 |
|     Anemia (hemoglobin level $< 10$ g/dl with iron supplement) | 5 |
|     Premature labor, controlled | 4 |
|     Diabetes mellitus, class A or B | 3 |
|     Primigravida aged $< 16$ or $> 34$ years | 3 |
|     Multiple pregnancy | 2 |
|     Hydramnios | 1 |
|     Family history of genetic or metabolic disease | 1 |
|     Cervical incompetence | 0 |
|     Significant drug/ethanol intake | 0 |
|     Rh immunization | 0 |
|     Renal disease | 0 |
|     (Recommendation: Consultation should be obtained and the patient should usually be transferred to the regional hospital for delivery) | |
| C: High risk | |
|     Premature labor (at 36 weeks or less of gestation), uncontrolled | 14 |
|     Prolonged rupture of membranes (before labor, requiring induction or augmentation) | 9 |
|     Severe fetal growth retardation (growth at $<$ the tenth percentile) | 5 |
|     Antepartum hemorrhage, continuing | 4 |
|     Premature rupture of membranes (at $< 36$-weeks' gestation) | 3 |
|     Hypertension with superimposed preeclampsia | 3 |
|     Severe preeclampsia | 2 |
|     Diabetes mellitus, class C, D, F, or R | 0 |
|     Renal disease with hypertension | 0 |
|     Heart disease | 0 |
|     (Recommendation: Whenever possible, the patient should be transferred to the regional hospital for intensive care and delivery) | |

Table 14-6. (continued)

| Grade of Risk and Risk Factor[a] | Number of patients[b] |
|---|---|
| N: Newborn at risk | |
| Previous severe respiratory distress syndrome, seizure disorders, Hirschsprung's disease, cystic fibrosis, congenital anomalies (Recommendation: Delivery in a high-risk center should be considered.) | 5 |

[a] Definitions are given in parentheses. None was provided in the Newfoundland and Laborador Prenatal Record.
[b] Some patients had more than one risk factor.
[c] NA = not applicable.
From Casson, R. I., and Sennett, E. S. Prenatal risk assessment and obstetric care in a small rural hospital: Comparison with guidelines. Can. Med. Assoc. J. 130:1311, May 1984. With permission.

involved are short and delivery is not believed to be likely to occur imminently.

3. Helicopter or fixed-wing aircraft is indicated, if available, when the patient is considered at high risk and the estimated time of ambulance transport to the Level III hospital is more than 30 minutes. Examples of this patient category are mothers with premature labor and premature rupture of membranes, premature labor with cervical dilation over 4 cm, or severe preeclampsia.

### Contraindications to Maternal Transport

Any condition that renders the mother's cardiovascular system unstable is a contraindication to transport until stability can be achieved. Examples of these conditions include severe preeclampsia or eclampsia before the mother has received adequate therapy to control her blood pressure. Another example is heavy vaginal bleeding such that the mother is in shock or impending shock. In addition, if there is any reasonable prospect that delivery may occur during the transport, it would be more beneficial for the mother and baby to remain at the original hospital for delivery. Generally, these are patients who present with advanced cervical dilation. Because it is impossible to perform a cesarean delivery in any type of transport vehicle presently in use, fetal distress is also a contraindication to transport. In some circumstances (usually only when hospitals are in very close proximity), it may be possible for a perinatologist or neonatologist, or both, from the Level III hospital to be present to assist with either the stabilization of the mother before her delivery or with immediate stabilization of the neonate for transport. However, because of the unpredictability of the time of delivery in most cases, it is not feasible for a regional transport program to offer this type of service as a routine, unless they have considerable backup resources (i.e., more than one transport vehicle and adequate personnel to staff for concurrent transports).

## Summary

It intuitively makes sense that, when specialized perinatal services are needed, the outcome is better when the fetus is transferred in utero rather than delivered and then transported as a neonate. Anecdotal experience, in conjunction with the albeit largely uncontrolled observations that have been published to date, would tend to support this concept.

The most common indications for transport are premature labor and premature rupture of membranes, but many maternal transports are also done for severe pregnancy-induced hypertension, maternal diabetes, or bleeding. The major contraindications to maternal transport are lack of sufficient time before delivery, maternal instability, and fetal distress. The importance of early assessment of risk and timely decision making cannot be overemphasized.

## References

1. Anderson, C. J., Aladjem, S., Ayuste, O., et al. An analysis of maternal transport within a suburban metropolitan region. *Am. J. Obstet. Gynecol.* 140:499, 1981.
2. Bose, C. L., Kochenour, N. K., and Brimhall, D. C. *Current Concepts in Transport . . . Neonatal Maternal Administrative.* Columbus, OH: Ross Laboratories, 1982.
3. Casson, R. I., and Sennett, E. S. Prenatal risk assessment and obstetric care in a small rural hospital: Comparison with guidelines. *Can. Med. Assoc. J.* 130:1311, May 1984.
4. Cho, S., Christman, C. M., Floyd, P. S., et al. Outcome of 201 maternal transports compared with newborn transports and infants born at the tertiary perinatal center. *Birth Defects* 18(3A):199, 1982.
5. Crenshaw, C., Payne, P., Blackmon, L., et al. Prematurity and the obstetrician: A regional neonatal intensive care nursery is not enough. *Am. J. Obstet. Gynecol.* 147(2):125, 1983.
6. Elliott, J. P., O'Keefe, D. F., and Freeman, R. K. Helicopter transportation of patients with obstetric emergencies in an urban area. *Am. J. Obstet. Gynecol.* 143:157, 1982.
7. Goodwin, J. W., Dunne, J. T., and Thomas, B. W. Antepartum identification of the fetus at risk. *Can. Med. Assoc. J.* 101:458, 1969.
8. Harris, B. A., Jr., Wirtschafter, D. D., Huddleston, J. F., et al. In utero versus neonatal transportation of high-risk perinates: A comparison. *Obstet. Gynecol.* 57:496, 1981.
9. Harris, T. R., Isaman, J., and Giles, H. R. Improved neonatal survival through maternal transport. *Obstet. Gynecol.* 52:294, 1978.

10. Hobel, C. J. Hyvarinen, M. A., Okada, D. M., et al. Prenatal and intrapartum high-risk screening. *Am. J. Obstet. Gynecol.* 117(1):1, 1973.
11. Kanto, W. P., Jr., Bryant, J., Thigpen, J., et al. Impact of a maternal transport program on a newborn service. *South. Med. J.* 76(7):834, 1983.
12. Knox, G. E., and Schnitker, K. A. In-utero transport. *Clin. Obstet. Gynecol.* 27(1): 11, 1984.
13. Lamont, R. F., Dunlop, P. D. M., Crowley, P., et al. Comparative mortality and morbidity of infants transferred in utero or postnatally. *J. Perinat. Med.* 11: 200, 1983.
14. Levy, D. L., Noelke, K., and Goldsmith, J. P. Maternal and infant transport program in Louisiana. *Obstet. Gynecol.* 57:500, 1981.
15. Miller, T. C., Densberger, M., and Krogman, J. Maternal transport and the perinatal denominator. *Am. J. Obstet. Gynecol.* 147:19, 1983.
16. Nesbitt, R. E. L., Jr., and Aubry, R. H. High-risk obstetrics. *Am. J. Obstet. Gynecol.* 103:972, 1969.
17. Rehm, N. E. Indications for Maternal Transport—The Utah Experience. In C. L. Bose, N. K. Kochenour, and D. C. Brimhall (eds.), *Current Concepts in Transport. . . . Neonatal, Maternal, Administrative.* Columbus, OH: Ross Laboratories, 1982.

# 15

# The Maternal
# Transport Team—
# Personnel and
# Equipment

Nancy E. Rehm
Neil K. Kochenour

*15A. Front view of Perot and Company's
improved medical wagon. (Reproduced from*
Description of Perot and Co's Improved Medical Wagon. *Philadelphia:
J. T. Morris Perot and Co., 1864.)*

*Contents of drawer number 9:
Three lbs. Ceratum Adipis
Twenty-four oz. Cinchona Sulph.
Six lbs. Sinapis Nig. Pulv.
Ten lbs. Farina
Twelve lbs. Sugar, white crushed
Four lbs. black tea*

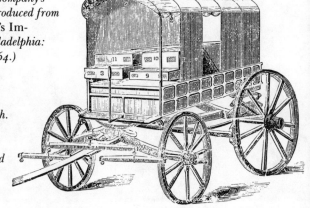

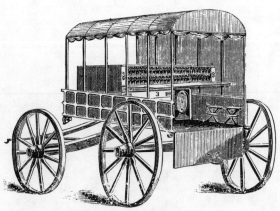

*15B. Back view of Perot and Company's im-
proved medical wagon. (Reproduced from*
Description of Perot and Co's Improved Medical Wagon. *Philadelphia:
J. T. Morris Perot and Co., 1864.)*

The structure and composition of a maternal transport team are determined by the needs of the geographical area served and the level of perinatal care provided by the hospitals within the region. Maternal transport teams vary in their organization but are similar in their goals, that is, the safe transport and optimal care of the perinatal patient.

Primary care (Level I) hospitals serve patients from a relatively circumscribed area and may have limited capability to supply other than emergency care to high-risk patients. Financial resources may be limited and fewer highly skilled personnel may live within the area. For these and other reasons, small community hospitals rarely have the resources to adequately meet the needs of all perinatal patients. However, many Level I hospitals do maintain an effective system for the transport of high-risk mothers. Ideally, such a transport system is one part of a regionalized health care system that matches the needs of each patient with the available facilities [1].

The individual differences that distinguish one hospital from another in the same region are reflected in the diverse ways in which they organize and staff their transport teams. In many communities the needs of the obstetrical patient are met by the same transport personnel who attend to the needs of all other transported patients. Regardless of the level of the hospital, the team that responds to calls is usually composed of at least two persons. Small hospitals frequently employ only two persons, who are on call for 24 hours, rather than use a pool of transport team members from which a team can be selected to meet the medical needs of the individual patient. The level of training and skill of the team members varies also, often related to the level of expertise and training provided by the parent hospital.

Only the larger medical centers, frequently those associated with medical schools and medical research institutions, can financially support the highly specialized facilities, equipment, and personnel required by some perinatal patients. These centers have service areas with the following characteristics:

1. A geographical area with a stable and adequate patient population, or
2. A large enough population to justify expensive and specialized facilities, such as a large metropolitan area, and
3. A population large enough from which to draw the skilled persons needed to staff such a facility.

The University of Utah Medical Center serves patients from an area encompassing all or part of eight states with approximately 78 hospitals. Between 300 and 350 obstetrical patients are transported annually, approximately 130 by air. The annual total for nonobstetrical transports by air is ap-

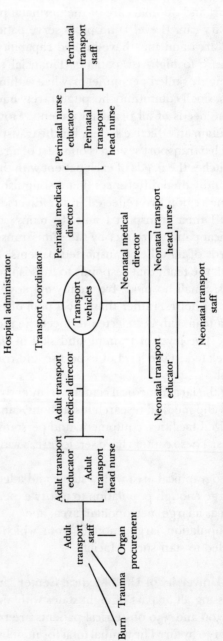

Fig. 15-1. A specialized multi-functional transport system. Maternal, neonatal, and adult teams each have their own administrative structure and share transport vehicles. Coordination among the teams is provided by an overall transport coordinator.

proximately 1300. A similar hospital in a large metropolitan area could successfully serve a smaller geographical area, with perhaps fewer referral hospitals, but with greater population density.

In considering the organization and composition of a maternal transport team, it is essential that the reader remember the diversity of the institutions that the maternal transport teams represent. It is only possible here to describe some of the elements with which they meet the needs of the perinatal patient. In this chapter we will discuss some of the important factors that have direct impact on team structure and function.

## Maternal Transport Team Personnel and Responsibilities

In a large medical center the maternal transport team may be a component of a comprehensive transport service, sharing overall administrative duties, vehicles, and basic equipment; this type of service is illustrated in Fig. 15-1. In a smaller hospital, the transport team is generally staffed from the emergency room personnel, or emergency medical technicians (EMTs) may be used. Figure 15-2 depicts this basic service. Level II hospitals will be somewhere on the continuum between these two, possibly using the local ambulance service but providing labor and delivery nurses as transport personnel. Regardless of the size of the service and although the team members may not have titles identical to those used in this chapter, the following roles and responsibilities must be fulfilled in order to provide an optimal transport service to obstetrical patients.

### MEDICAL DIRECTOR

The medical director (Table 15-1) of the maternal transport team is responsible for determining the policies and procedures, standards of medi-

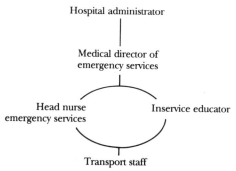

Fig. 15-2. A basic multi-functional transport system. The possible organization of a general patient transport service.

*Table 15-1. The role of the medical director*

Is a board-certified obstetrician or perinatologist
Sets standards for medical practice during transport
Sets safety standards for patient care during transport
Develops and updates written policies, procedures, and protocols with the transport coordinator
Oversees major equipment purchases
Reviews cases with team members (including a hospital administrator and those responsible for the supply and servicing of vehicles) for quality control.
Assists in developing a marketing strategy
Works closely with the transport coordinator to maintain optimal teamwork and follow-up and to correct problems

cal practice, and safety and medical protocols for transport of the high-risk obstetrical patient. The director oversees the activities of all staff providing medical care during transport and is consulted concerning major equipment purchases. He or she cooperates and collaborates with the hospital administrator responsible for the transport service, the outreach coordinator, the perinatal clinical specialist, and the head nurse of the maternal transport team, as well as with all members of the transport team. It is the medical director's responsibility to review transported cases on a regular basis to maintain the quality of care. This position should be held by a board-certified obstetrician who is hospital based within the institution providing the transport service.

TRANSPORT COORDINATOR
The transport coordinator (Table 15-2) is responsible for orienting the transport team members to their individual roles. This person may also be responsible for coordinating the other transport teams within a comprehensive transport system. The coordinator is responsible for regularly reviewing transport equipment and equipment inventory lists and for cooperating and collaborating with the medical director, hospital administrators, transport head nurse, and other transport team members in reviewing the policies, procedures, and standards of care for the transport system. He or she is responsible for the follow-up and correction of problems and concerns regarding the availability of all transport vehicles, for equipment function, and for referring any educational needs that are identified to the perinatal nurse educator. It is the coordinator's responsibility to ensure that the qualifications specified are consistently met by all team members and that ongoing critiques and quality assurance evaluations of the perinatal transport system are completed, in conjunction with the nurse educator and the medical director. The coordinator, together with the

head transport nurse, is responsible for reviewing and revising transport policies and procedures and ensures that the on-call schedule is adequately covered at all times. The coordinator is also responsible for providing continuing education for team members. This person may also act as the perinatal clinical specialist responsible for continuing in-service education of the perinatal staff.

TRANSPORT HEAD NURSE

In systems where there is more than one specialized transport team, there should be an administrative head of each team, that is, a head nurse (Table 15-3) for the maternal transport team, the neonatal transport team, and the adult transport team. The responsibilities of the transport head nurse include working closely with the transport coordinator in reviewing policies, procedures, and standards of care for the maternal transport system. This individual is also charged with the responsibility for helping to select and train transport nurses, for preparing the call schedule and, usually, for

*Table 15-2. The role of the transport coordinator*

IN A MULTIDISCIPLINARY TRANSPORT PROGRAM
Is a senior nurse with experience in a critical care field
Has recent hands-on experience with patient transport
Has excellent management and interpersonal skills
Has a means of updating his or her clinical knowledge base
Works with the medical director and head nurse of the obstetrical transport team
   to ensure that all aspects of the team function optimally
Coordinates the activities of the maternal transport team with those of the other
   specialty teams

IN AN AUTONOMOUS MATERNAL TRANSPORT TEAM
Is a senior nurse with experience (preferably recent) in high-risk obstetrics
Has recent (preferably ongoing) experience with the transport of high-risk
   obstetrical patients
Has excellent management and interpersonal skills
Sets standards for nursing care during transport
Reviews transport equipment and equipment inventory lists regularly
Collaborates with the medical director, hospital administrator, and other team
   members to review policies, procedures, and standards of care
Is responsible for the follow-up of problems and concerns regarding availability of
   vehicles and equipment function
Collaborates with the medical director in correcting problems
Refers identified outreach educational needs to the nurse educator
Ensures that team members have the specified qualifications
Works with the perinatal nurse educator to develop a training and continuing
   education program for team members
Ensures that all essential paperwork is completed by team members

*Table 15-3. The role of the transport head nurse*

Has recent experience in high-risk labor and delivery
Has recent (preferably ongoing) experience with maternal transport
Has excellent management and interpersonal skills
Works closely with the transport coordinator to review policies, procedures, and
    standards of care.
Assists in selecting and training transport nurses
Prepares the call schedule
Serves as the representative of the maternal transport team to an overall coordi-
    nating committee

*Table 15-4. The role of the perinatal nurse educator*

Has recent experience in high-risk labor and delivery
Has excellent interpersonal skills
Has a means of updating his or her clinical knowledge and skills
Maintains constant liaison with the maternal transport team and has in-depth
    knowledge of the program
Collaborates with the medical director and transport coordinator in reviewing
    program equipment, function, and the overall standard of care
Is innovative and understands the unique aspects of adult peer education
Develops ongoing outreach and in-house educational programs in collaboration
    with the medical director and transport coordinator
Ensures that the lines of communication between the referring and receiving hos-
    pitals are optimally maintained and developed

serving as the representative of the maternal transport team to an oversight
committee that coordinates all transport activities.

PERINATAL NURSE EDUCATOR (OUTREACH COORDINATOR)
The perinatal nurse educator (Table 15-4) cooperates and collaborates with
the medical director, the hospital administrator, the transport coordinator, the perinatal clinical specialist, the head nurse of the perinatal unit,
and the transport team members in reviewing the policies and procedures
and the standards of care of the maternal transport system.

The educator is responsible for the follow-up of problems or concerns
regarding the care of the patient prior to transport. He or she should place
an emphasis on continuing education at all levels and, in collaboration with
the medical director, organize programs to meet the educational needs of
the staff at both the receiving and the referring hospitals, as identified by the
transport team. The outreach education effort should include cooperation
with the state health department to organize training programs for EMTs.
Ensuring that direct lines of communication are maintained with the refer-

ring institutions, along with good rapport, are also important outreach responsibilities.

TRANSPORT NURSE

The selection criteria for a maternal transport nurse include (1) demonstrated experience, knowledge, and skill in the areas of labor, delivery, and the care of high-risk perinatal patients, (2) certification in advanced life support, (3) the ability to scrub for cesarean sections, and (4) the ability to assess the high-risk perinatal patient. Training requirements and continuing education performance standards include (1) annual recertification in life support, (2) attendance and continuing education in life-support workshops, and (3) a yearly evaluation of labor and delivery skills, including emergency delivery procedures. Yearly clearance by a physician is required if there is a positive history of a medical problem, for example, a heart condition that might interfere with flight tolerance or ability to survive an air-crash in mountainous terrain.

The requirements for a maternal transport nurse at the University of Utah Medical Center include (1) current licensure to practice as a registered nurse in Utah; (2) a minimum of 2-years' experience in nursing, with a minimum of 1-year's experience within the last year at a tertiary level perinatal center working in the labor and delivery area; (3) a minimum of 4 hours of training in altitude physiology; (4) a passing grade at a 90 percent competency level in a written test administered by the transport head nurse; (5) annual reverification of clinical expertise by an obstetrician, the head nurse of the perinatal unit, or the head nurse of the transport team; or a combination of these, (6) appropriate responses to oral questions on situations that could occur within the framework of transport responsibilities; (7) attendance at in-service training on emergency delivery and demonstrations of the skills necessary for a vertex delivery; (8) qualifications for scrubbing in at a cesarean section; (9) demonstrated leadership and management skills and professional behavior as demonstrated by keeping credentials and skills current by attending monthly transport and staff meetings, by giving one in-service presentation per year for nursing staff (as designated by the head nurse or assistant head nurse), and by being a role model in actions, dress, and philosophy for other staff RNs; and (10) attendance at the annual maternal transport workshop.

FLIGHT NURSE

The flight nurse position has the same requirements as the transport nurse but includes the addition of an in-depth knowledge of maternal air physiology and of flight safety. This knowledge can be acquired through an orientation course, with periodic update in the form of continuing education. The flight nurse must also be very familiar with the vehicles in use for patient transport and with the capabilities of individual aircraft.

## OBSTETRICIAN/PERINATOLOGIST

A designated obstetrician at the referral facility should be involved in the appraisal and care of each perinatal patient who is transported and should also be involved in the decision-making process when there is a question about the appropriateness of transport. He or she should be available on a 24-hour basis for consultation regarding transport and stabilization or other patient management decisions.

## EMERGENCY MEDICAL TECHNICIAN

The certification process for EMTs [2] is usually undertaken by the health department within each state and is awarded for a specific period of time after the successful completion of a training program. The training program consists of a minimum number of hours training and experience in the field and satisfactory completion of a certification examination. Patient care in the clinical areas of the emergency department; the intensive care unit; the coronary care unit; and the delivery, operating, and recovery rooms are included in the hospital training. The amount of time EMTs spend in the delivery room is minimal; therefore, it is imperative that stabilization of the perinatal patient is accomplished prior to transport, thus minimizing the possibility of a change in the patient's condition and the need for clinical decision making during a transport conducted by EMTs. Receiving perinatal centers may elect to offer more advanced training and in-depth experience for EMTs who are frequently involved in transporting perinatal patients.

## *Factors Affecting the Composition of the Transport Team*

### MEETING PATIENT NEEDS

Successful transport of the perinatal patient demands that the maternal transport team meet the needs of the specific patient to be transported (Table 15-5). This "customized" care can be achieved only by properly classifying the perinatal patient into a risk category prior to transport (see also Chap. 17). In most instances, an assessment of the patient's condition in relation to the time factor involved in the transport is the most reliable way to grade the risk. Making this assessment will also be of help in making a decision regarding the best transport vehicle, the skills required of the transport personnel, and the choice of team members to be sent.

*Table 15-5. Guidelines for determining the composition of the obstetrical transport team based on patient needs*

| Condition of mother | Members of transport team |
|---|---|
| Stable, not in labor (e.g., early rupture of membranes without labor)* | No transport team (patient may travel by automobile over short distances without medical personnel) |
| Not in labor but condition requires some stabilization (e.g., mild preeclampsia, stable third trimester bleeding) | Referring hospital personnel (obstetrical nurse or physician) if timely transport is available |
| Early labor that has stopped with tocolysis | Referring hospital personnel if timely transport is available |
| Not in labor but requires extensive stabilization (e.g., severe preeclampsia) | Maternal transport team from regional center |
| In labor | Maternal/neonatal transport team from regional center |

*Patients with a fetus in breech position and premature rupture of membranes should not travel in a sitting position because of the risk of prolapse of the umbilical cord.

Low-risk patients are those patients for whom time is not a critical factor, for example, a patient with premature rupture of membranes, without either the presence of labor or an abnormal presentation. The patient's condition is stable; therefore, an obstetrically trained attendant is not necessarily required during transport.

A patient at medium risk is one for whom time is a factor although the mother's condition is currently stable, and delivery is not anticipated prior to arrival at the receiving hospital. A professional attendant is required to administer and supervise intravenous infusions and to measure vital signs. If ground transport time is longer than the time for which the patient's condition is expected to remain stable, then consideration should be given to transporting the patient by air ambulance.

High-risk patients are those whose maternal condition can be stabilized but possibly may deliver the infant, although it is unlikely, within the transport time. If these patients are transported, they must be accompanied by professional attendants who are able, if necessary, to assist in delivery and resuscitate the neonate. An example of this type of patient is one who is in premature labor and is receiving tocolytic agents to stop contractions. Transport time is critical for this type of patient, and specialized personnel must be in attendance and equipped to deal with any obstetrical or neonatal emergency.

The ultra–high-risk patient is one for whom prediction of the time of delivery is difficult or whose condition is so unstable that decisions about transport might have to be changed by the time that the transport team arrives at the referring institution. Examples include patients with advanced premature labor, patients with significant maternal hemorrhage in whom the vital signs are unstable or blood volume replacement is not complete, and patients with significant medical conditions such as septic shock.

## LEVEL OF CARE PROVIDED BY PARENT HOSPITAL

The policies of the institution providing the transport capability will influence the composition of the team provided. A referring hospital that provides transport for its patients to a medical center with more capabilities than its own is more likely to have a single team that provides transport for all medical and surgical patients. This type of hospital operates a one-way transport system. The large medical center is more likely to have a dedicated maternal transport team and usually provides a two-way type of transport service. A discussion of one- and two-way transport is in Chap. 2.

The maternal transport team that responds to an individual transport call is usually composed of a minimum of two persons and may include obstetrically trained physicians, R.N.s, and paramedical personnel. The team is usually staffed from the obstetrical area or the emergency room. In cases involving risks to both mother and newborn, a neonatal specialist is often included. In practice, smaller hospitals often employ the minimum number of individuals to man the transport team and require only training in basic life support, in addition to general nursing or medical training. At the other end of the scale, depending on patient needs, teams dispatched from medical centers may include highly trained specialists. Usually the team includes an obstetrician or obstetrical resident and a high-risk labor and delivery nurse, unless the condition of the patient requires the presence of other specialists.

## NEED FOR OBSTETRICAL JUDGMENT

As the distances involved and the length of time required for transport increase, the importance of appropriate obstetrical management decisions also increases. Unlike trauma patients, who are often initially transported to a primary care facility, obstetrical patients are usually inpatients at a primary medical facility when the need for transport is recognized. The primary medical need with trauma patients is to transport them to a medical facility as rapidly as possible. However, with perinatal patients, stabilization of the clinical condition prior to transport assumes priority, that is, appropriate medical care at the referring hospital is usually preferable to emergency care rendered during transport (see also Chap. 17). Situations exist in which a maternal transport may be contraindicated because of patient instability at the time of the request, for example, a patient with severe third-trimester bleeding who is showing evidence of fetal distress, or a patient with preterm labor with rapidly progressing cervical dilation who is at a hospital some distance from the referring hospital. The decision whether or not to transport can often not be made by the transport team until they assess the patient at the referring institution.

Prudent obstetrical judgment is extremely important for any maternal transport team. Ideally, this judgment is provided by the member of the team who can best assess the patient and make the decision regarding the advisability of transport; this decision should always be made in conjunction with the referring physician. To make this decision, the transport team may need to consult by telephone with the perinatal consultant or the medical director of the team. In such instances it is extremely important that there be someone on the transport team who can accurately describe the patient's condition so that the appropriate decision can be made.

GEOGRAPHICAL CONSIDERATIONS
In the western United States geographical factors often determine the mode of patient transport, that is, whether by land or air and, if by air, by fixed- or rotary-wing aircraft (Fig. 15-3). These decisions, in turn, affect the composition of the transport team. Throughout the United States seasonal

*Fig. 15-3. The area covered by the University of Utah Patient Transport System.*

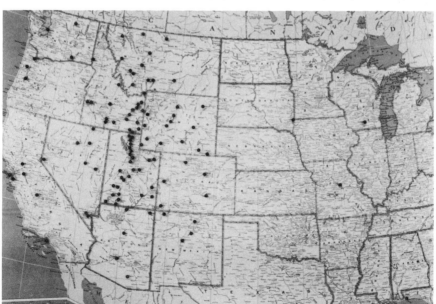

weather patterns, coupled with geographical factors, complicate the decision regarding the transport vehicle. Winter storms and mountainous terrain can close mountain passes to ground transport and make transport
conditions of any kind generally unsafe. Fog is another hazardous weather
condition that can significantly complicate transport. These weather conditions demand serious attention when making a decision regarding the
method and safety of patient transport.

The terrain to be covered often determines the time involved in transport, as well as the equipment needed. The shorter the duration of a transport, the fewer decisions need be made in transit, for there is less opportunity for the condition of the patient to change. Since the mode of transport
may be dictated primarily by distance and terrain, this will secondarily dictate any additional training, such as in flight safety and physiology, that
team members may require. Three case histories follow that will illustrate
some of these considerations.

## Case Studies

These studies illustrate the importance of stabilizing the patient prior to
transport and the need for flexibility in staffing for the transport of high-
risk obstetrical patients.

CASE 1
*History*
The obstetrical service at the University of Utah Medical Center (UUMC)
receives a call from a board-eligible obstetrician at a Level I center in a community in southern Idaho, approximately 1-hour's flight time from Salt
Lake City. A gravida VIII mother is in labor at 29-weeks' gestation, with a
cervical cerclage in place. She is 2-cm dilated, 80 percent effaced, and has
been placed on ritodrine. The referring physician requests a maternal
transport.

*Response*
A resident in obstetrics and a labor-and-delivery nurse go to the Level I
hospital by fixed-wing aircraft. On arrival at the hospital, examination of
the patient shows the cervix is unchanged, the cerclage appears to be tearing the cervix posteriorly, and the membranes are bulging. Contractions
are occurring approximately every 7 to 8 minutes and are mild to moderate in intensity.

The referring physician and the obstetrical resident confer with the perinatal consultant by telephone, and a decision is made to transport the pa-

tient. Because the cervix has not changed significantly during the past 90 minutes and the contractions are mild to moderate in intensity, it is decided not to remove the cerclage prior to transport. The tocolytic agent is continued.

*Outcome*
The patient arrives safely in Salt Lake City, with the cerclage in place. The suture is then removed, and the patient delivers a 1300-g infant within an hour. The infant subsequently does well.

*Discussion*
It is extremely helpful to have a member of the transport team with enough clinical judgment and experience to make a decision regarding the safety of patient transport, especially when long distances and time are involved. The decision whether or not to remove the cerclage prior to transport had to be made. Because the cerclage appeared to be tearing loose, the patient was observed and reexamined. The decision to leave the cerclage in place subsequently proved to be correct; the patient did not deliver during the transport.

CASE 2
*History*
The obstetrical service at UUMC receives a call from a board-certified obstetrician at a Level I hospital in a community in southern Utah. A gravida II mother with unknown dates, but at approximately 29-weeks' gestation by ultrasound, is in active labor. Her previous infant was delivered by a classical cesarean section. This fetus is in a breech presentation, and a repeat cesarean section had been planned because of the previous surgery. The membranes had ruptured 12 hours prior to the call. Flight time to Salt Lake City is approximately 2 hours. This community has minimal hood oxygen, blood gases, and open warmer capabilities.

*Response*
After consultation with the neonatal service, it is decided that the mother cannot be safely transported but that the neonate can be delivered safely at the referring hospital. A neonatal team is mobilized to attend the delivery.

*Outcome*
The mother is delivered of a 29-weeks' gestation 1100-g male infant with the neonatal team in attendance. Apgar scores are 3 at 1 minute and 6 at 5 minutes, with early onset respiratory distress syndrome. The infant is stabi-

lized, including intubation, and transported to the UUMC on a ventilator; the infant subsequently requires 1 week of ventilatory support. After 4 weeks of hospitalization, the infant is returned to the community hospital.

*Discussion*

This case illustrates the value of a flexible response to a request for transport. In this instance, because the patient had had a previous classical cesarean section, it was deemed unsafe to transport the mother while she was in labor. The alternative was to deliver the baby at the community hospital and transport the baby after initial stabilization. However, it should be noted that, although ideal in this case, the capability of a tertiary level center to send a team from the neonatal service to attend a delivery depends on their ability to staff and financially support a backup team and vehicle for this purpose so that availability of the transport service is not compromised.

CASE 3

*History*

The obstetrical service at the UUMC receives a call from a family physician at a community hospital on the eastern border of Utah, regarding a 19-year-old gravida I patient at 31-weeks' gestation, with a blood pressure of 190/120 mm Hg and 2+ proteinuria. The physician requests a maternal transport.

*Response*

The consultant at the UUMC recommends the initiation of magnesium sulfate for preeclampsia and hydralazine hydrochloride therapy for hypertension. A team consisting of an obstetrical resident and a labor-and-delivery nurse is dispatched by air. On arrival at the community hospital, the patient's blood pressure is 170/110 to 116 mm Hg. Reflexes are 2+, urine output is adequate, and fetal heart rate is 140/minute. Additional hydralazine is given until the patient's blood pressure is lowered to approximately 160/90 to 100 mm Hg.

*Outcome*

The patient is then transferred by air to the UUMC where labor is induced. She is delivered of a 1270-g infant, who subsequently does well.

*Discussion*

This case illustrates the importance of adequate preparation and stabilization of the patient prior to transport. At the recommendation of the consultant, the patient was begun on magnesium sulfate and antihypertensive therapy prior to arrival of the transport team. When the transport team arrived, however, the patient's blood pressure was still elevated and additional therapy was required prior to transport.

## Equipment for Maternal Transport
The vehicle and equipment chosen for a transport are determined by the needs of the specific perinatal patient to be transported, geographical factors, and the weather conditions expected at the time of the request.

SPECIFICATIONS FOR EMERGENCY TRANSPORT VEHICLES
Some general specifications for an aircraft used to transport the obstetrical patient and the transport team are included in Table 15-6 (see also Book Appendix 8). The specifications for ground emergency vehicles are stipulated in *Federal Specifications No. KKK-A-1822 B*. Washington, D.C.: General Services Administration, 1985.

The configuration of the space within the transport vehicle should allow for the easy installation and removal of a patient on a stretcher or in an isolette. The patient should not have to be tilted excessively when loaded

*Table 15-6. Aircraft specifications—basic considerations for patient transport*

HELICOPTER*
1. Size—larger craft require larger hangars and helipads, are more expensive to operate, and make more noise
2. Range—maximum range (no reserve) varies with model from approximately 250 nautical miles (nm) to approximately 500 nm
3. Hover characteristics
4. Useful load
5. Lift—particularly important to consider when operating at higher altitudes
6. Cruising speed at maximum load under local temperature and altitude conditions

FIXED-WING AIRCRAFT
1. Number, type, and power of engines (single-engine aircraft are not large enough to accommodate the personnel and equipment necessary to care for a critically ill perinatal patient)
2. Pressurization ratio ≥ 6.3 psi
3. Cruising speed at maximum load
4. Cruising range relative to geographical characteristics of area to be covered
5. Height above ground of the main door (this can significantly affect the ease of patient loading)

*Refer to Book Appendix 8.

into the vehicle. The working space should be sufficient to allow reasonably unrestricted access while in transit by at least two transport team members to at least two patients. In addition to the requirement that the storage space for the medical supplies and equipment be adequate, access to the supplies and equipment should also be convenient. The frame of the vehicle should allow for the secure anchoring of a transport stretcher, incubator, air/oxygen tanks, ventilators, and monitoring equipment. The vehicle must have a way for providing air and oxygen to the patient-care portion of the vehicle, with one air and one oxygen outlet for each patient. Outlets must be of the standard hospital type (or appropriate adapters should be available), and the system should be capable of supplying 50 psi of air and 100 percent oxygen at 15 liters/minute for approximately 5 hours of operation. Suction capabilities must be available in the working area of the vehicle; a suction unit of a standard hospital type should be able to supply a minimum vacuum of 20 mm of mercury to each outlet. There should be one outlet available per patient stretcher. Intravenous holders capable of supporting at least two intravenous lines for each patient must be available.

EMERGENCY TRANSPORT EQUIPMENT
The equipment carried for maternal transport is determined by several factors: (1) the equipment needed for the specific patient being transported, (2) the standard equipment needed by the transport team (Table 15-7), and (3) the equipment that is required by state laws for ambulance services in general. Basic and advanced life support equipment is usually required by law and is carried routinely in ground ambulances and both rotary-wing and fixed-wing air ambulances. The American Society of Hospital-Based Emergency Air Medical Services also makes recommendations concerning transport team equipment [3, 4].

The UUMC maternal transport team chooses supplies and equipment so that, in addition to the equipment required by law, team members can adequately manage a high-risk patient during transport including, when necessary, delivery en route or any other unanticipated emergency. This supplementary equipment is divided into three separate bags: one for maternal equipment, one for neonatal equipment, and one for essential drugs. A digital blood pressure machine is also available. Intermittent fetal monitoring can be done en route using a Doppler machine or a fetoscope. Electronic fetal monitoring might be preferable because it may be difficult to hear the fetal heart above the background noise in the transport vehicle. However, the monitoring equipment that is currently available is very heavy and occupies considerable space so that it is rarely used on transport.

*Table 15-7. Basic equipment for maternal transport**

Doppler for fetal heart monitoring, preferably with earphone capability
Medications to treat the mother
IV infusion pump and supplies
Oxygen
Suction machine
Surgical pack for emergency delivery
Neonatal resuscitation equipment

*Refer to Chapter Appendix I for a comprehensive list.

The Bureau of Emergency Medical Services within the Utah State Department of Health has determined that certain minimum quantities of supplies and equipment shall be carried on each air ambulance vehicle, in accordance with the air ambulance service licensure level [5]. Most states have similar regulations. The list may be modified at the discretion of the Department of Health as other needs are recognized and new methods become known. The basic equipment required by law for ambulance services, whether air, ground, or water based varies very little; availability of other equipment is determined by the level of licensure of the ambulance service. For example, a ground ambulance service carrying only EMTs with basic EMT-1 training would not be required to carry equipment for intravenous infusion because EMT-1 personnel are not allowed by law to administer intravenous solutions.

Chapter Appendixes I, II, and III list the equipment and drugs required on each air ambulance vehicle in accordance with the air ambulance service licensure level, beginning with basic life support through advanced life support and including obstetrical specialty life support. Chapter Appendix IV lists the equipment and drugs carried by the maternal transport team regardless of the vehicle being used. This equipment is stored in two soft-sided bags (one multicompartment size 18 × 11 × 9 inches and one single compartment size 18 × 9 × 6 inches) in the labor and delivery area. The medications are kept in a fish tackle box (Fig. 15-4). All equipment must be stored or secured in such a manner as to prevent movement during a crash, and all medications must be stored according to the manufacturer's recommendations.

The charting forms listed in Chapter Appendix IV are always taken on each transport call. The patient and any accompanying family member are asked to sign permit forms for transport. This is necessary before the patient can legally be transported. A booklet describing the newborn in the intensive care unit is left with the family.

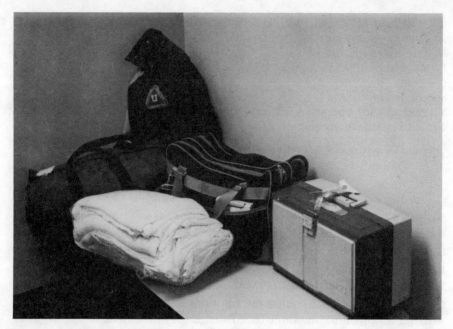

*Fig. 15-4. Transport equipment ready for the next maternal transport.*

## Equipment Maintenance and Availability

After each transport it is the responsibility of each transport nurse to replace in the transport bags any equipment and medication used. The
transport head nurse is responsible for checking the equipment twice a
month and is also responsible for resterilizing and updating equipment as
required. This inspection serves as a double check, to ensure that the appropriate equipment is in the proper transport bag. The medical director
and coordinator/head nurse of the transport team are responsible for reviewing the equipment needs annually or more frequently if indicated. At
this time decisions are made concerning the purchase of new or replacement equipment and medications.

## Summary

There is no particular approach to establishing a maternal transport unit
that is best. Institutional needs, the geography of the area to be served, and
the distances and time involved will usually dictate the type of system that is
needed. Transport systems serving a large number of patients are able, to
some extent, to tailor staffing to the needs of the individual patient. Institu-

tions with a small number of perinatal patients can usually support a single small team whose members have broader training and experience.

## References
1. Boehm, F. H., and Haire, M. F. One-way maternal transport: An evolving concept. Inpatient services. *Am. J. Obstet. Gynecol.* 134:484, 1979.
2. Powell, J. P. Training for EMT paramedics in perinatal care and transport. *J. Tenn. Med. Assoc.* 75:133, February 1982.
3. Specialty Care Team, American Society of Hospital-Based Emergency Air Medical Services. *Fixed-Wing Criteria.* American Society of Hospital-Based Emergency Air Medical Services, October 17, 1985.
4. Specialty Care Team, American Society of Hospital-Based Emergency Air Medical Services. *Rotorcraft Criteria.* American Society of Hospital-Based Emergency Air Medical Services, October 16, 1985.
5. State Emergency Medical Services Committee. *Air Ambulance Rules.* Title 26, Chap. 8, Utah Emergency Medical Services System Act, October 1985.

## Chapter Appendix I: Required Basic Life-Support Service Equipment (Utah)

GENERAL EQUIPMENT
1 patient litter or stretcher, with approved restraints
1 sheet
2 blankets
1 pillow with vinyl cover
1 emesis basin or bag
2 towels
1 map of geographical areas for which service is provided

AIRWAY EQUIPMENT
1 bulb syringe (neonatal size)
1 portable or fixed suction apparatus, with wide-bore tubing and rigid pharyngeal suction tip
1 self-inflating resuscitation bag, with adult-, child-, and infant-size masks; ventilation units must be capable of use with an oxygen supply
1 portable oxygen apparatus capable of metered flow, with adequate tubing and with semi-open, valveless, transparent masks and nasal cannula, with adult and pediatric sizes; the apparatus must be capable of delivering oxygen at a rate of 10 liters/minute

EQUIPMENT FOR MONITORING VITAL SIGNS
1 electronic Doppler device
1 stethoscope
1 adult blood-pressure cuff

1 set of pediatric blood pressure cuffs or doppler blood pressure machine
1 thermometer

DRESSINGS AND SUPPLIES
2 cardboard or air splints, or equivalent, in arm and leg sizes
9 tongue depressors
1 flashlight
1 sound suppressor
2 mouth gags or padded tongue depressors
1 roll each adhesive tape, sizes ½ in., 1 in., 2 in., and 3 in.
2 trauma dressings
24 sterile gauze pads (4 × 4 inches)
6 nonsterile gauze pads
2 triangle bandages
2 × three (3)-in. elastic bandages
2 × four (4)-in. elastic bandages
15 band-Aids, various sizes
4 rolls of gauze bandages
several pairs of sterile gloves
3 vaseline gauze pads
1 box adhesive bandages
2 wrist restraints
3 large safety pins

TRAUMA EQUIPMENT
1 pediatric compartmentalized pneumatic anti-shock trousers (CPAST)
1 adult CPAST
1 traction splint
1 small, medium, and large cervical collar
1 short spine board or its equivalent

---

From State Emergency Medical Services Committee. *Air Ambulance Rules.* Title 26, Chap. 8, Utah Emergency Medical Services System Act, October 1985. Pp. 11–12.

## Chapter Appendix II: Required Advanced Life-Support Services Equipment (Utah)[a]

---

AIRWAY EQUIPMENT
1 laryngoscope, with curved and straight blades, sizes for adult, pediatric, and neonatal patients; spare batteries, bulbs, and adapters for attaching endotracheal tube to oxygen supply
1 each, endotracheal tubes, sizes 9, 8.5, 8, 7.5, 7, 6, 5, 4, 3.5, 3, 2.5
1 magill forceps, pediatric and adult
1 esophageal obturator airway, with gastric suction capability
2 chest darts with one-way valves

1 each, chest tubes, 32, 28, 20, 12, 10
1 roll umbilical tape, 30 inches
1 stylet
1 each, oral airway for adult, child, infant
1 each, nasal pharyngeal airway, sizes 32F, 25F, 22F

CARDIAC EQUIPMENT
1 portable, battery-powered cardiac monitor with strip-chart recorder
6 spare ECG electrodes for each lead
1 spare roll of ECG recording paper
1 portable, battery-powered defibrillator, with 4 conductive pads and conductive gel; the defibrillator may be a unit in the cardiac monitor

INTRAVENOUS FLUIDS[b] AND EQUIPMENT
3 each, 500 ml 5% D/W, 3000 ml Ringer's lactate (RL), or 5% dextrose in Ringer's lactate, or normal saline (NS)
10 alcohol and 10 povodine-iodophor preps
2 each, "butterfly," or equal, needles, sizes 25, 23, 21, and 19 gauge
2 each, over-the-needle catheters, sizes 14, 16, 18, 20, 22, 23, 25 gauge
1 each, central line intracaths, sizes 12, 14, 16, 19, 21 gauge
3 blood administration sets
3 IV air-pressure infusion pumps
3 microdrip sterile tubing
4 extension tubing, sterile
1 safety razor
1 pair bandage scissors
2 each, syringes, tuberculin and insulin, 3 ml, 5 ml, and 6 ml
3 each, needles, 18, 19, 20, 22, 25 gauge
1 bottle povodine-iodine, 30 ml
1 30-ml bacteriostatic water
2 arm boards, two different sizes

MISCELLANEOUS EQUIPMENT AND SUPPLIES
1 set adult three-compartment pneumatic trousers
1 set pediatric three-compartment pneumatic trousers, when appropriate
1 each, nasal gastric tube, sizes 8F, 10F, 14F, 18F, 16F
1 scoop stretcher or long board
1 each, cervical collars, large, medium, and small
1 Foley catheter set
1 femur traction splint, adult and pediatric
1 suture kit
1 Kendrick extrication device or its equivalent
1 needle holder
3 sutures with curved needles, 3.0 suture material
1 Kelly clamp
1 pick-up forceps
1 hypothermia thermometer
1 bottle reagent strips for glucose (Dextrostix[c])
1 viscous lidocaine hydrochloride, 2%, 15 ml
1 tube surgical lubricant, 15 ml

DRUGS
3 mg atropine
100 mg diphenhydramine
3000 mg bretylium tosylate
3 g calcium chloride
100 mg dexamethasone
200 mg meperidine
2 mg adrenalin, 1 : 10,000
4 mg adrenalin, 1 : 1000
800 mg dopamine
2 mg isoproterenol
200 mg furosemide (Lasix)
260 mg phenobarbital
20 mg morphine sulfate
50 mg promethazine hydrochloride
300 mEq sodium bicarbonate
40 mg diazepam (Valium)
50 mg lidocaine, 1% without epinephrine
50 g mannitol, 25%
100 ml 50% D/W
20 mg naloxone hydrochloride
10 mg trinitroglycerine
30 ml bacteriostatic water
500 mg dimenhydrinate (Dramamine)
30 ml bacteriostatic normal saline

[a] All equipment and supplies listed for basic life support, plus the equipment listed here, are required.
[b] Fluids shall be in compressible plastic containers unless not available.
[c] Ames Division, Miles Laboratories, Inc. Elkhart, IN 46515.
From State Emergency Medical Services Committee. *Air Ambulance Rules.* Title 26, Chap. 8, Utah Emergency Medical Service System Act, October 1985. Pp. 12–13. With permission.

## Chapter Appendix III: Required Specialized Life Support Service Equipment: Maternal-Fetal Life Support Equipment (Utah) [a]

GENERAL EQUIPMENT [b]
2 each, endotracheal tubes, sizes 2.5, 3.0, and 3.5
1 silver Swaddler or plastic wrap
1 bulb syringe
2 suction catheters, 6, 8, 10 for newborn
2 No. 8 French infant feeding tubes
1 each, laryngoscope blades, oo and 1
1 self-inflating newborn bag for assisted ventilation

1 obstetrical kit, disposable, which includes scissors, 2 Kellys, 2 cord clamps, basin, cord blood tubes
2 baby blankets
1 Porta-warm mattress[c]

ADDITIONAL DRUGS SPECIFICALLY FOR OBSTETRICAL CARE
2 g ampicillin
100 mg gentamycin
1 ml ampules of oxytocin, 10 units/ml, 4 ampules
25 mg ephedrine sulfate
Two 0.2 mg/ml, ergotamine tartrate
100 mg hydralazine hydrochloride (Apresoline)
25 g $MgSO_4$, 50%
1 mg glucagon
50 mg ritodrine hydrochloride
Three 1 mg terbutaline sulphate ampules
1 10-ml vial, epinephrine, 1:10,000
30 mEq sodium bicarbonate, 4.2%
1 20-ml vial of 10% D/W
0.02 mg/ml naloxone hydrochloride, one 2-ml vial

[a]In addition to the equipment supplies specific for the basic life support and advanced life support services, the obstetrical transport team is required to have this equipment available, as set forth by the State Emergency Medical Services Committee. *Air Ambulance Rules.* Title 26, Chap. 8, Utah Emergency Medical Services System Act, October 1985. P. 18.
[b]Refer to Book Appendix 6 for a detailed list of equipment required for neonatal transport.
[c]Porta-warm mattress. American Hospital Distributors K-Laboratories, P.O. Box 81571, 1660 Hotel Circle North, Suite 620, San Diego, CA 92138.

## Chapter Appendix IV: Equipment Additions Made by the University of Utah Maternal Transport Team

MEDICATIONS
Potassium chloride, 30 ml/60 mEq
Xylocaine, 2%, 20 mg/ml, 20-ml vial
Sodium citrate, 30 ml, 0.3 M
$MgSO_4$, 500/ml, 5 mEq/ml, mini-jet
Diphenhydramine hydrochloride (Benedryl), 50 mg/ml, 1-ml steri-dose syringe
Dramamine, 50-mg tablets
Oxymetazoline hydrochloride[a] (Afrin) nasal spray, 15 ml
Prochlorperazine (Compazine), 2 ml/10-mg vial
Calcium gluconate, 10%, 10 ml for IV use
Ammonia capsule
Digoxin (Lanoxin), 0.5 mg/2-ml ampule
Lasix, 2 ml/20 mg, 2 ml IM/IV

Promethazine hydrochloride (Phenergan), 25 mg/ml, 1 ml
Heparin flush, 10 units/ml
Ergotamine tartrate, 0.2 mg/ml
Ephedrine, 25 mg/ml

EQUIPMENT: MATERNAL BAG
*Routine Maternal Care Supply Section of Bag*
1 blood pressure cuff with scope
2 each, sterile gloves of all sizes
Examination gloves No. 8
Lubricating gel
1 emesis basin
1 green plastic adult mask
3 absorbent bed pads
2 perineal pads
Nitrazine paper
*IV Therapy/Lab Work Section of Bag*
2 tourniquets
1 wrist board, adult
2 culturettes
1 each, adhesive tape, ½ × 1 in., nylon; clear tape, ½ × 1 in.
2 scalp vein needles, 25 gauge
3 each, blood tubes, red, purple, blue, grey
12 alcohol swabs
6 each, Betadine prep swabs and ointment
Syringes, 1 ml (TB), 3 ml, 5 ml, 10 ml
2 each, angiocaths, 16, 18, 20, 23 gauge
IV tubing, additive main (2), secondary (2), blood (Fenwall) (1), extension (2), volu-
    trol (1), blood administration cuff (1)
*IV Solutions*
1 each, liters Ringer's Lactate, normal saline
*Adult Resuscitation and Foley Section of Bag*
1 laryngoscope, adult size (scope, blades (2), spare bulbs (several), syringe, endo-
    tracheal tubes (No. 6.0−9.0) with scissors, stylets, airways in an emergency kit)
2 batteries
Lubricating gel
Oral airways of varied sizes
1 Hope II resuscitation bag, adult size, rubber masks No. 4 and 5
1 green plastic adult mask
1 flashlight with batteries
1 each, suction catheters No. 5, 8, 18 with tubing
1 Foley 14 French with plug and clamp
Reagent strips for urine Ph, glucose, protein, and blood
*In Outside Pockets of Bag*
1 box of facial tissues
10 measuring tapes
*Linen Pack*
2 thermal blankets

2 bath blankets
1 each, pillow case and pillow
*Charting Forms*
1 complete chart with delivery record
1 obstetrical transport record[b]
2 copies of transfer permit (one copy is left with the patient)
2 copies of transport permit for accompanying family member
Nursing protocols for patient care
Equipment list
1 newborn ICU booklet for family

INFANT BAG[c]
*Emergency Delivery Kit*
2 cord blood tubes
1 curved scissor
1 straight scissor
1 medium needle holder
1 ring forceps
1 pick-up forceps, plain
1 solution bowl
1 linen pack
    4 delivery room towels
    1 double half
    12× (4 × 4) gauze sponges
    2 baby blankets
*Delivery (Miscellaneous Supplies Bag)*
3 absorbent bed pads
2 perineal pads
3 disposable diapers
1 vaginal prep set
2 bulb syringes
2 cord clamps, single wrap
1 bubble bag (plastic air cap insulation material cut into a wrap for the infant)
Sutures
    2 chromic 3 degrees
    1 each, 2 and 4 degrees
    1 package umbilical tape
    1 sanitary belt
*Infant Resuscitation Bag*
1 infant resuscitation bag capable of delivering 100% oxygen
1 laryngoscope, infant size
2 batteries
2 blades, size 0 and 1
Several spare bulbs
7 endotracheal tubes, sizes No. 2.5–4.0
4 oral airways, varied sizes
2 DeLee suction
2 suction catheters, sizes 6.5 and 8 Fr

1 gauze swab (4 × 4) in a package of 10
1 roll each of gauze bandage 3 × 6 in.
2 each three-way stopcock
3 infant feeding tubes, No. 8 and 5
3 infant-size resuscitator
1 mask, full-term size
1 mask, premature size
1 250-ml 5% D/W
1 250-ml 10% D/W IV solution
1 pediatric Metriset
2 each, butterfly No. 23 and 25
2 tongue blades

---

[a] Nasal stuffiness and sinus conditions may be exacerbated by pressure changes during air transport.
[b] See example of obstetrical transport record on page 312.
[c] For a more comprehensive list, see Book Appendix 6.
From University of Utah Medical Center Policy and Procedure Manuals, Revised May 1984.

# 16

# The Mechanism of
# Maternal Transport

Patricia A. Payne

16A. Evans' ambulance wagon, interior view. Interior has been arranged for recumbent and sitting patients. A class 4 sick transport conveyance (conveyance drawn by animals). "That the system which I propose for the transport of the wounded is itself faultless, I do not claim; that it is a step foreward, that it is an improvement upon any other known system, I fully believe. . . ." (Reproduced from Evans, T. W. History and Description of an Ambulance Wagon Constructed in Accordance with Plans Furnished by the Writer. Paris: E. Briere, 1868.)

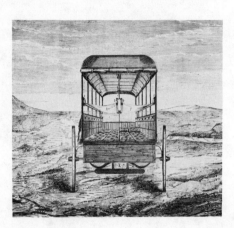

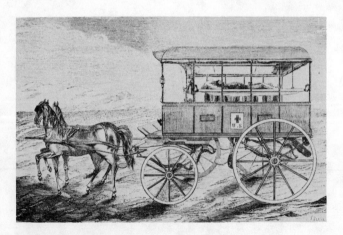

16B. Evans' ambulance wagon, lateral view. A class 4 sick transport conveyance (conveyance drawn by animals). (Reproduced from Evans, T. W. History and Description of an Ambulance Wagon Constructed in Accordance with Plans Furnished by the Writer. Paris: E. Briere, 1868.)

"A safe transport of the perinatal patient requires skilled personnel, appropriate equipment, and effective communication between the hospital facilities of the region" [3]. For a transport system to work smoothly, everyone who has contact with the transported patients or referring physician should be thoroughly familiar with each step in the referral process. This process includes the consultation, referral, transport, and paperwork. Most important, involved personnel must recognize the need for prompt action when a consultation or referral is requested. New employees should undergo a detailed orientation to the transport system. Hospital staff (physicians and nurses) should receive a regular update on changes in the system, as well as statistics on perinatal outcome. This update ensures that the information conveyed is as accurate and consistent as possible.

The mechanism of transport will be discussed in order of occurrence during an actual transport (Fig. 16-1) including:

1. initial phone call
2. consultation
3. arranging a transport
4. patient records
5. receiving staff response
6. follow-up communication

### Initial Phone Call

If the system is well planned and publicized, the referring physician will have ready and immediate telephone access to a perinatal center. This contact may be through a central publicized statewide number or by direct contact with the closest perinatal center. The referring physician should then be able to consult, without delay, with an individual who can provide immediate feedback as to the availability of beds, appropriateness of transport,

Table 16-1. Basic information the referring physician should provide to the consultant

1. Name and location of referring hospital and phone number of referring physician
2. Patient's name, age, parity, expected date of confinement, and reason for consultation
3. Maternal and fetal status and treatment to date (to include vital signs, laboratory data, interpretation of fetal monitor tracings, and findings on cervical examination)
4. Other relevant information that may affect the decision to transport, such as extreme maternal distress at the prospect of transfer

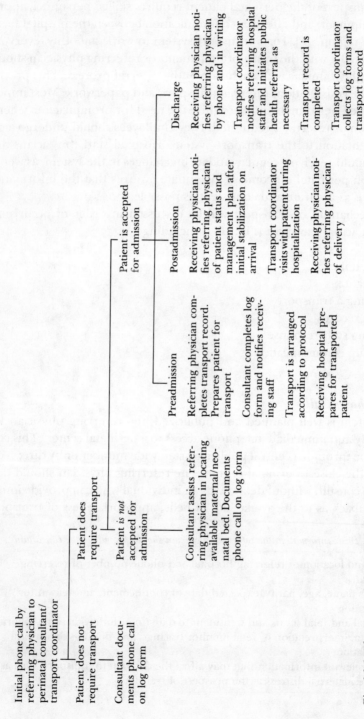

Fig. 16-1. Flow pattern of maternal transport.

**Initial phone call by referring physician to perinatal consultant/transport coordinator**

**Patient does not require transport**

**Patient does require transport**

Consultant documents phone call on log form

**Patient is not accepted for admission**

Consultant assists referring physician in locating available maternal/neonatal bed. Documents phone call on log form

**Patient is accepted for admission**

**Preadmission**

Referring physician completes transport record. Prepares patient for transport

Consultant completes log form and notifies receiving staff

Transport is arranged according to protocol

Receiving hospital prepares for transported patient

**Postadmission**

Receiving physician notifies referring physician of patient status and management plan after initial stabilization on arrival

Transport coordinator visits with patient during hospitalization

Receiving physician notifies referring physician of delivery

**Discharge**

Receiving physician notifies referring physician by phone and in writing

Transport coordinator notifies referring hospital staff and initiates public health referral as necessary

Transport record is completed

Transport coordinator collects log forms and transport record and any special stabilization treatment and precautions necessary prior to or during transport. It is important that the referring physician provide basic and accurate information regarding the patient's status, which will expedite the consultation and transport (Table 16-1).

Every phone call should be documented. The log forms are used for ongoing evaluation of referral patterns, patient disposition, and reasons for denial.

## Consultation

At each perinatal center, there should be an identified mechanism for receiving phone calls, including a posted schedule for consultants. The consultant should be a member of the attending staff or a trained nurse coordinator, who is familiar with referral patterns, management practices, and the capabilities of referring physicians and institutions in the region. He or she should also have rapid access to up-to-date information on bed availability for both maternal and neonatal care. Many maternal transfers do not result in the use of a neonatal bed; however, the ones that do will tend to produce small sick babies [1]. Many of the decisions related to transport can be made on an individual basis. However, there are some management decisions that cannot be made optimally without input from staff in the neonatology department or hospital administration and in-depth knowledge of departmental policy. Resident obstetricians may be quite capable of making clinical management decisions regarding patients in their own institution; however, they do not always know all of the details that are necessary to provide appropriate consultation. They are also often not well accepted by physicians working in the community, who prefer to consult with an attending physician.

The purpose of consultation is to answer the following questions:

1. *Does the patient require transport?*
   The referral call may result in a telephone consultation without patient transfer, an outpatient referral, or an inpatient transfer. Each transport program should establish guidelines with indications for maternal transport, which will assist the referring physician and perinatal consultant in making a joint decision. However, each clinical situation must be carefully considered and the required action may not exactly follow established guidelines. In many states, the shortage of neonatal beds may necessitate transport of a mother to a referral center where a neonatal bed is not available. The mother is transported and stabilized, and the infant is

delivered. She or her baby, or both, may then be transported to a hospital where neonatal beds are available. Ideally, transport should be reserved for acute situations that could not have been predicted (i.e., when possible, early consultation and transfer of care is preferable to emergency transport).

2. *Where is the most appropriate referral site?*
The best receiving hospital may be dictated by maternal or potential neonatal conditions that require the expertise of medical specialists such as a cardiologist, nephrologist, or pediatric surgeon.

3. *What special precautions should be taken prior to or during transport?*
The answer to this question requires a thorough knowledge of the capabilities of the transport personnel, transport distance, and duration and mode of transport. The referring physician and perinatal consultant should discuss stabilization prior to transport, as well as medications that may be used during transport. Each transport system should have written guidelines for basic patient management during transport that are specific to the clinical condition of the patient, for example, patients in preterm labor should have intravenous fluids prior to and during transport. The use of tocolytics during transport, however, may vary with the current management practices in each region.

4. *How will the patient be transported?*
In some cases, the consultant may have no choice as to the mode of transport; in others, the decision may depend on individual considerations, for example, clinical status, weather or availability of aircraft.

Once a decision is made to transport a patient, the perinatal consultant should notify appropriate staff, including the transport team, nursing staff, clerical staff, and resident staff. The responsibility of each of these individuals in the transport process should be clearly established and posted in the labor area.

## Arranging a Transport
Protocols for transportation of a perinatal patient must be clearly established prior to the actual transport of patients. When a transport team exists, they can immediately prepare for transport. In a one-way transport,

*Table 16-2. Basic information included in a maternal transport referral form*

1. Patient's name, age, parity, expected date of confinement, and next of kin
2. Referring physician and institution
3. Prenatal care provider
4. Payment source
5. Significant clinical information
6. Indications for referral
7. Mode of transport

the referring hospital staff is responsible for the initial instructions to the EMTs on the specifics of patient care. Guidelines must be available for the consultant and for EMS personnel so that conflicts will not occur. These should include information on response time, use of medications, and the capabilities and responsibilities of the members of the EMS team. The perinatal consultant must have immediate telephone access to the EMS system and be aware of pertinent regulations related to the transport of perinatal patients. If a decision regarding ground versus air transport is to be made, the perinatal consultant and referring physician must collaborate to make the best decision for the patient.

### Patient Records
When a patient is transported, the transfer package should include copies of the prenatal record, relevant portions of fetal monitor tracings (if significant to future care), and a standardized transport referral form. The transport referral form serves a dual purpose: It provides immediate access to patient information for the receiving staff and allows for ongoing data collection for the regional program. The form should be short and easy to read, as well as provide specific instructions for communication and referral (Table 16-2). This will expedite the transport process for those individuals who are infrequently involved in preparing patients for transport or who cannot easily locate the guidelines in the middle of the night.

Ideally, the transport referral form will also include outcome information (see p. 109). The form serves an educational purpose by correlating status, management, and outcome information. When a patient is discharged, the outcome section is completed and copies are given to the transport coordinator. The coordinator keeps copies for statistical purposes and sends one to the staff at the referring institution.

During transport the patient's clinical status and any medical interventions necessary are carefully documented at regular intervals.

## The Receiving Staff Response

Pertinent staff at the receiving hospital should be notified as soon as the decision is made for a patient to be transferred. These staff members include the charge nurse in labor and delivery; the chief obstetrical resident; and personnel in the intensive care nursery, admitting office, security department, and emergency room. The first priority is to identify the personnel who will receive the patient and at what location in the hospital. Transported patients usually enter the hospital through the emergency room; therefore an estimated time of arrival (ETA) should be established and a physician and nurse from labor and delivery sent to meet the patient. If transport is by air, it may be necessary to dispatch an ambulance with appropriate personnel to receive the patient and transport her from the landing area. In the event that an unexpected delivery has occurred or is imminent, a doctor or nurse from the neonatal unit should accompany the team. The list of priorities and identification of the team leader should be clear so that confusion does not occur while preparing to receive the patient.

## Follow-up Communication

One of the most critical steps, and often the one receiving the least attention in the transport process, is follow-up communication. Private physicians are, understandably, very skeptical of a system that does not provide them with feedback. In fact, the incidence of future referrals may be inversely proportional to the number of instances of failed communication.

A minimum of three (two if the patient does not deliver) follow-up phone calls should be made by the physician caring for a transported patient to the referring physician. The first call is made as soon as the patient is stabilized and the management plan is established, the second when the patient delivers, and the third when the patient is discharged. Written follow-up communication may be in the form of a hospital summary, maternal transport summary (see Chapter Appendix I) or a personal letter from the referring physician. When the patient is discharged from the receiving hospital, communications are optimized if the transport coordinator contacts a member of the delivery room staff at the referring hospital and sends them a copy of the transport record.

Any regional program should expect a small percentage of unnecessary referrals [1]. The number can be minimized by bringing examples to the attention of the referring physician and discussing the reasons why they might have occurred, in a positive and constructive manner.

## Summary

"The transport of pregnant women and newborn infants between hospitals is recognized as an essential component of regionalized perinatal care" [2]. Careful planning of each step in the transport process should provide high-quality care for mothers and babies, and encourage ongoing support of the regional program.

## References

1. Kanto, W., Bryant, J., Thigpen, J., et al. Impact of a maternal transport program on a newborn service. *South. Med. J.* 76:7, 1983.
2. Modanlou, H. D., Dorchester, W. Freeman, R. K., et al. Perinatal transport to a regional perinatal center in a metropolitan area: Maternal versus neonatal transport. *Am. J. Obstet. Gynecol.* 138:1157, 1980.
3. *Tennessee Perinatal Care System Guidelines for Transportation.* Tennessee Department of Health and Environment, Maternal and Child Health Section, September 1985.

## *Chapter Appendix I: Maternal Transport Summary*

**MATERNAL TRANSPORT SUMMARY**

| DATE | PATIENT NAME | | HISTORY NUMBER |
|---|---|---|---|

| REFERRING M.D. / INSTITUTION | RECEIVING M.D. AND INSTITUTION |
|---|---|

TRANSPORTATION TO RECEIVING HOSPITAL VIA:
☐ AMBULANCE    ☐ PRIVATE VEHICLE   ☐ HELICOPTER

| ADMISSION DATE | ADMITTING DIAGNOSIS |
|---|---|
| DISCHARGE DATE | DISCHARGE DIAGNOSIS |

HOSPITAL COURSE

| DELIVERY INFORMATION | BIRTHWEIGHT | SEX | APGAR |
|---|---|---|---|
| ☐ SVD ☐ CESAREAN | _____ GMS | ☐ MALE ☐ FEMALE | _____ |

| NEWBORN STATUS AT DISCHARGE | REMAINS IN | | FETAL DEATH/ |
|---|---|---|---|
| HOME WITH ☐ MOTHER | ☐ NEWBORN NURSERY | ☐ ICN | ☐ STILLBORN |

DISCHARGE INSTRUCTIONS / FOLLOW-UP CARE
☐ NEONATAL DEATH

ADDITIONAL COMMENTS

Thank you for referring this patient to us. Feel free to contact our department if we can be of further assistance.

_____
SIGNATURE

_____
PRINTED NAME AND PHONE NUMBER

cc: Transport Coordinator

830211 (04-83) ☆ ⊕                                                    1313

# 17

# *Stabilization and Management of the Pregnant Patient Prior to Transport*

Larry G. Dennis

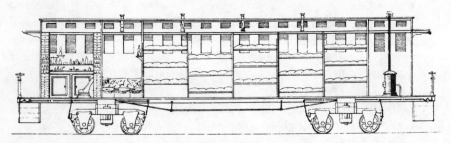

*17A. A type 5 sick transport conveyance (conveyance moved by steam power). Hospital rail wagon holding 30 wounded. (Reproduced from Doin, O. [ed.].* Transport par Chemins de Fer des Blessés et Malades Militaires. Paris, 1885.)

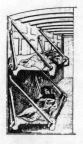
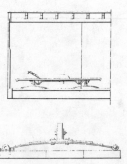

*17B. Rail wagons modified for medical transport, with diagrams of the modified suspension systems installed for the benefit of the patients. (Reproduced from Doin, O. [ed.].* Transport par Chemins de Fer des Blessés et Malades Militaires. Paris, 1885.)

The indications for maternal transport have been discussed in Chapter 14. In this chapter I will describe the evaluation and stabilization of the pregnant patient prior to and during the transport process. Since the goal of transporting a mother and fetus is to obtain more intensive care than would have been available at the referring hospital, it is very important that those patients appropriate for transfer are identified, expedited, and provided with the necessary care to effect stabilization of the maternal-fetal unit.

In a recent review of the indications for maternal transports to the George Washington University Hospital it was found that the majority were for either premature rupture of membranes (45%) or preterm labor (35%). The other indications included preeclampsia, pregnancy-induced hypertension, intrauterine growth retardation, third-trimester bleeding, oligohydramnios, placenta previa, fetal anomalies, facility-related indications (such as lack of available beds, insufficient number of ventilators), and mechanical problems (such as lack of heat or water).

The first step in organizing a maternal transport occurs before the transport team is called. This step is the initial evaluation of the patient by her physician to determine whether it is necessary and safe to move the patient to another hospital. The importance of rapid and effective stabilization of the maternal-fetal patient prior to transport cannot be overemphasized. Appropriate treatment of the mother prior to transport may be the key factor in achieving an eventual successful outcome of the pregnancy instead of a disastrous transport and obstetrical course. By providing outreach education, personnel at the tertiary care center can assist the referring physician and other hospital staff well in advance of any transport. Educational conferences can provide information about services available, how patients can be referred (including the names and phone numbers of key personnel), which patients should be transported, when they should be transported, how to prepare patients for transport, and what records, blood specimens, so forth, should accompany the patient. Finally, it is important to maintain lines of communication with the referring hospitals, even at times when no mothers are being transported, so that the referring physician will feel comfortable calling the tertiary care center to arrange a transport when indicated.

A less formal opportunity to provide outreach education occurs during consultation or while arranging a transport. While the transport team is in transit, the perinatologist should gather information from the referring physician and make recommendations regarding the optimal management of the patient. If such communication is made in an appropriate fashion, the patient's condition should be optimally stabilized on arrival of the transport team or, when indicated, for one-way transport by the referring hospi-

*Table 17-1. Steps involved in transport*

1. Patient evaluation
2. Transport decision
3. Change IV
4. Treatment
5. Transport

tal (see Chap. 2). Confusion and unnecessary delay can be minimized by such an approach.

A two-way transport process is divided into several steps, as shown in Table 17-1. When the team arrives at the referring hospital, the first step is evaluation of the patient. The primary question to be answered is "Is it safe to transport this patient?" The essential areas to be evaluated include

1. Medical and surgical status of the mother
2. Fetal status, including gestational age
3. Is delivery imminent or likely to occur during the transport?
4. Status of obstetrical problems

If, after evaluation of the patient, the transport team agrees that transfer is appropriate, they then proceed with the third step. However, the team may feel that it is not safe to transport the patient at that point in time. If there is a clinical problem that can be stabilized, then this should be done and the patient then transported. Rarely, the team will find that it is not appropriate to transport the patient. In such a case, the team leader, after telephone consultation with the consultant attending physician at the receiving hospital, should inform the referring physician of the decision and the logic involved in reaching it. Optimally, the referring physician should be actively involved throughout the decision-making process.

The third step is to change the bottle of intravenous fluids. Even with optimal communication between medical personnel, a bottle of intravenous fluid may be mislabeled—the drug or the dose being administered may be different from that stated. This confusion could be disastrous (e.g., if oxytocin (Pitocin) is mislabeled as ritodrine) during transport.

The fourth step involves treatment and stabilization of the patient, if such measures are necessary. In the majority of cases, very little pretransport therapy will be necessary.

The remainder of this chapter will outline the basic steps involved in the pretransport stabilization of obstetrical patients.

## Evaluation of the Medical/Surgical Status of the Mother

GENERAL PRINCIPLES

Initial assessment of the medical status of the patient should include hemo-dynamic status, especially in patients who have a history of significant blood loss. Those patients who appear unstable should have rapid correction of hemodynamic balance to ensure adequate uterine perfusion (Table 17-2). Hypovolemia should be corrected initially with Ringer's lactate, followed by type and Rh-specific blood (preferably whole or reconstituted blood). Pregnant patients with evidence of shock have lost at least 25 to 35 percent of their total blood volume [1]. When calculating the patient's total blood volume, 25 percent or more should be added to the standard volume for a nonpregnant patient of the same height and weight to replace the normal blood volume expansion that occurs during pregnancy. Vasopressors should be avoided during pregnancy although, in extreme circumstances when fluids and blood replacement do not correct a severe hypotensive episode, vasopressors may be required. The drug of choice in such a case is ephe-drine (10–15 mg intravenously) because it causes the least decrease in uterine blood flow when compared to other vasopressors. Dopamine may also be useful, although its effect on uterine vasculature has not been thoroughly studied. If the patient is supine and blood loss is minimal, displacement of the uterus from compressing the vena cava is a simple, effective means of restoring blood return to the right side of the heart and may restore a normal blood pressure. Displacement of the uterus can be achieved by turning the patient onto her left side or by merely pushing the uterus to the left. Pneumatic antishock garments (PASGs) can be used during pregnancy; however, only the trousers should be inflated, not the abdominal portion of the garment.

In contrast to the hypovolemic patient, there is a possibility of fluid overload in patients who have been treated with beta-adrenergic drugs, particularly when ritodrine hydrochloride is used in conjunction with steroids [3, 5, 6]. Assessment of the patient for possible fluid overload includes ex-

*Table 17-2. Guidelines in the treatment of shock in pregnancy*

1. Remember patient has lost at least 25–35% of total blood volume
2. Insert two large-bore IV lines
3. Immediately resuscitate with Ringer's lactate solution
4. Displace the uterus off the vena cava
5. Transfuse type and Rh-specific whole blood
6. Apply pneumatic antishock garment (PASG) trousers
7. Administer vasopressors (ephedrine, 10–15 mg IV as a bolus, or dopamine) as a last resort

*Table 17-3. Guidelines in the management of fluid overload*

1. Monitor fluid intake and urine output
2. Restrict fluid
3. Administer diuretic therapy—Furosemide, 10–40 mg IV
4. Administer sedation—Morphine, 5–15 mg IV or subcutaneous
5. Intubate and ventilate, if necessary

amination of the heart and lungs and review of fluid intake and urine output. Possible signs and symptoms may include dyspnea, tachypnea, tachycardia, wheezing, and cough with or without a frothy sputum. Further evaluation by chest x ray, ECG, and arterial blood gas analysis may be helpful. Management of this problem includes close monitoring of fluid intake and urine output, fluid restriction, assessment of cardiopulmonary function, diuretics, and providing adequate oxygenation. Mechanical ventilatory support may be necessary. Sedation with morphine (5–15 mg intravenously or subcutaneously) will help decrease patient anxiety, but it should not be used when respiration is depressed. Furosemide (10–40 mg intravenously) will usually provide rapid, effective diuresis (Table 17-3).

Occasionally a pregnant patient is transported for general surgical indications. In such a circumstance it is necessary to determine whether the patient has a condition that may necessitate immediate surgery, and thus transport may be contraindicated. An acute surgical abdomen is such a condition. Otherwise, stabilization and management are similar to that described for medical problems.

A review of all maternal medical conditions that may make a transport necessary is beyond the scope of this text; however, several of the more serious medical problems will be discussed.

DIABETIC KETOACIDOSIS
Diabetic ketoacidosis is one of the most severe complications of diabetes to occur during pregnancy and can be fatal to both mother and fetus. It is caused by a severe insulin deficiency that often is precipitated by some acute illness, commonly infection. This results in a significant increase in blood glucose and ketone levels. Diuresis leads to dehydration, electrolyte imbalance, and metabolic acidosis. Since glucose and ketones both readily cross the placenta, the fetus is presented with very high blood levels of glucose and ketones and cannot adequately respond.

The diagnosis can be confirmed by the presence of maternal hyperglycemia (usually a blood glucose level > 300 mg/100 ml) and ketonemia. Other abnormal laboratory findings may include elevated serum potas-

*Table 17-4. Laboratory studies helpful in the management of diabetic ketoacidosis*

Blood glucose and ketone levels
BUN
Electrolytes
Urinanalysis
Complete blood count
Arterial blood gases

sium, increased hematocrit due to hemoconcentration, and evidence of a metabolic acidosis. Laboratory studies to determine the severity of the disease should include blood glucose and ketone levels, blood urea nitrogen (BUN), electrolytes, urinanalysis, a complete blood count, and arterial blood gas measurements (Table 17-4).

Treatment must be prompt to optimize the outcome for both mother and fetus. The items that need rapid correction and continued assessment include (1) blood glucose levels, (2) fluid status, (3) serum potassium levels, (4) serum bicarbonate levels, and (5) fetal status. The management as outlined below is adapted from Porte and Halter [9].

1. Insulin: 20 to 30 units (0.4 U/kg) of regular insulin should be given intravenously as a bolus, followed by an infusion of 5 to 10 U/hour of regular insulin. The infusate is prepared by adding 100 U of regular insulin to 1000 ml of normal saline. If the infusion is run at 50 ml/hour, then 5 U of insulin will be administered in an hour. The dose per hour can then be adjusted according to blood glucose levels.

2. Fluids: The patient may have a fluid deficit of 6 to 10 liters. Thus rapid initial fluid replacement is essential, especially if the patient is hypotensive. One to two liters of normal saline should be infused in the first hour of therapy. After this, 150 to 200 ml/hour should be given. When sodium levels are less than 155 mEq/liter, 0.5 normal saline solution should be used. When blood glucose is less than 250 mg/dl, a 5% glucose solution should be used. Placement of a Foley catheter may be necessary to measure renal output, especially if the patient is comatose.

3. Potassium: If serum $K^+$ is low or normal, begin infusing potassium chloride at 20 to 30 mEq/hour as needed to maintain normal serum $K^+$ levels. If serum $K^+$ is high, potassium chloride should not be infused until adequate urine output has been established. Once urine output is adequate, infuse potassium chloride at 20 mEq/hour as necessary to maintain normal serum $K^+$ levels.

4. Bicarbonate: It is not usually necessary to treat with bicarbonate. How-

ever, if the pH is less than 7.1, then 44 mEq of sodium bicarbonate may be infused intravenously over 1 to 2 hours as needed.

5. Fetal status: The presence or absence of fetal heart tones should be documented as early as is practical. If fetal heart tones are present and the gestational age is greater than 24 weeks, then the fetal heart should be checked frequently, at least every 15 to 30 minutes. When the patient reaches the receiving hospital, continuous fetal monitoring should be instituted.

6. Further monitoring: Hourly studies of blood glucose, electrolytes, arterial blood gases, and urine output should be done and the results recorded on a flow sheet. While central venous pressure measurement is a useful adjunct, a central venous line is best placed after the patient reaches the receiving hospital. A nasogastric tube should be placed in those patients who are comatose.

Prompt management of all abnormalities and meticulous record keeping of patient progress will help to ensure an optimum outcome for both fetus and mother.

SEVERE CARDIOPULMONARY DISEASE WITH FAILURE
The diagnosis of cardiac disease during pregnancy may be difficult because many clinical signs and symptoms are common to both pregnancy and heart disease. A prior history of heart disease should alert the physician to the possibility of cardiac failure. Those signs and symptoms that are suggestive of cardiac disease include dyspnea; syncope with exertion; palpitations; hemoptysis; paroxysmal nocturnal dyspnea; exercise-induced chest pain or limited physical activity, or both; cyanosis; finger clubbing; increasing and unanticipated edema; pulmonary edema; atrial arrhythmia; diastolic murmur; or a loud, harsh systolic murmur. Since there are ECG and chest x-ray changes associated with a normal pregnancy, it is important to differentiate these changes from pathological findings. When there is pre-existing cardiac disease, the physiological changes that occur during pregnancy can be sufficient to cause cardiac failure that may be somewhat insidious in onset. Other precipitating factors include infection, anemia, hypervolemia, thyrotoxicosis, arrhythmias, an increase in physical activity, and obesity.

Initial evaluation of the patient with cardiac failure should include a history with pertinent questions seeking the symptoms listed above and a search for precipitating events. Physical examination should include a careful assessment of cardiopulmonary function. An ECG, chest x ray, arterial

*Table 17-5. Guidelines for treatment of heart failure*

1. Administer oxygen
2. Intubate and ventilate, if necessary
3. Administer morphine—5–15 mg IV
4. Administer furosemide—40–80 mg IV
5. Normalize serum electrolytes
6. Administer digoxin—0.5 mg IV initially, then 0.25 mg IV every 2–4 hours
7. Ascertain fetal status

blood gases, complete blood count, and serum electrolyte measurements are necessary for a complete clinical evaluation.

Management should include oxygenation and, if necessary, endotracheal intubation and mechanical ventilation. Morphine, 5 to 15 mg intravenously, is useful to reduce anxiety. In the acute phase of cardiac failure, prompt diuresis is one of the cornerstones of therapy. Furosemide, 40 to 80 mg intravenously, and repeated as necessary, is the drug of choice. Serume electrolyte levels should be followed and abnormalities treated. Digitalization may be useful in some patients, especially those with a supraventricular arrhythmia with a rapid ventricular response. In patients who have not had any digitalis in the preceding 2 weeks, a loading dose of 0.5 mg of digoxin can be given intravenously, followed by maintenance doses of 0.25 mg every 2 to 4 hours (Table 17-5).

Meticulous control of fluid intake, with fluid restriction, is essential. Serum electrolyte levels and the clinical response of the patient will direct further therapy. Fetal status should be determined as soon as it is practical. Invasive monitoring may be necessary, but in most circumstances, it is preferable to place the required catheters at the receiving hospital. The diagnostic studies and therapeutic maneuvers needed prior to transport will vary for each patient. However, as in all transfers, the patient must be medically stable enough to be moved. Thus, enough evaluation and treatment must be accomplished to ensure a safe trip for the mother and fetus.

RENAL FAILURE

Renal failure is an unusual indication for obstetrical referral. Most of these patients are sufficiently stable to tolerate transport with minimal stabilization. In the obstetrical patient, acute renal failure most commonly occurs secondary to an episode of hypotension. Because hypotensive episodes are more likely to occur during the intrapartum or postpartum periods, renal failure is more likely to occur in the postpartum period than in the antepartum period.

There are three major classifications of renal failure:

1. Prerenal—due to insufficient renal perfusion
2. Renal structural disease—from ischemia, nephrotoxic drugs, or congenital abnormalities and
3. Postrenal causes—which are obstructive in nature

On initial evaluation of a patient with renal failure, the history will usually lead to a classification of the disease. Physical examination often provides little useful information, although the presence of costovertebral angle tenderness or low back pain, or both, may suggest a renal infection or acute ureteral obstruction. A urine specimen via a catheter should be obtained to look for evidence of infection (white blood cells), trauma to the urinary tract (hematuria), and to assess renal function (concentration of urine electrolytes and osmolality). Serum electrolytes should also be determined.

The majority of patients will not require any special therapy prior to transport. Abnormal levels of serum electrolytes should be treated as necessary. Fluids should be provided as indicated. In patients with renal failure caused by hypotension, rigorous treatment with intravenous fluids and blood is essential. Assessment of fetal status should be accomplished and documented.

### Evaluation of Fetal Status

Evaluation of fetal status should commence with an estimate of gestational age. This estimate can be best accomplished by reviewing available data. Review of prenatal records and ultrasound examinations, discussion with the patient as to date of conception and method of contraception, measurement of fundal height, and determination of an estimated fetal weight are all helpful (Table 17-6). Once these data have been collected, consideration of the probable gestational age should be included in the decision whether or not to transport the patient. If the fetus is previable (see under Evaluation of Obstetrical Status) with good dating, then transport may not be appropriate.

Further evaluation should include assessment of fetal heart tones and the presence or absence of fetal compromise. Test results useful to review include the results of nonstress tests, oxytocin challenge tests, and fetal biophysical profiles.

Finally, ultrasound and other reports (such as chorionic villus sampling or genetic amniocentesis results) should be reviewed to rule out significant fetal abnormalities that might be lethal and significantly alter the management of the patient. It would seem appropriate not to transport those patients in whom a known lethal fetal anomaly is present, assuming there are

*Table 17-6. Evaluation of gestational age*

1. Last menstrual period
2. Type of contraception
3. Fetal heart tones first heard with a fetoscope
4. Fundal height
5. Uterine size at first examination
6. Time of first fetal movement
7. Ultrasound reports
8. Review of prenatal records

no associated maternal complications. However, the referral of such a patient may be necessary due to difficulty on the part of the referring physician in dealing with patients who have a fetus with a severe anomaly. His or her anxiety may be due to a psychological inability to handle the emotions of the parents or a lack of secure knowledge regarding any further evaluation that might be required or recommendations that should be made.

Maternal transport may be indicated because the neonate will require surgery soon after delivery. The consulting obstetrician and transport team must ensure that the appropriate pediatric surgical staff have been informed of the case and will be available when the patient arrives at the receiving center. Great care should be taken to ensure that these patients will not deliver during the transport. Preferably these patients should be handled by consultation and transfer well before the onset of labor.

## Evaluation of the Stage of Labor

The primary question to answer is "Will this patient deliver while being transferred?" Determination of the presentation of the fetus and effacement and dilatation of the cervix must be accurate. If the cervix is effaced or dilated, then further evidence of labor should be looked for, such as the strength, duration, and frequency of contractions and the presence of ruptured membranes. A patient who is in labor can be safely transported if labor can be stopped, or if the transport team can be certain that neither delivery nor any other complication will occur during the transport. These criteria are discussed in detail in the following sections.

## Evaluation of Obstetrical Status

Three basic areas will be covered, because these represent the most common reasons for transport of the pregnant patient. They include premature rupture of the membranes, preterm labor, and preeclampsia.

PREMATURE RUPTURE OF MEMBRANES

Premature rupture of membranes (PROM) is the reason for transfer in approximately one-half of all patients transported to the George Washington University Hospital. The main reasons for transferring a patient with PROM include prematurity and presumed evidence of fetal infection.

At George Washington University Hospital the philosophy has been to accept all patients when the referring hospital/physician is not comfortable about his or her ability to provide optimal care. The indication varies from hospital to hospital, but most referrals are at less than 34-weeks' gestation. It is difficult to determine a cutoff at the lower gestational ages. There is some variability from hospital to hospital as to what is considered the youngest fetus that has potential for reasonably intact survival. A gestational age of 20 weeks or less is an absolute criterion for nonintervention and, in the event of PROM, termination of pregnancies of less than 24-weeks' gestation may be indicated. The problem is compounded in those cases where there are uncertain dates. We tend to transfer the patient if the gestational age of the fetus is in doubt.

Between 24- and 36-weeks' gestation the management of a patient with PROM prior to transport is usually straightforward. First, rupture of the membranes must be confirmed. This evaluation can be done by examining fluid obtained from the posterior vaginal vault and looking for evidence of ferning, a positive nitrazine test, vaginal pooling of amniotic fluid, or a combination of these. Once PROM has been confirmed, the status of the cervix should be ascertained.

The decision whether or not to transport requires consideration of the distance and time involved. In patients with cervical dilatation to greater than 3 to 4 cm, transport may not be appropriate unless immediate helicopter transport is available. If there is evidence of labor, it must be ascertained as far as possible that delivery will not occur during the transport. While tocolytics are not routinely recommended for patients with PROM, it is appropriate to provide tocolysis to prevent delivery during a transport. The presentation of the fetus should be determined and prolapse of the umbilical cord ruled out. Following this, attention should be turned to the fetus, looking for evidence of fetal distress and signs of fetal infection.

PRETERM LABOR

In our experience this complication accounts for over one-third of maternal transports. The patient should have a pelvic examination to determine the extent of cervical dilatation and effacement; fetal presentation; and the presence of complications, such as a prolapsed umbilical cord. Since PROM often occurs in these patients, a sterile speculum examination is essential. In patients who have uncomplicated labor without PROM, management should include transport via stretcher and treatment with a tocolytic agent. The use of three tocolytic agents, ritodrine hydrochloride, magnesium sulfate, and terbutaline sulphate, will be discussed.

*Ritodrine Hydrochloride*
One hundred fifty mg ritodrine hydrochloride (three ampules) mixed in 500-ml fluid will give a concentration of 0.3 mg/ml. The ritodrine should be mixed with 0.9% sodium chloride solution, 5% dextrose solution, 10% dextran 40 in 0.9% sodium chloride solution, Ringer's lactate solution, or Hartman's solution, as clinically indicated.

The intravenous dosage should start at 0.05 mg/minute and be increased every 10 to 30 minutes by 0.05 mg/minute until either (1) a maximum dose of 0.35 mg/minute is reached, (2) labor stops, or (3) evidence of maternal toxicity occurs, as indicated by symptoms such as chest pain, heart rate greater than 150 bpm, apprehension, and hypotension. Serious toxicity can result in pulmonary edema [2, 3, 8].

If there is difficulty safely maintaining a constant intravenous infusion rate during transport, intramuscular administration of ritodrine may be preferable to intravenous administration:

1. Administer ritodrine 10 mg intramuscularly.
2. Subsequent doses of 5 to 10 mg may be given every 2 to 4 hours prn.
3. Intravenous ritodrine is initiated on arrival at the tertiary center.

*Magnesium Sulfate*
Magnesium sulfate should be given slowly as a 4-g intravenous bolus, followed by a maintenance dose of 2 to 3 g intravenously per hour. The lowest effective maintenance dose should be used in order to avoid hypermagnesemia, which may be toxic to both mother and fetus. The loss of the patellar reflexes is evidence that toxic levels of magnesium sulfate have been reached. The most serious complication of magnesium therapy is respiratory depression.

*Terbutaline Sulfate*
Terbutaline can be given intravenously. However, in the acute case, our protocol is to use it either intramuscularly or subcutaneously, with oral maintenance doses once labor has been stopped. The usual intramuscular or subcutaneous dose is 0.25 to 0.50 mg every 3 to 4 hours. If used intravenously, it can be infused at a rate of 0.01 to 0.08 mg/minute, depending

Table 17-7. Drugs used to treat preterm labor

| Method of administration | Ritodrine hydrochloride | Terbutaline sulfate | Magnesium sulfate |
|---|---|---|---|
| IV | 0.05–0.35 mg/min | 0.01–0.08 mg/min | 4-g bolus, then 2–3 g/hr |
| IM | 5–10 mg every 2–4 hrs | 0.25–0.50 mg every 3–4 hrs | |
| PO | 10–20 mg every 2–4 hrs | 2.5–5.0 mg every 2–4 hrs | |

on the frequency of uterine contractions. Oral terbutaline can then be given every 2 to 4 hours in doses of 2.5 to 5.0 mg (Table 17-7).

Combination drug therapy for preterm labor is not usually recommended because the incidence of therapeutic complications is significantly increased [4].

SEVERE PREECLAMPSIA AND ECLAMPSIA

Occasionally it is necessary to transport a patient with severe preeclampsia or, rarely, overt eclampsia. The stabilization of such patients for transfer is similar to the standard treatment of the hospitalized patient. The therapeutic priority in dealing with an eclamptic patient is to control convulsions using intravenous magnesium sulfate. The protocol used at Parkland Memorial Hospital is outlined in Table 17-8 [10].

When convulsions occur in a patient who is already on magnesium sulfate, another anticonvulsant agent may be used. Drugs such as Valium, 5 mg, or a short-acting barbiturate such as pentobarbitol, 125 mg, can be given intravenously. As with magnesium sulfate therapy, there is a risk of respiratory depression. Medical staff should be prepared to treat this complication with endotracheal intubation and mechanical ventilation until spontaneous respiration is restored.

Patellar reflexes should be followed to help adjust the amount and frequency of maintenance doses of magnesium sulfate, and urine output should be followed. Dosage adjustment must be done with particular care in patients with impaired renal function. Minimal adequate urine output is 25 to 30 ml/hour. If significant respiratory depression occurs, mechanical ventilation should be initiated immediately and the patient treated with calcium gluconate, 10 ml of a 10% solution given intravenously over 3 minutes [7].

The next therapeutic priority includes the control of hypertension and determination of fetal status. Maternal blood pressure greater than 160/110 mm Hg should be treated with an antihypertensive agent. Hydralazine in

5- to 10-mg doses can be given intravenously at 15- to 20-minute intervals, until adequate blood pressure control is demonstrated. The dose of hydralazine can then be adjusted as necessary to maintain appropriate blood pressure levels. The aim should not be to normalize the blood pressure, but rather to maintain systolic pressure below 160 mm Hg and diastolic pressure between 90 and 110 mm Hg.

Appropriate monitoring should include ongoing measurement of the fluid intake (the patient should not be receiving anything by mouth), urine output (a Foley catheter should be in place), and blood pressure (maintain blood pressure < 160/110). Fetal heart tones should be checked periodically, preferably every 15 minutes until continuous fetal monitoring can be done.

The protocol for patients with severe preeclampsia without convulsions is the same as outlined in Table 17-8, with the omission of step 3.

Diuretics should be avoided in the management of preeclampsia and eclampsia. Intravenous fluids should be limited to no more than 150 ml/hour, and invasive monitoring techniques are best delayed until the patient reaches the receiving hospital. Other laboratory studies, which may be helpful in determining the severity of the disease but are not essential prior to transfer, include a platelet count, fibrin split products, plasma fibrinogen, and serum glutamic-oxaloacetic transaminase.

*Table 17-8. The Parkland Memorial Hospital protocol for treatment of preeclampsia and eclampsia with magnesium sulfate\**

---

STEP 1

Four g of magnesium sulfate as a 20% solution is given intravenously over 4–5 minutes. At the same time, 10 g of magnesium sulfate as a 50% solution is injected IM in two divided doses deeply in the upper outer quadrants of the buttocks.
If the convulsions have stopped, then proceed with step 3. However, if the convulsions do not cease promptly, then proceed with step 2.

STEP 2

Two g of magnesium sulfate as a 20% solution is given IV over 2 minutes. Repeat the dose if needed, especially if the patient is large.
Once convulsions have stopped, proceed with step 3.

STEP 3

Five g of magnesium sulfate in a 50% solution is given IM deeply in the upper outer quadrants of alternate buttocks every 4 hours. Alternatively, maintenance doses of magnesium sulfate may be given intravenously at a rate of 1–3 g/hour.

---

\*From Pritchard, J. A., Cunningham, L. E., and Pritchard, S. A. The Parkland Memorial Hospital protocol for treatment of eclampsia: Evaluation of 254 cases. *Am. J. Obstet. Gynecol.* 148:951, 1984.

In summary, the management essentials for these patients prior to and during transport include

1. Avoiding convulsions
2. Avoiding delivery during the transport
3. Assessment of fetal status

### Problems Encountered During Transport

Optimum care for the maternal-fetal unit must continue during the transport. Normal vital signs must be maintained and medications continued as indicated. All patients must have an intravenous line started prior to transport if they are bleeding or if there is any possibility that medications will have to be given during transit. The environment in an ambulance, medevac helicopter, or airplane is very different from that of the labor room. Patient management in a very confined space can be complex. It is not usually possible to provide optimum delivery care for the high-risk mother or fetus in an ambulance. It is virtually impossible to perform some procedures, such as a cesarean section, forceps or vacuum delivery, in such a confined area. Even a simple procedure, such as repair of an episiotomy, is a major undertaking in a transport vehicle. Thus, it is imperative that, whenever possible, delivery or other complications be avoided during the transport.

The limited amount of equipment available during a transport is another constraint on the capabilities of the transport team. It is essential to be familiar with the equipment available on an individual transport vehicle. The team should bring with them any special equipment needed for a particular patient.

The amount of noise and movement present in a transport vehicle should not be underestimated. These factors are most significant in a small helicopter. In these vehicles, the amount of working space available is extremely limited, the noise from the engines and rotors may be so excessive that even to determine blood pressure may be impossible, and unanticipated movement of the aircraft can occur in any direction or in several directions at once. Similar problems are experienced in small fixed-wing aircraft. If distance considerations and the clinical condition of the patient allow, road transport offers the advantage that an ambulance can stop on the side of the road if necessary, and thus allow emergency procedures to be performed on a stable platform. In a ground ambulance a little room can be gained by opening the doors.

Finally, it should be remembered that as an aircraft ascends, the atmospheric pressure decreases, except in aircraft that have pressurized cabins.

Most commercial and military aircraft maintain a cabin pressure approximately equal to the atmospheric pressure that would be found at an elevation of 7000 ft above sea level. Since most nonpressurized transport aircraft do not exceed a maximum height of 3000 ft, the decrease in atmospheric pressure is not a problem except in some special cases such as the patient with cardiopulmonary disease, a pneumothorax (which may expand as the atmospheric pressure decreases), or sickle cell disease (a decrease in atmospheric pressure, with resulting decrease in blood $PO_2$, may precipitate a hemolytic crisis). It is imperative to have adequate oxygen supplies and equipment on board. It should also be remembered that in aircraft capable of high-altitude flight, such as commercial jets, which typically cruise at 30,000 to 40,000 ft above sea level, there is a remote possibility of total loss of cabin pressure. For example, this could occur if a door should open unexpectedly in flight. If a drop in atmospheric pressure might prove disastrous to a patient, a risk-benefit determination should be made and an alternative method of transport considered.

## References

1. *Advanced Trauma Life Support Course for Physicians.* Chicago: American College of Surgeons, 1984. P. 305.
2. Beall, M. H., Edgar, B. W., et al. A comparison of ritodrine, terbutaline, and magnesium sulfate for the suppression of preterm labor. *Am. J. Obstet. Gynecol.* 153(8):854, 1985.
3. Bendetti, T. J. Maternal complications of parenteral-sympathomimetic therapy for premature labor. *Am. J. Obstet. Gynecol.* 145(1):1, 1983.
4. Ferguson, J. E., Hensleigh, P. A., and Kredenster, D. Adjunctive use of magnesium sulfate with ritodrine for perterm labor tocolysis. *Am. J. Obstet. Gynecol.* 148:166, 1984.
5. Jacobs, M. M., Knight, A. B., and Arias, F. Maternal pulmonary edema resulting from betamimetic and glucocorticoid therapy. *Obstet. Gynecol.* 56:56, 1980.
6. Kauppilov, A., Tuimala, R., Ylikorkala, O., et al. Effects of ritodrine and isoxsuprine with and without dexamethasone during late pregnancy. *Obstet. Gynecol.* 51:288, 1978.
7. McCubbin, J. H., Sibai, B. M., Abdella, T. N., et al. Cardiopulmonary arrest due to acute maternal hypermagnesemia. *Lancet* 1:1058, 1981.
8. Nimrod, C. A., Beresford, P., et al. Hemodynamic observations on pulmonary edema with a beta-mimetic agent: A report of two cases. *J. Reprod. Med.* 29:341, 1984.
9. Porte, D., Jr., and Halter, J. B. The Endocrine Pancreas and Diabetes Mellitus. In R. H. Williams (ed.), *Textbook of Endocrinology.* (6th ed.). Philadelphia: W. B. Saunders, 1981.
10. Pritchard, J. A., Cunningham, L. E., and Pritchard, S. A. The Parkland Memorial Hospital protocol for treatment of eclampsia: Evaluation of 245 cases. *Am. J. Obstet. Gynecol.* 148:951, 1984.

# VI

# *Transport of the High-Risk or Sick Neonate*

# 18

# Defining the Indications for Neonatal Transport in a Perinatal Referral Network

Albert L. Bartoletti

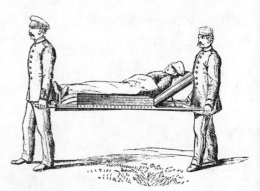

*18A. Contrivance used as a hand litter designed for conveying a recumbent patient in a compartment of a first-classs railway carriage. "This form of litter is stated to have been found very useful during the war of 1866 on the Baden Railways, especially for the transport of wounded officers." (Reproduced from Longmore, T. A* Treatise on the Transport of Sick and Wounded Troops. *London: Her Majesty's Stationery Office, 1869.)*

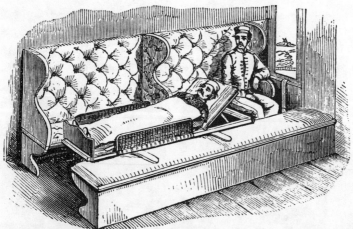

*18B. The contrivance shown in 18A in use within the carriage. A type 5 sick transport conveyance (conveyance moved by steam power). ". . . Its expense, however, not simply as regards the cost of the stretcher itself, but also in respect to the amount of space occupied by it, for there would only be room in the compartment of the carriage for an attendant beside the patient, would probably mitigate against its adoption for the general purposes of military transport; still for occasional special cases its use may be found desirable." (Reproduced from Longmore, T. A* Treatise on the Transport of Sick and Wounded Troops. *London: Her Majesty's Stationery Office, 1869.)*

The transport of high-risk obstetrical patients and neonates to regional care centers is considered an essential component of optimal perinatal care in the United States. Review of statistics from the Albany Medical Center, the sole perinatal/neonatal tertiary care center for a 20-county region of northeastern New York State, reveals that as the number of maternal transports has steadily increased, the number of neonatal transports has also increased. Although these trends seem contradictory, the following conclusions can be drawn:

1. The number of seriously ill neonates delivered at Level I or II hospitals because of sudden onset, life-threatening maternal/fetal conditions that preclude maternal transport remains significant.
2. Many neonates are transported for management of anomalies that are not detected prior to birth.
3. Obstetrical transport remains underused.
4. The indications for neonatal transport have changed. Infants previously considered too small for survival or too sick to transport and those with problems formerly managed at the community hospital (e.g., various respiratory problems, infections, and exchange transfusions) are now being transported.

There is no doubt that multispecialty, optimally staffed, well-equipped tertiary care centers offer advantages to high-risk obstetrical and very sick neonatal patients that Level I and II hospitals cannot provide. However, tertiary care resources are limited, and every effort must be made to use these scarce resources efficiently.

Defining the indications for neonatal transport is difficult because each referral region, hospital, and patient is, in some way, unique. The process of developing guidelines for obstetrical and neonatal consultation and referral, with emphasis on optimal communication between referring and receiving hospitals, will be discussed in this chapter.

### The Consultation and Transfer Agreement

The decision to transport a patient should be made when the patient's problem requires a level of care greater than that which can be provided by the referring institution. Conditions that require patient transport from one institution do not necessarily apply for another. Circumstances within an institution can change from one day to the next with the presence or absence of highly motivated, well-trained physicians, nurses, or respiratory therapists; however, it should be recognized that the level of care designated for an institution is based on the presence of a complete team of skilled professionals who are present to provide that level of care 24 hours per day.

It is not possible to formulate an extensive list of conditions requiring referral that is applicable to all hospitals. Instead, an agreement that establishes guidelines for obstetrical or neonatal consultation and transfer can be devised by staff at the regional center with the cooperation of representatives from each of the referring hospitals. The agreement should address all aspects of transport as they apply to each institution. In its final form it should include the following:

1. Statement of purpose
2. Composition of the transport committees representing each institution
3. Mechanisms for evaluating standards of care
4. Guidelines for consultation and transfer
5. Methods for accomplishing consultation and transfer
6. Provisions for continuing medical education
7. Consideration of general issues such as liability, reimbursement, resolution of disputes, and duration of agreement

The purpose of an interhospital consultation and transfer agreement for high-risk obstetrical and neonatal patients is to ensure the availability of optimal care for all such patients served by either institution. Optimal care can best be accomplished by establishing effective communication between the institutions.

TRANSPORT COMMITTEE
Representatives at each hospital should participate in a transport committee whose purpose is to review all aspects of interhospital care. The committee should consist of physicians and nurses representing obstetrics and pediatrics, or in the case of the regional center, the perinatal and neonatal services, and representatives from respiratory therapy, discharge planning, and social services, the ambulance companies, and the administrations of each hospital.

In addition to serving as a means for improved communication, other functions of the transport committee include

1. Evaluation of services provided by each institution
2. Establishment of guidelines for perinatal/neonatal evaluation and transfer
3. Organization of educational and training programs related to interhospital care

4. Collection of data relating to the transport process as it applies to the network in general and to each institution in particular

The importance of each of these functions is obvious and yet, without a formal transport agreement, they are rarely realized. The transport committee serves as fact finders. The contents of the consultation and transport agreement are based on conclusions concerning the availability of pertinent resources at each institution.

Each representative (e.g., physician, nurse, or respiratory therapist) on a transport committee must establish communication with counterparts serving on other transport committees in the referral network, for the purpose of defining limits of care. One defines limits of care by identifying and quantifying essential resources including nonhuman resources (equipment, laboratory and x-ray support, patient care facilities) and the availability of competent physicians, qualified nurses, respiratory therapists, social workers, and other ancillary personnel.

The availability of nurses and physicians competent to provide care to neonates is the most important factor in defining the limits of care. The American Academy of Pediatrics and the American College of Obstetricians and Gynecologists' *Guidelines for Perinatal Care* [1] suggests that at least one registered nurse be available for each high-risk obstetrical patient and for each critically ill neonate. This requirement alone is often beyond the staffing capabilities of hospitals with small obstetrical services. In addition, the nurses must be skilled in providing neonatal care.

For intermediate level care of neonates, one registered nurse must be available for every three to four patients during all shifts. These nurses must also be skilled in neonatal resuscitation, estimation of gestational age, physical diagnosis of neonatal illness, gavage feeding, and oxygen monitoring.

The guidelines for physicians are not as easily defined. Knowledge of neonatal resuscitation, fluid and electrolyte administration, respiratory management, and nutritional support is essential. In addition, technical skills such as endotracheal intubation, insertion of peripheral intravenous lines, blood sampling, thoracentesis, and umbilical vessel catheterization are important. Many of these skills require frequent application to maintain proficiency.

Ancillary services such as respiratory therapy, blood banking services, blood gases, and other essential laboratory services must be available on a 24-hour basis. These services are required for the provision of even the most basic emergency neonatal care. Thus, in circumstances where they are not available, it is strongly recommended that maternal transfer be accomplished as soon as a high-risk factor is recognized that could result in the birth of a critically ill infant.

GUIDELINES FOR CONSULTATION AND TRANSFER
Sometimes transport of the mother before delivery cannot be safely accomplished because of certain circumstances. These include nonmedical conditions that would jeopardize the safety of the mother or fetus during transport (e.g., inclement weather, mechanical breakdown, or lack of patient cooperation). Under these circumstances preconceived emergency measures must go into effect. These include mobilization of appropriate medical experts to be present at delivery, and, if time permits, communication with the tertiary center most likely to become involved with the infant's postnatal care. A review of the principles of neonatal stabilization with the consult, including respiratory and pharmacological support, thermoregulation, and fluid administration may be helpful under these circumstances. Once birth occurs, and while the transport team is en route, additional consultative advice can more specifically address those neonatal problems that exist.

All consultative calls should be documented by the physician initiating the call and by the neonatologist receiving the call at the regional center. A central registry of telephone consultations should be maintained at both institutions and should be reviewed at least annually by a neonatologist and perinatologist during an on-site visit.

A list of medical and surgical conditions that commonly require consultation and possible transfer to a regional center is given in Table 18-1. Transfer is initiated by a consultative discussion between the primary physician at the referring hospital and a neonatologist or postdoctoral fellow in neonatology at the regional center. Any call concerning the care of a neonatal patient should be considered a consultative call until agreement is reached that transport is indicated. At no time should a neonatal transport occur without a telephone consultation and discussion of the treatment to be rendered prior to and during the transport. The means of accomplishing transport and the type of personnel necessary to accompany the patient should be determined by the consultant or the medical director of transport at the regional center.

OTHER COMPONENTS OF THE TRANSPORT AGREEMENT
Appropriate patient history data, laboratory and radiological data, specimen samples, and a summary of the infant's course at the referring hospital should be furnished to the neonatal transport team. Additionally, the referring hospital should agree to:

*Table 18-1. Some abnormalities in the neonate for*
*which consultation with a neonatologist is recommended*

1. Infants with severe perinatal asphyxia
    a. Apgar scores of 3 or less at 5 minutes
    b. Requirement for ventilation greater than 15 minutes in the delivery room.
       (Ventilation is defined as by ambu bag and mask and/or by endotracheal
       intubation with ambu bag or ventilator assistance.)
    c. Infant's clinical condition not stable by 1 hour of age because of conditions
       such as:
        1. Unstable blood pressure
        2. Severe metabolic acidosis
        3. Abnormal neurological examination
        4. Seizures
        5. Apnea or bradycardia, or both
        6. Persistent cyanosis or hypoxia
2. Infants with respiratory problems
    a. Meconium below the vocal cords
    b. Premature or term infants with immediate symptoms of respiratory dis-
       tress or who require supplemental oxygen for more than 2 hours
    c. Premature or term infants delivered after 24 (> 12 hours if associated with
       labor) or more hours of ruptured membranes or delivered of mothers with
       symptoms of bacterial infection, or both
    d. Infants with congenital anomalies or air block complications resulting in
       symptoms of respiratory distress, or both
3. Premature infants less than 34-weeks' gestation
4. Infants who weigh less than 1800 g
5. Infants with central nervous system defects, injury, or infection, which may
   include:
    a. Microcephaly
    b. Hydrocephalus
    c. Myelomeningocele
    d. Meningitis
6. Infants with major congenital anomalies diagnosed within the first 28 days of
   life
7. Infants with a congenital intrauterine infection or an acquired infection
8. Infants who require an exchange transfusion for hyperbilirubinemia or
   polycythemia
9. Infants with persistent direct bilirubin level of greater than 3.0 mg/dl during
   the first 28 days
10. Infants with a positive metabolic screen
11. Infants of mothers taking hazardous drugs
12. Perinatal or neonatal blood loss or bleeding diathesis
13. Infants of diabetic mothers
14. Infants with symptoms of bowel obstruction or inflammation

1. Ensure that written, informed parental permission for transfer is obtained by the referring physician or a designee.
2. Ensure that the physician's order for transfer is written in the chart.
3. Provide records documenting all medical and nursing care rendered to the patient prior to arrival of the transport team.
4. Cooperate with the transport team on arrival; the attending physician and appropriate nurses should remain present until departure of the transport team from the facility.
5. Facilitate x-ray and laboratory services.
6. Provide cord blood, maternal blood, and other specimens (e.g., the placenta) requested by the transport team.
7. Maintain ongoing communication with the neonatal unit at the regional center.

The regional center should agree to:

1. Provide an exclusive telephone line for neonatal referrals.
2. Depart for transport within 30 minutes of receiving the request whenever possible.
3. Organize, train, and maintain personnel and equipment necessary for patient transport, in accordance with state, hospital, and other pertinent codes.
4. Take all necessary measures to ensure the safety of transport vehicles.
5. Provide periodic interim reports on the status of transported patients to the referring hospital and referring medical personnel.
6. Provide feedback or educational sessions in the form of transport review conferences every 4 to 6 months [2].

Through the coordinated efforts of the transport committees representing both the regional center and the referring hospital, a list of conditions, such as those listed in Table 18-1, for which consultation is recommended, should be developed and reviewed periodically during site visits. From this list a subgroup of conditions automatically indicating transport can be formulated. If agreement on these conditions cannot be reached by all referring physicians, the formal transport agreement should list those conditions that a majority of the involved physicians would consider indications for transfer (Table 18-2). The referring nursery should keep a record of consultative calls, transports, and infants who met the guidelines for transport but were not transported.

*Table 18-2. Conditions in the neonate for which transfer should be
considered from all level I and most level II hospitals in the United States*

Gestational age < 30–32 weeks (35–36 weeks for a Level I hospital)

Birth weight < 1250 g (1750–2000 g for a Level I hospital)

Respiratory problems anticipated to require mechanical ventilation for > 24 hours
   (> 1 hour in the case of a Level I hospital)

Major congenital anomalies (unless components of a readily recognizable lethal
   condition)

Neonatal seizures (transfer from a Level II hospital will depend on severity, duration, and local diagnostic facilities)

Conditions requiring surgical correction

Hemorrhage or bleeding diathesis[a]

Hyperbilirubinemia requiring exchange transfusion[a]

Asphyxia with multisystem involvement such as central nervous system, pulmonary, renal, gastrointestinal or hematological compromise (unless prognosis
   does not indicate aggressive therapeutic intervention)

Infants with persistent cyanosis/hypoxia

Septic or hypovolemic shock[b]

Persistent hypoglycemia[a]

[a]Level II hospitals with a large enough patient population to ensure that staff maintain the
required skills do not necessarily refer these infants.
[b]Infants with suspected or confirmed sepsis or meningitis should automatically be transferred
if the facility cannot provide continuous intravenous access.

BACK TRANSPORT OF INFANTS

When appropriate, infants should be transferred back to the referring hospitals for convalescent care. Through the efforts of the transport committees, a list of conditions compatible with back transport should be compiled
that is individualized to the capabilities of each referring hospital. The procedure for organizing the return transport is identical to that for transfer
to the regional center. Parental consent must first be obtained. (This is facilitated if the possibility of back transport is presented to the parents early in
the infant's hospitalization.) The physician who is to provide ongoing convalescent care is contacted directly by the neonatologist, fellow, or a designee from the regional center. A summary of the infant's course is provided, which details current therapy, anticipated long-term problems, and
recommended follow-up appointments. Acceptance by the physician is obtained, along with confirmation of bed availability, from the hospital to
which the infant is to be transported.

   The means of transport and the personnel necessary to accompany the
patient should be determined by the neonatologist or a designee at the regional center, following conversation with the physician assuming care.

CONTINUING MEDICAL EDUCATION
The content of the outreach educational program should be planned in consultation with the coordinator and medical director of the transport program and should include review of:

1. The management of patients transferred from the referring hospital to the regional center
2. Infants who met the requirements for consultation or transfer, or both, but remained in the community hospital
3. Management of return transports from the regional center

During outreach sessions, nursery and obstetrical units can be visited and patient care and transport protocols can be reviewed and updated.

GENERAL PROVISIONS OF THE
INTERHOSPITAL TRANSFER AGREEMENT
The transfer agreement must include a mechanism to resolve disputes. A mediation committee, consisting of representatives from the regional center and the referring hospital, can be established to consider the issues in dispute.

The transport agreement should be reviewed at least annually, with the understanding that it can be modified in writing at any time by mutual agreement of both parties. Formal communication should occur through the chairperson of each transport committee.

## Summary

Each regional center and referring hospital is unique in terms of the resources available for providing care. Thus, it is necessary that a means of establishing optimal communication between the two institutions be developed to achieve an efficient transport system. To accomplish this necessary objective, it is suggested that hospitals each develop transport committees that are charged with the task of reviewing all aspects of patient transport. By doing so, communication is established between physicians, nurses, respiratory therapists, and other personnel who play vital roles in accomplishing the safe transport of seriously ill obstetrical and neonatal patients.

## References

1. Brann, A. W., Jr., and Cefalo, R. C. (eds.). *Guidelines for Perinatal Care.* American Academy of Pediatrics/The American College of Obstetricians and Gynecologists, Evanston, Ill. 1983.
2. Philip, A. G. S., Little, G. A., and Lucey, J. F. *The transport conference as a teaching strategy. Perinatol-Neonatal.* 8 : 63–68, 1984.

# 19      *The Drama of Neonatal Transport*

Judith A. Cannon
Marilea K. Miller

*19A. Stretchers adapted to form part of the equipment of bearers. French soldier, equipped and armed. One of the traverses of the stretcher is carried on the knapsack. Half the sacking of the stretcher is worn around the waist. The scabbard that receives the iron part of the lance when the latter is used as one of the stretcher poles is at the soldier's side (right). The same soldier seen from behind. The legs of the traverse are received into two leather sheaths at the sides of the knapsack (left). A traverse separated from the knapsack (bottom). (Reproduced from Longmore, T.* A Treatise on the Transport of Sick and Wounded Troops. *London: Her Majesty's Stationery Office, 1869.)*

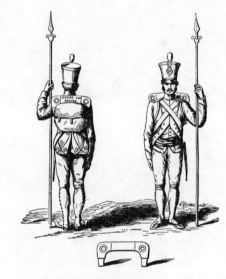

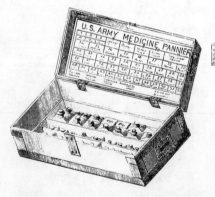

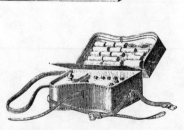

*19B. Portable medical supplies used during the Civil War. "The medicine chest and bulky hospital supplies were transported in wagons of the supply train, and were often inaccessible when most urgently required. To obviate this inconvenience, panniers were provided containing the most necessary medicines, dressings and surgical appliances." (Reproduced from* Reports on the Extent and Nature of the Materials Available for the Preparation of a Medical and Surgical History of the Rebellion. War Department, Surgeon General's Office, Circular No. 6, Nov. 1, 1865. Philadelphia: J. B. Lippincott, 1866.)

Smooth neonatal transports are like well-rehearsed plays or musicals. Clarity of communication, focus of resources, and repeated practice by experienced participants lead to polished performances and enhanced outcomes. Cooperation by group participants is essential, while individuals must remain receptive to direction and guidance. Occasionally, improvisation may be necessary; however, more often than not, a solid understanding of the role and the problems that must be confronted as well as prior study of the script or protocols will stand the cast and crew in good stead. Flexibility in the field is requisite and is an art.

Many hands work behind the scenes to enhance the production, to provide appropriate and safe props or equipment for the principals, and to keep the scenes moving and the vehicles ready for action. Considerable organization and forethought are needed by the support staff to provide these elements in a timely and safe fashion.

In this chapter we will discuss certain aspects of the drama of neonatal transport. We will focus on the mechanism and communications while describing the cast, crew, and the equipment and supplies needed for modern neonatal transports. In addition, we will emphasize the importance of the script or protocol book and the directors and their roles.

## *Orchestration and Choreography*

A well-established system is required to handle requests for the transfer of critically ill neonates from referring hospitals to neonatal intensive care units (NICUs). Effective communications, efficient dispatch of incoming calls, and determination of the mode, personnel, and equipment required cannot be left to chance or hurriedly arranged or assembled at the time of the call.

PATIENT REFERRAL

Referral calls requesting the transport of sick neonates may be received in several ways. In well-regionalized areas the telephone number of a regional perinatal dispatch center (RPDC) is distributed to all potential users of the transport system [10]. Funding for start-up costs of an RPDC may be sought from various grant agencies, whereas ongoing maintenance costs may be supported by participating hospitals (see Book Appendix 1 for a sample request for funds to initiate an RPDC). This RPDC number is usually toll free and has 24-hour accessibility. Other systems use direct phone-line connections between nurseries, computer linkups, or speed-call dialing systems. Regardless of the method used, incoming calls to the NICU must be answered promptly by someone who can screen the call, collect pertinent data, and immediately refer the call to an appropriate resource for further data collection, consultation, advice, and dispatch of a transport team, if indicated. For the system to work smoothly and efficiently, institutions or organizations providing neonatal transport services must have skilled personnel and appropriately equipped vehicles available 24 hours a day, 7 days a week.

Data collection begins with the initial call. The patient's name and location, names and telephone numbers of the referring hospital and referring physician, and nature of the primary problem can usually be obtained and documented by secretarial personnel. The caller can then be immediately referred to an appropriate contact person for further data collection. This contact person may be an appropriately oriented transport nurse, neonatologist, neonatology fellow, senior resident, neonatal nurse practitioner (NNP), charge nurse of the NICU, or other designated person depending on individual circumstances. To aid in data collection it is advisable to orient contact personnel and to use a standard form to collect information in an orderly manner (see Chapter Appendix II in Chapter 4). If referring hospitals are provided with copies of the standard form in advance, personnel there can assemble the required information prior to making the referral call. Important data or information to obtain for neonatal transports are listed in Table 19-1. After reviewing this information, the neonatologist can decide whether transfer is indicated and the caller may be advised on further interim management of the patient. The advice given should be carefully documented in case questions arise later concerning these recommendations.

MOBILIZATION OF THE PRIMARY CAST—THE TRANSPORT TEAM
Once the neonatologist has accepted a transfer and has given initial advice concerning further stabilization, the transport team must be promptly dispatched. Prompt dispatch is best accomplished if a designated transport team is available. The composition of the team will be determined by local resources, the mode of transport (air or ground), and how critically ill the infant is.

In many regions neonatal transport nurses, experienced NICU nurses who have received additional specialized training in the stabilization and management of sick neonates, are successfully used as team leaders [1, 4, 8, 9]. Job descriptions for the transport nurses are written to delineate their qualifications and duties (see Book Appendix 2). Their work requires periodic review by an expanded roles committee, the transport coordinator, and the medical director of the transport program. They are expected to study and to follow the carefully constructed scripts or protocols from

*Table 19-1. Basic information to obtain from referring hospitals*

Patient name
Birth date and time of birth
Location of patient (including floor and unit in hospital, city, and state)
Name of referring hospital and nursery telephone number
Name of referring physician and telephone number
Name of obstetrician
Caller's name and title
Mother's perinatal history
Neonate's gestational age
Birth weight
Type of delivery
Complications during labor or delivery
Apgar scores
Delivery room resuscitation required
Problems and subsequent medical management postdelivery
Vital signs
Blood glucose determination
Respiratory status including oxygen requirements, type of assisted ventilation, if
    any, and settings
Sites, types, and rates of parenteral infusions
X-ray results
Laboratory reports

which they work, under the direction of a designated physician. The protocols stipulate the limits of care that may be rendered independently and when consultation with the supervising physician is necessary.

Most transports require a two-person team. The second team member may be a second transport or NICU nurse, a neonatal nurse practitioner, a respiratory therapist, or a specially trained emergency medical technician (EMT) or paramedic. If available, an appropriately trained and well-oriented respiratory therapist (RT) can be very valuable, particularly when the neonate requires assisted ventilation. The RT is responsible for checking all respiratory support equipment before the team leaves the receiving hospital. His or her focus is on maintaining airway patency and providing adequate oxygenation and ventilation for the neonate during transport. If the respiratory equipment malfunctions during transport, the RT can troubleshoot and often correct the problem. In the absence of an RT on the transport team, the nurse team leader assumes this role.

A physician is not needed on every transport but may be required to accompany the team when the neonate is extremely unstable or requires medical skill not possessed by other team members. Some centers send a physician on all transports, often more for public relations, marketing, or staffing reasons than from actual necessity dictated by the condition of the patient. During the transport, it is extremely important that the transport team be able to contact the supervising neonatologist at all times by radio or telephone.

Team members involved in air transports should receive special training in flight physiology, safety, and survival. Ideally, they should be provided with flame-resistant uniforms. Knowledge of the effects of altitude and air transport on sick patients is essential as are their efforts to minimize the risks to the patient (see Chaps. 11 and 13).

PROPS, EQUIPMENT, AND SUPPLIES

To ensure safe transports and to properly treat and monitor patients, certain props, equipment, and supplies are necessary (Fig. 19-1). These include the following major items:

1. Transport incubator
2. Monitor(s) to continuously assess respiratory rate, heart rate, temperature, and arterial blood pressure
3. Parenteral infusion pumps
4. Transcutaneous monitors for the measurement of $PO_2$ and $PCO_2$, or a pulse oximeter, or all of these
5. Inspired oxygen concentration monitor
6. Ventilator
7. Oxygen tanks, hood, and tubing
8. Oxygen blender
9. Air compressor or air tanks
10. Heated humidification system for oxygen delivery
11. Suction apparatus
12. Bag and masks for assisted ventilation
13. Equipment for intubation, umbilical vessel catheterization, and chest tube placement
14. Tackle box or, preferably, soft-sided storage packs for medications and other supplies
15. Transport forms and permits kept on a clipboard or in a folder or notebook

At times the transport team may need and want to transport more than one neonate at a time. Under such circumstances two incubators and twice the amount of certain equipment will be needed.

Drugs or medications and supplies carried by the neonatal transport team should be kept to the minimum necessary for potential emergencies.

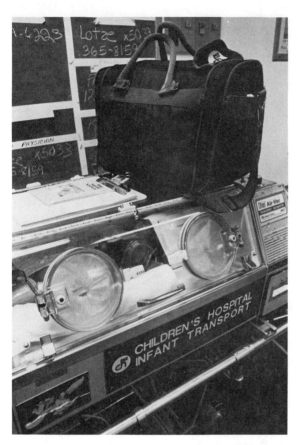

*Fig. 19-1. Transport equipment ready for use. (Copyright © 1987, David W. Wooddell. Reproduced with permission.)*

Careful consideration, however, must be given to the total time needed to complete the transport and to resources available at referring hospitals. The drugs and supplies should be systematically checked for disappearance or use by the transport nurse after each transport, and also daily for outdating (Fig. 19-2). Medications proposed for use during transport should be approved by the hospital pharmacy. As a rule narcotics are not stocked for use on neonatal transports but, if needed, may be requested at the referring hospital. Certain medications that should be kept refrigerated, such as pancuronium, or that are rarely used, such as prostaglandin $E_1$, may be taken on transports if there are specific indications. To keep medications cool during transports, they may be placed in a plastic bag or covered container on ice. (Lists of supplies and drugs carried by a typical busy neonatal transport service are listed in Chap. Appendix I and Book Appendix 6.)

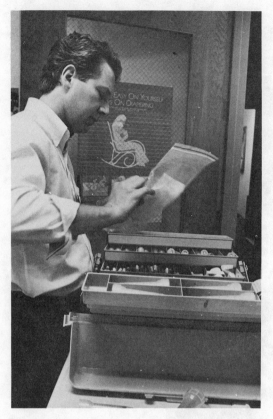

Fig. 19-2. A transport nurse checks the medication box
on completion of a transport. (Copyright 1987, David W.
Wooddell. Reproduced with permission.)

All vital equipment must be kept in good working condition, clean, and
readily available for use. This requires a dedicated and coordinated effort
and is often a source of bickering and quarrels. Specific individuals must be
assigned responsibility for the various aspects of preventive maintenance,
repair, preparation, and cleaning of equipment. If a piece of equipment
malfunctions, repair should begin immediately. In general, biomedical engineers will be needed and willing to perform major repairs and preven-
tative maintenance, but they will not always do so in the time frame that
transport team members may desire. Thus, certain pieces of equipment
should have backups in stock, so that transports will still be possible while
the original is repaired.

It is logical and prudent to assign the task of upkeep of the transport incubator and associated respiratory equipment to respiratory therapists or other personnel (e.g., cleaning technicians), but this step is not always possible. Contingency plans for cleaning major equipment have to be made for nights and weekends. Often, unfortunately, these tasks fall by default to the transport nurse.

The person who is responsible for each specific role in the preparation of the transport equipment should be asked to complete and sign a checklist to document thorough completion of the task. If there are problems later, the responsible individual can be directly counseled.

MODE OF TRANSPORT
The infant's condition, location, and the resources available at the referring hospital help to determine the mode of transport. There are advantages and disadvantages to all methods. Ground transport ambulances are usually most economical, but the time required to reach the patient must be determined and must not be excessive. Helicopters have the advantages of speed and ability to land at virtually all sites but have problems with space, noise, and vibration, and are unable to fly in certain weather conditions [7]. Helicopters are also expensive, unless used frequently. Fixed-wing aircraft that are pressurized and equipped to handle transport equipment are useful when traveling distances over 100 miles. They are not as noisy as helicopters, usually allow more room to work in, but must land at airports and require arrangements for connecting transportion (see Chaps. 4, 11, and 13) [1].

INITIATION OF TRANSPORT
An orderly dispatch system should exist to follow through with the organization of the transport vehicle and to provide details (e.g., estimated time of arrival) while the medical personnel plan the patient care aspects of the transfer.

Prior to leaving on a transport, the transport team should review all information and data collected from the referring hospital and develop a patient management plan with the neonatologist. All equipment should be checked to ensure adequate operation and sufficient supplies. A transport team member should call the referring hospital just before leaving to obtain updated information on patient status and to advise the referring hospital of the expected time of arrival.

THE TRANSPORT TEAM AT THE REFERRING HOSPITAL
On arrival at the referring hospital the transport team should introduce themselves to the personnel caring for the neonate, listen to a report of the

patient's condition following the last telephone contact, review all laboratory and x-ray data, check the neonate's identification band, and make a thorough physical assessment of the infant.

By assuming previously agreed on roles and responsibilities, transport team members will be able to "divide the labor" and save precious time (e.g., one transport team member may prepare and move the patient into the mobile intensive care module with the aid of staff at the referring hospital, while the other transport team member talks with the family). This coordination promotes speedy turn around time, which is especially important for air transports. Prolonged elapsed ground time is expensive and takes vehicles out of service, making them unavailable for other emergency transports.

Team members may occasionally need to work together to properly prepare the transport equipment or to do certain procedures to stabilize or prepare the infant for transport. Any stabilization required should be promptly but thoroughly performed to ensure a safe transport (see Chap. 20). During stabilization, attention must be given to maintaining adequate oxygenation of the neonate. A transcutaneous electrode or pulse oximeter may be applied to the infant for continuous monitoring, if indicated. Maintenance of normal body temperature is essential. This maintenance may require careful warming and the use of adjuncts such as caps, heat shields, and warming mattresses, in addition to a neutral thermal environment. Patients transported by air require particularly careful evaluation for and management of trapped gases, hypoxemia, and hypothermia. Specific measures to deal with these problems must be taken prior to flight [6].

While stabilizing the patient, it is essential that members of the transport team communicate effectively with the staff at the referring hospital. The transport nurse should inform the referring hospital nurse exactly when he or she is taking over aspects of the patient's care. Transport team members should be considerate and tactful when requesting help, medications, or supplies from referring hospital personnel. A demanding or disrespectful demeanor is extremely detrimental to referral relationships and rapport. Direct criticisms should be avoided, although alternative approaches may be diplomatically suggested. Clinical assessments and reasons for interventions should be explained. A transport team member can be an effective educator. If disagreements concerning management arise, direct phone contact between the referring physician and the supervising neonatologist is in order.

Equipment at the referring hospital may be used on request and serves the dual purpose of conserving transport supplies while allowing referring staff to see that they do have the means necessary to stabilize a similar neonate should the need arise again. After stabilization of the infant, all supplies (e.g., drugs and fluids) that are anticipated to be needed during transport should be prepared and secured for easy accessibility inside the transport incubator.

Transport personnel must also communicate with the family. Every effort should be made to allow parents to see and touch the infant prior to transport. Equipment in use should be explained to them, prior to viewing the neonate. A photograph of the infant is usually appreciated. The family should receive an honest appraisal of the neonate's condition and the short-term management plans. Any questions that the family have should be answered as completely as possible. They should be given both written and oral information concerning where the neonate will be taken, including directions to the receiving hospital. In addition, pertinent phone numbers and the names of personnel who will be caring for the neonate at the receiving medical center should be provided. If possible, a booklet describing the NICU, its equipment, medical terminology, and staffing hierarchy should be given to the parents. Information required from the parents includes family medical history, certain aspects of perinatal history, method of payment, and pertinent telephone numbers. Permission for the transport and for admission to the receiving NICU must also be obtained.

Just prior to leaving the referring hospital, the transport team should contact the receiving NICU to give an updated report on the neonate's condition, equipment and other needs on arrival, and the estimated time of arrival. Further consultation with the neonatologist can also be made to update the management plan during transit.

When the neonate is placed in the transport unit, care must be taken to secure the neonate and all equipment (Fig. 19-3). A final assessment should be made to ensure correct tube placements, patency of lines, and availability of emergency equipment. In most circumstances, a copy of the neonate's chart, a copy of the mother's chart, a tube of the mother's blood (for crossmatching purposes at the receiving hospital), and copies of x rays and laboratory results should be taken with the neonate. Many transport systems also request the placenta (which should not be placed in formalin) and a cervical culture from the mother. Gross and microscopic examination of the placenta may be helpful, particularly in cases of suspected intrauterine infection, hydrops fetalis, or multiple congenital anomalies.

THE TRANSPORT TEAM IN TRANSIT

Continuous monitoring of the neonate during transport is required. Ideally, parameters to be assessed include temperature, heart rate and rhythm, res-

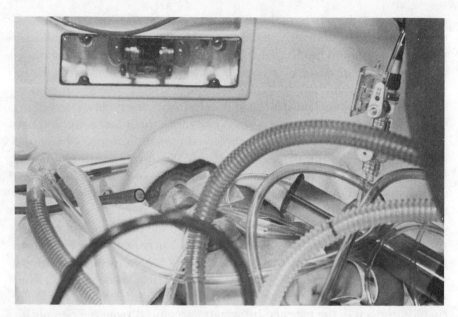

*Fig. 19-3. The principal character. A small premature infant leaving a referring hospital in a neonatal transport module. (Copyright ©1987, David W. Wooddell. Reproduced with permission.)*

piratory rate, blood pressure, ventilator settings (when in use), the concentration of oxygen administered, transcutaneous oxygen or pulse oximetry, and intravenous infusion rates. If stabilization at the referring hospital has been complete, little intervention will be required during transit. If transcutaneous monitoring or pulse oximetry is in use, adjustments to ventilatory support systems and fraction of inspired oxygen ($FiO_2$) can be made as indicated [3, 6]. Documentation of all assessments, monitoring, interventions, and reasons for such intervention should be made frequently on forms that become part of the infant's permanent hospital record on admission to the NICU (see examples in Chap. Appendixes II and III).

During transit, a telephone or radio communication system is required to advise the receiving NICU of any changes in the neonate's clinical status or to discuss management of unforseen complications not responsive to routine management, or both.

### ARRIVAL AT THE RECEIVING INSTITUTION

On arrival at the receiving NICU the neonate's condition should be immediately reassessed. Vital signs and, if appropriate, an arterial blood gas should be checked prior to removal from the transport unit, to document the patient's condition on admission and the response to transport. The transport team should assist the receiving staff in moving the neonate from the transport module to the bed, being careful not to dislodge any tubes. Once the neonate is settled, the transport team should give a thorough oral report to the physicians and nurses who are assuming care of the neonate. This report should include the perinatal history, medical management of the neonate prior to arrival of the transport team, clinical assessment and management by the transport team, all medication and fluids given, laboratory and x-ray results, the family's understanding of the neonate's condition, and any other pertinent data. All questions from receiving personnel should be answered. Copies of the written documentation of the transport care administered should be completed and placed in the neonate's medical record at the receiving hospital.

After the neonate is settled in the receiving bed, a telephone call should be made to the referring hospital staff and to the family to advise them of the infant's condition on arrival. All transport equipment and supplies should then be cleaned and restocked, in preparation for subsequent transports. Any problems encountered with equipment or the carrier should be documented, and appropriate action to correct problems should be taken immediately.

RETURN OR "BACK" TRANSFERS
Tertiary care level NICU beds can be best used when convalescent neonates are back transported to community hospitals (Fig. 19-4)[2,5]. Such transfers are facilitated when ongoing communication regarding the neonate's progress has occurred between the community hospital, the referring physician, and the NICU and when families have been prepared for the possibility from the outset. Assessment of candidacy for back transfer must take into account the abilities and limitations of the individual community hospital. An annually updated registry of criteria for back transfer, appropriate to each individual referring hospital, may be compiled by surveys taken of nurses and physicians at referring hospitals. In addition, the transport team can often be of help in determining which neonates can be safely back transferred, based on their direct knowledge of the personnel and equipment available at individual community hospitals.

Once a candidate for back transfer has been selected, the physician responsible for the neonate's care should call the referring physician at the community hospital to discuss future care needs and contact the parents to inform them of the plan. Once agreed on, the back transport can be optimally organized using a systematic completion checklist (see Chap. Appendix IV). A complete nursing summary (see Chap. Appendix V) and a

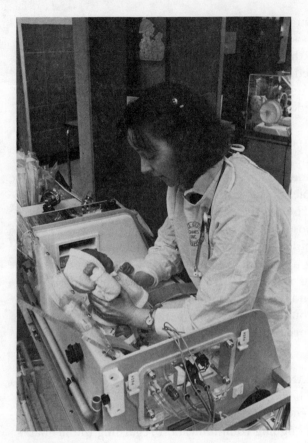

Fig. 19-4. A baby is prepared for back transfer to her hospital of birth.

physician's discharge summary should accompany the infant. In addition, copies of significant x rays and laboratory reports should be sent.

IN-HOUSE TRANSPORTS
When transport team members are not picking up neonates at referring hospitals, their expertise is frequently used to transport patients within the home base hospital (Fig. 19-5). Such transports are for procedures such as fluoroscopy, body imaging studies, cardiac catheterization, or surgery. The same careful approach to assessment, stabilization, and constant monitoring of the neonate's condition should be practiced as for any other transport. Particular attention should be paid to thermoregulation, patency of the neonate's airway, maintenance of endotracheal tubes in proper alignment and position, and adequacy of oxygenation. The use of transcutane-

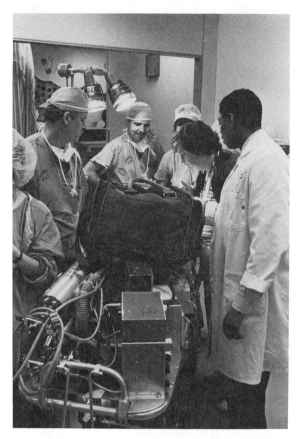

*Fig. 19-5. Intrahospital patient transport. The equipment and expertise of the newborn transport service is used to ensure optimal homeostatis for a premature infant during transport between the ICN and the operating room. (Copyright ©1987, David W. Wooddell. Reproduced with permission.)*

ous $PO_2$ and $PCO_2$ monitors or of oximeters during in-house transport is particularly helpful.

The advent of advanced life support techniques, such as extracorporeal membrane oxygenation (ECMO), has made many transport programs recognize a need to secure portable battery packs that can be used to support the considerable needs for electrical power that advanced forms of cardiopulmonary life support, such as an ECMO pump, demand during in-house transport. When relying on battery-operated equipment, transport personnel must meticulously check that batteries are fully recharged prior to each transport use. During procedures, such as surgery or radiographic studies, the apparatus should be plugged into the main electrical supply to conserve the battery power.

FOLLOW-UP AND QUALITY ASSURANCE

Regular oral and written reports regarding the status of transported neonates should be provided by tertiary care nursery personnel to nurses and physicians at referring hospitals, to the pediatrician, and, ideally, to the mother's obstetrician. Initially, at least, direct telephone communications are in order. Weekly written interim reports are also desirable but may be tedious and difficult to accomplish unless data and diagnoses are computerized. Transport team personnel's access to word processors may considerably lighten the load.

Regular follow-up staff meetings of the team members, the transport nurse coordinator, and the medical director for neonatal transports should include a review of recent difficult or interesting transports and should be structured to identify and correct any deficiencies in the transport mechanism or communications.

Case reviews should be performed to demonstrate both positive and negative approaches and results. Cases to be reviewed should meet certain selection criteria that might include (1) having educational merit, (2) exhibiting a repetitive problem or serious incident, (3) demonstrating a positive outcome, or (4) resulting in mortality or significant morbidity for the patient. Case reviews should include the initial information available to the receiving hospital, the response times, the initial assessment of the patient by the transport team, the clinical stabilization necessary, and the outcome (including autopsy findings, if pertinent). Additional aspects of care that should be addressed are adequacy of communications, equipment function or malfunction, and psychosocial issues. Important questions to be answered during case reviews are What went well?; What was unavoidable?; and What could have been improved during the transport? Documentation of the case reviews can be submitted for quality assurance purposes and should include the problem and issues, discussion, recommendations, actions taken, and follow-up plans (see Book Appendix 4).

In addition to case reviews, transport staff meetings may also include instruction on x-ray interpretation and differential diagnosis; discussion of feedback from transport reviews or families; development of new policies, procedures, or protocols and revision of previous ones; ventilation of feelings and impressions regarding overwhelming incidents that occurred during transport; equipment updates; reminders of the responsibilities of transport personnel regarding checks of equipment and follow-up commu-

*Table 19-2. Transport team performance—questionnaire for referral hospitals*

1. Was there an acceptable response time?
2. Were communications appropriate?
3. Did transport team members introduce themselves?
4. Did transport team members receive a report on the patient from referring hospital personnel?
5. Did transport team members stabilize the neonate prior to transport?
6. Were transport team members effective?
7. Were referring hospital personnel involved in stabilization of the patient?
8. Were questions of the referring hospital personnel answered appropriately?
9. Were families well informed about the problems of infant and short-term management plans?
10. Do you have any recommendations for future transports?

*Table 19-3. Transport team performance—questionnaire for families*

1. Did the transport team member explain the indications for transport of your infant?
2. Were you told by the transport team member what your infant's problems were thought to be and what procedures might be necessary to treat your infant?
3. Were you given information regarding visiting policies, telephone numbers, and directions to the receiving hospital nursery?
4. Were your questions answered?
5. Were you allowed to see the infant before the transport team left?
6. Do you have any recommendations for the transport team?

nications; and troubleshooting regarding interdepartmental or personnel disputes related to transport.

Close liaison of transport team members with the outreach education program will help to ensure that staff at referring hospitals receive appropriate educational input and appropriate praise when indicated.

As part of the quality assurance effort, questionnaires may be distributed to referring hospitals and families to receive their impressions of the adequacy of transport team performance. Items appropriate to such questionnaires are outlined in Tables 19-2 and 19-3.

Further quality assurance review is possible with the aid of monthly and annual transport statistics compiled by the transport team. This review will enable the program director to advise the hospital of communication problems, poor response times, shortages of personnel or vehicles, deficiencies in carrier performance, the lack of adequate numbers of neonatal beds, changing patterns for referrals, or needs for formalizing relationships or contracts for service with referring hospitals. Samples of monthly data kept by a busy neonatal transport service are given in Book Appendix 5. Computerization of the transport data and statistics allows for quick updates, retrieval, and analysis.

## The Script

Just as a script is essential for a play and the actors, so is a protocol manual essential for a neonatal transport program and the team members. If transport personnel are to serve in expanded roles and perform procedures or administer medications without a physician physically present, then the neonatal protocol manual becomes their guide and sanction for doing so. For medicolegal reasons, the protocol manual must be reviewed and be acceptable to the hospital administration, and it may require review by an expanded roles committee. The manual should include sections that delineate the following:

1. How to handle incoming transport calls
2. Physician supervision for the transport team
3. Determination of who goes on which transports
4. Management of return or back transfers
5. Protocol for general transport management
   a. General approach to the transport of neonates
   b. Transport care log
   c. Transport progress notes
6. Protocol for the care of premature infants
   a. General approach to the transport of premature infants
   b. Thermoregulation considerations
   c. Assessment of gestational age
7. Fluid management
8. Management of hypoglycemia
9. Oxygen administration and ventilatory support
10. Resuscitation of the neonate
11. Drug dosages and administration
12. Acid-base balance
13. Management of shock
14. Protocols for management of specific problems
    a. Hyaline membrane disease
    b. Transient tachypnea of the neonate
    c. Pulmonary hemorrhage
    d. Asphyxia
    e. Meconium aspiration

     f.  Persistent pulmonary hypertension
     g.  Seizures
     h.  Sepsis and meningitis
     i.   Hemolytic disease and hydrops fetalis
     j.  Congenital heart disease
     k.  Intestinal obstruction
     l.   Abdominal wall defects (gastroschisis and omphalocele)
     m. Tracheoesophageal fistula and esophageal atresia
     n.  Diaphragmatic hernia
     o.  Choanal atresia
     p.  Neural tube defects (meningomyelocele or meningocele)
     q.  Multiple congenital anomalies (genetic cases)
15. Protocols for procedures
     a.  Intravenous line placement
     b.  Umbilical vessel catheterization
     c.  Intubation of the trachea
     d.  Arterial puncture
     e.  Emergency evacuation of a pneumothorax

Standard operating procedures, which the transport nurse may initiate during stabilization and prior to consulting the supervising physician, may be denoted with an asterisk or other symbol in the transport protocol manual.

### *Directors*

The directors of the neonatal transport team are key individuals. If they are committed, knowledgeable, and enthusiastic, they foster the growth, depth, and quality of the program. Usually there are two directors for a neonatal transport program: the nurse coordinator and the medical director.

The transport nurse coordinator (see Book Appendix 3 for job description) is usually professionally responsible to the clinical unit nursing coordinator for the nurseries, while clinically responsible to the medical director of neonatal transport. The nurse coordinator is supervised during transport by the attending neonatologist on-service or on-call. He or she is usually an experienced registered nurse with advanced training, who has excellent management and interpersonal skills, practices as a transport nurse, and is the supervisor of the other transport nurses. He or she helps set standards for nursing care during transport, reviews transport equipment and equipment inventory lists regularly, and addresses problems and concerns regarding the availability of vehicles or equipment malfunction. He or she serves on the front line to settle disputes between transport personnel. The transport coordinator has responsibility for many administrative aspects of the infant transport system including preparing work and call schedules for transport nurses; maintaining monthly and yearly statistics for the transport system; evaluating the clinical performance of transport nurses; planning and participating in the orientation of new transport nurses; attending transport committee meetings; collaborating with the medical director, hospital administrator, and other team members to review policies, procedures, and standards; and helping prepare the transport budget. In addition, the transport nurse coordinator is the liaison for the outreach educators to identify the training needs of referring hospitals and with in-house nurse educators to ensure that ongoing educational programs are available for transport team members. The job is challenging, very demanding, and requires considerable maturity and remarkable organizational skills.

The medical director for neonatal transport, a neonatologist, works closely with the nurse coordinator. He or she sets standards for medical practice and safety during transport; participates in the development and updating of policies, procedures, and protocols in the transport manual; helps oversee major equipment purchases; and aids in correction of problems. He or she works with hospital administrators to develop a transport budget, promote cost containment, monitor safety, and delineate a marketing strategy. The medical director reviews new equipment available for neonatal transports and encourages replacement of old equipment prior to obsolescence or breakdown. The medical director participates in case reviews and helps teach team members; he or she is their mentor.

The directors of the transport program shape the dimensions and scope of the work that can be accomplished which requires long-range vision. They may choose to meet monthly to discuss goals and to review problems and plans for improving neonatal transports. Other key members who might be asked to attend such an administrative transport committee meeting include a designated hospital administrator, the director of respiratory therapy services, a representative of the contracted carriers, and a biomedical engineer.

## Denouement

The correct mix of many elements is required to bring a play or musical to an exciting and satisfying finale. Similarly, a well-organized and effective neonatal transport service requires an adequate referral base, clear communications, well-tested mechanisms, skilled team members, safe and reliable vehicles, adequate supplies, and well-serviced equipment. A carefully constructed script or protocol manual, dedicated transport directors, as well as other receptive and responsible members of the hospital staff and administration are also essential. As a drama unfolds, refinements are necessary. As transports are accomplished, review and reevaluation are vital to ensure that each performance is more polished than the last.

## References

1. Bose, C. L., Jung, A. L., and Thornton, J. W. Neonatal transport. The practical issues. *Perinat.-Neonat.* 8(5):61–73, 1984.
2. Bose, C. L., LaPine, T. R., and Jung, A. L. Neonatal back-transport. Cost effectiveness. *Med. Care* 23:14–19, 1985.
3. Clarke, T. A., Zmora, E., Chen, J., et al. Transcutaneous oxygen monitoring during neonatal transport. *Pediatrics* 65:884–886, 1980.
4. Cook, L. J., and Kattwinkel, J. A prospective study of nurse-supervised versus physician-supervised neonatal transports. *J. Obstet. Gynecol. Neonatal. Nurs.* 12:371–376, 1983.
5. Jung, A. L., and Bose, C. L. Back transport of neonates: Improved efficiency of tertiary nursery bed utilization. *Pediatrics* 71:918–922, 1983.
6. Miller, C., Clyman, R. I., Roth, R. S., et al. Control of oxygenation during the transport of sick neonates. *Pediatrics* 66:117–119, 1980.
7. Parsons, C. J., and Bobechko, W. P. Aeromedical transport: Its hidden problems. *Can. Med. Assoc. J.* 126:237–243, 1982.
8. Pettett, G., Merenstein, G. B., Battaglia, F. C., et al. An analysis of air transport results in the sick newborn infant: Part I. The transport team. *Pediatrics* 55:774–782, 1975.
9. Thompson, T. R. Neonatal transport nurses: An analysis of their role in the transport of newborn infants. *Pediatrics* 64:887–892, 1980.
10. Vogt, J. F., Chan, L. S., Wu, P. Y. K., et al. Impact of a regional infant dispatch center on neonatal mortality. *Am. J. Public Health* 71:577–582, 1981.

## Chapter Appendix I: Neonatal Transport Supplies

VENTILATORY SUPPORT SUPPLIES
1 laryngoscope handle
1 size 0 laryngoscope blade with $O_2$ port
1 size 1 laryngoscope blade with $O_2$ port
1 cut $O_2$ tubing to adapt for laryngoscope blade oxygen delivery
2 batteries
2 extra bulbs for laryngoscope
1 endotracheal locator gun
Two 4.0 endotracheal tubes (with magnetic strip if available)
Two 3.5 endotracheal tubes (with magnetic strip if available)
Two 3.0 endotracheal tubes (with magnetic strip if available)

Two 2.5 endotracheal tubes with magnetic strip
2 stylets
1 package oral airways (premature and newborn)
1 roll 1 inch cloth tape
1 scissors
5 ampules benzoin
1 Laerdal bag with masks, CPAP adapter, manometer, tubing
1 venti mask or nonrebreathing mask
1 pack transcutaneous monitor supplies
2 pulse oximeter sensors
1 each—extra small, small, and large CPAP nasal prongs
2 CPAP hats with ties
1 extra ventilator circuit with exhalation valve
Two 8F suction catheters
Two 6.5F suction catheters
1 suction connecting tubing
4 vials of normal saline for suctioning
1 suction cannister
2 portable suction units
VASCULAR ACCESS SUPPLIES
1 umbilical vessel catheterization tray
Two 5F umbilical catheters
Two 3.5F umbilical catheters
1 steri-drape
1 scalpel with No. 11 blade
1 stopcock
One 60-ml bottle povidone-iodine (Betadine) solution
1 sterile umbilical tape
One 4.0 silk suture on needle
Two size 15 Luer-tip adapters
Two size 18 Luer-tip adapters
One 20-ml vial of normal saline for injection
1 vial heparin 1000 U/ml
1 tape measure
Syringes—assorted
Needles—assorted
Alcohol impregnated swabs
Two 24-gauge Jelco catheters
Two 24-gauge Quick catheters
Two 22-gauge Quick catheters
Two 23-gauge butterfly needles
Two 25-gauge butterfly needles
2 arm boards
Rubber bands
1 razor
2 T-connectors
2 IV infusion plugs (heplock)
2 Y-connectors

3 extension sets, transducer sets
3 preheparinized syringes
Assorted blood tubes for micro-method and regular tests
Two packs of 2 × 2 inch sterile gauze sponges
2 Op-site dressings[a]
Syringe pumps
PNEUMOTHORAX SUPPLIES
2 10F chest tubes with trocars
2 12F chest tubes with trocars
2 steri-drapes
2 vaseline gauze dressings
2 Op-site dressings
2 5-in-1 adapters
2 Y-connectors
2 Heimlich valves
1 suction connecting tubing
2 C-clamps
2 18-gauge Jelco catheters or 2 Fox Pneumotap devices[b]
2 T-connectors
2 stopcocks
2 povidone-iodine (Betadine) swabs
1 roll cloth tape
1 portable transilluminator
MISCELLANEOUS SUPPLIES
1 8F nasogastric tube
1 5F nasogastric tube
1 10F Levin tube
Monitor patches, leads, temperature probes
BP transducer, cuffs
Ace bandages
Adaptic dressings
Porta-warm mattresses
Parent information books, permits, maps
Charts
Protocol manual
Camera and film
DRUGS
3 NaHCO$_3$ 1 : 1 Bristojets
1 epinephrine 1 : 10,000 Bristojet
1 atropine 0.1 mg/ml Bristojet
1 vial calcium gluconate
1 vial dopamine
1 vial dobutamine
1 vial tolazoline (Priscoline) with filter
2 vials 10% D/W vials
One 250-ml bottle 5% albumin
2 vials ampicillin
1 vial gentamicin

1 vial phenobarbitol
1 vial phenytoin (Dilantin)
1 vial heparin
1 vial furosemide (Lasix)
1 vial naloxone (Narcan)
1 vial pancuronium bromide (Pavulon)
1 vial $PGE_1$
Needles
Syringes
Medicine labels
IV labels
10 meclizine hydrochloride (Antivert) tabs (for staff)

---

[a]T. J. Smith and Nephew, Ltd., Hull, England. Distributed in the United States by Acme United Co., Bridgeport, Conn. 06609.
[b]MDI, Inc., West Conshohocken, Penn. 19428.

## Chapter Appendix II: Neonatal Transport Progress Notes

Transport Assessment Management Form

Patient's name _____

Date:          Time:                    ID Band ☐ ✔ if on patient

Resident/Attending Comments

(circle one)
Wt.      gms;   Length      cm;   H.C.      cm;   EGA      wks;   SGA, AGA, LGA

PE:        (✔ no abnormality; x abnormal; 0 not done)

General Appearance:                              Color:
HEENT:
    Head, fontanelle, sutures:
    Nose, mouth, palate:

CR:
    Chest, lungs, heart, pulses:

Abdomen:

Neurological:
Skin:

Extremities:
Other significant findings:

Lab, X-ray Data:

| Transport Problem List | Management Based on Protocols | Time | Outcome/ New Data |
|---|---|---|---|
| 1. | | | |
| 2. | | | |
| 3. | | | |
| 4. | | | |
| 5. | | | |

| Problem Number | Alteration in Management Based on M.D. Order | Time | M.D. Name | Outcome/ New Data |
|---|---|---|---|---|
| | | | | |
| | | | | |
| | | | | |
| | | | | |
| | | | | |
| | | | | |

Signatures:   Transport nurse: _____
Supervisory M.D.: _____        Transport physician: _____

## Chapter Appendix III: Transport Care Log

CHILDREN'S HOSPITAL NATIONAL MEDICAL CENTER—NICU
111 MICHIGAN AVE. N.W. WASHINGTON, D.C. 20010
202/745-5275

**TRANSPORT CARE LOG**     (enter "?" if unknown)

ADDRESSOGRAPH

TRANSPORT DIRECTION (circle only one):
1. Primary (patient to CHNMC) From:
2. Return (backtransport) To:
3. Shunt (transfer for other institution) From:
8. Other (specify)                      To:

TYPE TRANSPORT (circle all that apply):
1. Fixed wing aircraft
2. Helicopter
3. Ambulance
8. Other

MAJOR CARRIER NAME

DATE _____

TIME

| | | |
|---|---|---|
| TRANS TEAM READY | | |
| CARRIER READY | | |
| TEAM LEFT CHNMC | | |
| TEAM RETURNED CHNMC | | |

TEAM:

Trans RN _____
RN#2/NNP _____
RT _____
MD on Trans _____
MD Supervising _____

IV FLUIDS:

#1 _____
#2 _____
#3 _____
#4 _____

Pt. Wt. _____ gms

| STA-TUS¹ | TIME | VITAL SIGNS | | | | | | | LAB | | IV's | | | | OUTPUT | | VENTILATION | | | | | | B.G. STATUS | | | | | | | | | COMMENTS |
|---|---|---|---|---|---|---|---|---|---|---|---|---|---|---|---|---|---|---|---|---|---|---|---|---|---|---|---|---|---|---|---|---|---|
| STATUS¹ | TIME (HRS) | AMB TEMP (°C) | TEMP (°C) | HEART RATE | RR | BP | Mean BP | DEXT (mg %) | HCT (%) | Site IV#1 | Site IV#2 | Site IV#3 | Site IV#4 | STOOL (-) (-) | URINE (-) (-) | FIO2 (%) | RATE | INSP TIME (SEC) | PRES LIM (cm H2O) | PEEP (cm H2O) | Tc CO2 | Tc O2 | pH | PCO2 | PO2 | BE (-) | TYPE BG² | COLOR³ | Procedures/Meds, Etc |

¹STATUS: (1) Arrive Ref. Hosp. (Back Transport-Pre Transport)  (2) Depart Ref. Hosp. (Depart Clinic)  (3) Arrive Final Destination
²TYPE BLOOD GAS: (1) Arterial,  (2) Capillary,  (3) Venous,  (4) Skin Sensor,  (8) Other,  (0) None
³COLOR: N-Pink (normal),  P-Pale,  D-Dusky,  C-Cyanotic,  M-Mottled

CHNMC 009 1

## Chapter Appendix IV: Return Transport Checklist

Patient name: _____

____ 1. Receiving hospital called to accept back transfer

____ 2. Transport order written

____ 3. Permit from parents signed

____ 4. Ambulance arranged   Date _____ Time _____

____ 5. Chart copied—includes

 ____ a. Fact sheet

 ____ b. Admitting data base

 ____ c. Progress notes

 ____ d. Transfer summary

 ____ e. All consults

 ____ f. Nursing care plan

 ____ g. Current IV sheets, day sheet, respiratory flow sheet

 ____ h. Nurse's summary

 ____ i. Current IV orders

 ____ j. Medication record

 ____ k. Laboratory data

Results

 ____ 1) Last H/H, CBC _____

 ____ 2) Last lytes _____

 ____ 3) Current or last bilirubin _____

 ____ 4) Metabolic screen (e.g., PKU, $T_4$) _____

 ____ 5) Other applicable laboratory results _____

____ 6. All original x rays sent with baby

____ 7. Copy of most recent chest x ray

____ 8. Follow-up appointments made

____ 9. Receiving hospital called with report on baby's condition, equipment needed, estimated time of arrival

____ 10. Personal belongings of patient packed

Signature _____

## Chapter Appendix V: Nurse's Summary for Return Transports

Name _____ Date _____
Birth date _____ Gestational age at birth _____
Birth weight _____ Current weight _____
Birth length _____ Current length _____
Birth head circumference _____ Current head circumference _____
                                  Current abdominal girth _____

*Current Vital Signs Ranges (last 24–48 hr)*
Infant temperature _____ Isolette temperature _____
Heart rate _____ Resp. rate _____
BP _____ Dextrostix _____
FiO₂ _____
Last blood gas:  pH _____ pO₂ _____ pCO₂ _____
              Site drawn _____
No. of episodes of apnea or bradycardia/24 hr _____

*Feeding*
Type _____ Volume _____ Frequency _____
Special considerations (e.g., type of bottle, nipple, position for feeding)
_____
_____
_____

*Urine Output*
Vol./24 hr _____ S.G. _____ Dipstick _____

*Stool*
No./24 hr _____ Description _____

*IVs*
No. 1 solution _____ Rate _____ Site _____
No. 2 solution _____ Rate _____ Site _____

*Chapter Appendix V (continued).*

*Medications*

| Name | Dosage | Route | Frequency | Schedule |
|------|--------|-------|-----------|----------|
| 1. | | | | |
| 2. | | | | |
| 3. | | | | |
| 4. | | | | |
| 5. | | | | |
| 6. | | | | |

*Special Treatments or Procedures* (e.g., Dressing changes, exercises)

| Treatment | Frequency | Schedule |
|-----------|-----------|----------|
| 1. | | |
| 2. | | |
| 3. | | |

*Parents and Follow-up Needs*

Mother:  Name _____   Home No. _____   Work No. _____
Father:   Name _____   Home No. _____   Work No. _____
Visiting/calling pattern  _____
Specific teaching done  _____

_____

Teaching needs  _____

Follow-up appointments  _____
Additional comments  _____

_____

Primary nurse at CHNMC  _____

# 20

# Stabilization of the High-Risk Neonate Prior to Transport

Gary Pettett
Gerald B. Merenstein

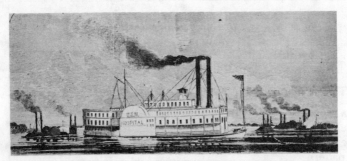

*20A. A type 5 sick transport conveyance (conveyance moved by steam power). The hospital steamer ship, "Red Rover," used during the Civil War.*

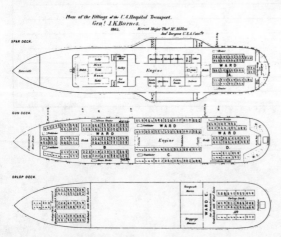

*20B. Reproduced from* Reports on the Extent and Nature of the Materials Available for the Preparation of a Medical and Surgical History of the War of the Rebellion. *War Department, Surgeon General's Office, Circular No. 6, Nov. 1, 1865. Philadelphia: J. B. Lippincott, 1866.)*

There are approximately 3.5 million births annually in the United States in over 5000 hospitals across the country. Only 15 percent of these infants are delivered in institutions with perinatal intensive care units [61]. The development of regional neonatal-perinatal programs in the United States and Canada has been associated with a significant reduction in neonatal morbidity and mortality within the referral area [5,51,54,61,64,67,68].

Regional programs are most effective when high-risk patients are identified in sufficient time to allow for planned obstetrical and neonatal care at an institution with appropriate clinical resources [7,8,29,40,52]. Both the presence of an intramural neonatal intensive care unit (NICU) and the antenatal referral of women with complicated pregnancies to a regional perinatal center have been associated with lower mortality rates than has neonatal transfer alone [15,27,41,43,53,67]. Unfortunately, antenatal screening identifies only 50 to 60 percent of infants who ultimately require neonatal intensive care [10,60]. A significant number of newborn are referred to a tertiary care center for complications that are not apparent until the late intrapartum or early neonatal period. These neonates require excellent care in the first minutes and hours of life. In the regional system the maintenance of the level of this care is partly the responsibility of the tertiary level center. This responsibility is fulfilled both through an educational outreach program and through the training of transport personnel with the required expertise to stablize a neonate's clinical condition to the fullest extent possible prior to transport.

In the past few years the development of new treatment methods and technology, such as extracorporeal membrane oxygenation (ECMO) and high-frequency ventilation, has led to the transfer of neonates who are extremely critically ill between tertiary-level neonatal centers. Transfer usually becomes necessary because the neonate has failed to benefit from the standard therapy for his or her condition. The care of these very sick and clinically unstable neonates during transport requires a very sophisticated level of knowledge and expertise on the part of the transport team. The transport itself may exacerbate the clinical instability, and the team must be able to maintain multiple life-sustaining treatments and initiate any emergency interventions required en route.

### Training Programs for Transport Personnel

The composition of the neonatal transport team may vary from region to region and from case to case [16,22,48]. In many regions, the majority of

The opinions expressed in this manuscript are those of the authors and do not necessarily represent the opinions of the Department of the Army or the Department of Defense.

neonatal transfers are performed by appropriately trained nurses with the assistance of ancillary support personnel such as respiratory therapists, emergency medical technicians, or flight nurses [1,17,48,63].

Prerequisites for functioning as a transport nurse include (see also Chap. 19 and Book Appendix 3) (1) licensed registered nurse, (2) neonatal intensive care experience (1 year), (3) leadership capabilities, (4) maturity, (5) organizational skills (ability to establish priorities), (6) good communication skills, (7) the ability to cope with stress, and (8) a commitment to perinatal transport and the team [65]. Completion of a formal training program and mastery of certain objectives (Table 20-1) are additional requirements at many regional perinatal centers [2,17,21,65]. The length of training varies from 2 to 12 months and includes formal didactic lectures, procedural skill sessions, and on-the-job intensive care experience. Graduates of the training program gain further practical experience by serving an internship with the transport team (under the supervision of a more senior transport nurse) and participating in regular nursery (NICU) conferences (rounds, case presentations). Team members involved in air transport should receive special training in flight physiology, safety, and survival (see Chap. 13).

In some programs, candidates may be required to pass a cognitive exami-

*Table 20-1. Objectives for the neonatal transport nurse educational program*

1. Obtain and record a complete perinatal history
2. Perform a thorough newborn physical examination including gestational age assessment
3. Learn the pathophysiology of newborn respiratory, cardiac, neurological, metabolic, infectious, and surgical disorders
4. Learn the indications for respiratory support
5. Learn the management of infants in shock and congestive heart failure
6. Identify problems affecting an ill newborn
7. Establish a management plan and initiate appropriate intervention
8. Stabilize the newborn prior to transport, including prevention or correction of hypothermia, hypotension, hypoxemia, hypercarbia, and acidosis
9. Skillfully perform and initiate the following procedures:
   a. Endotracheal intubation
   b. Respiratory support
   c. Umbilical vessel catheterization
   d. Pleural catheter placement
   e. Percutaneous arterial and venous puncture
   f. Peripheral IV line placement
   g. Cardiopulmonary resuscitation
10. Communicate and interact effectively with parents and health care team
11. Transport the infant and provide intensive care therapy
12. Identify own limitations in managing ill newborns

nation before they are accredited for transport service. Ongoing evaluation of both team and individual function is accomplished by regularly reviewing the care of all transported infants. Review sessions provide a source of continuing medical education for the transport team and a method of monitoring the changes in the quality of regional perinatal care.

## General Principles of Stabilization Prior to Transport

The primary objective of neonatal transport is to move the critically ill neonate from the referring hospital to a regional intensive care unit as quickly and safely as possible. How well this objective is met will depend on the adequacy of resuscitation (at birth) and the infant's management before (stabilization) and during transport. Any hospital with an active obstetrical service should have an organized and ongoing educational program for staff members in the standards and skills required for neonatal resuscitation and stabilization [62] (for detailed protocols, see Book Appendix 7).

The availability of a skilled transport service and a tertiary referral center does not diminish the importance of care during the immediate neonatal period. Hypothermia, hypotension, and acidosis during the pretransport period have a significant impact on neonatal morbidity and mortality [20, 31]. Chance et al. compared the outcome of infants stabilized and transported by trained and untrained personnel [11,12]. They reviewed 152 neonatal transports that occurred before an organized transport service was available (1972) [12]. Consultation concerning treatment rarely occurred before transport; 4 percent of the neonates arrived at the tertiary care center unexpectedly. Intravenous access was present in only 36 (23.7%) neonates but in the majority was nonfunctional on arrival at the center. Supplemental oxygen was inappropriately used and inadequately monitored. Facilities available during transfer were inadequate for the severity of the neonate's illness. Several neonates traveled without a secure airway, despite obvious indications for airway control prior to transfer. Medical attendants were not sufficiently trained and most lacked knowledge of their patient's condition or illness. Two neonates were transported with undrained pneumothoraces. Hypoxia, hypercapnia, hypotension, metabolic acidosis, and hypothermia were common findings when the neonates arrived at the center. Twenty-seven (47.4%) of the transported infants died.

In 1978 the authors repeated their study following the development of a trained transport team and increased efforts at outreach education [11]. Unlike neonates in the previous survey, those transported by the team had received an average of 42 ± 21.4 minutes of treatment and stabilization (by the transport team) before leaving the referring hospital. The results of neo-

374

Table 20-2. Outcome of regional neonatal transport before and after development of a regional transport team

| | 1972 [12] | | 1978 [11] | |
|---|---|---|---|---|
| | RDS < 1500 g | Uncomplicated < 1500 g | Conventional personnel | Transport team |
| Number of patients | 36 | 21 | 12 | 22 |
| Birth weight (g) | 1240 (690–1490) | 1060 (600–1500) | 1086 + 259 | 1167 + 258 |
| pH | 7.16 (6.90–7.47) | 7.28 (6.98–7.48) | 7.23 + 0.16 | 7.31 + 0.12* |
| $PCO_2$ (mm Hg) | 53.9 (25–92) | 39.4 (19–78) | 52.8 + 24.3 | 42.9 + 14.6 |
| BE | −10.4 (+0.9 to −22) | −7.0 (+1 to −18) | −7.9 + 4.8 | −5.7 + 3.6 |
| Rectal temperature (°C) | (D) 34.5 (31–36.4) | (D) 32.2 (31–36) | 35.0 + 1.6 | 36.5 + 1.0* |
| | (S) 35.6 (33–39.3) | (S) 34.7 (32–36.7) | | |
| Incubator temperature (°C) | (D) 30.5 (15–38.9) | (D) 31.6 (30–32.2) | 34.5 + 3.9 | 38.4 + 1.9* |
| | (S) 32.5 (26.7–35.6) | (S) 32.2 (23.9–40) | | |
| Deaths | 21 | 6 | 5 | 3* |
| Mortality (%) | 58.3 | 28.6 | 41.7 | 13.6 |
| NICU days | N/A | N/A | 28.6 + 17.3 | 19.1 + 21.8* |
| Hospital days | N/A | N/A | 62.4 + 23.6 | 37.9 + 20.7* |

(D) = died; (S) = survived; N/A = not available; numbers in parentheses represent range.
*Value significantly different from conventional group.
From Chance, G. W., Matthew, J. D., Gash, J., et al. Neonatal transport: A controlled study of skilled assistance. J. Pediatr. 93:662–666, 1978; and Chance, G. W., O'Brien, M. J., and Swyer, P. R. Transportation of sick neonates, 1972: An unsatisfactory aspect of medical care. Can. Med. Assoc. J. 109:847–852, 1973.

natal transport by the team were compared with those of neonatal transport performed by untrained (conventional) attendants who were used when the transport team was not available. Neonates transported by the team showed significant improvement in the proper maintenance of neutral thermal environment, rectal temperature, inspired oxygen concentration, blood pressure, pH, arterial $PO_2$, and arterial $PCO_2$. Stabilized neonates had a lower mortality rate and shorter hospitalizations than the conventional group. Table 20-2 shows the differences in the condition of infants less than 1500 g on arrival in the intensive care unit before [12] and after [11] the use of a trained transport team.

Many of the unsatisfactory aspects of neonatal transport [12] can be prevented by proper stabilization of the infant before leaving the referring hospital. Stabilization involves basic physiological support and is defined as the treatment or correction of those processes that, if not addressed, may eventually lead to a deterioration of the neonate's condition. The evaluation and treatment of high-risk neonates should begin before the transport team arrives and should focus on the following areas of clinical support:

Airway control
Oxygenation and ventilation
Acid-base balance
Thermal support
Metabolic support
Maintenance of vascular volume

AIRWAY CONTROL
The initial objective in stabilization and preparation of infants for transport is to secure an adequate and reliable airway. Direct laryngoscopic visualization and suctioning (DeLee apparatus, endotracheal tube) of the trachea and upper airway may be indicated in neonates with excessive secretions or those suspected of recent aspiration. Suctioning under direct visualization to prevent aspiration pneumonia is most effective when performed before the onset of gasping or vigorous respiratory efforts. Neonates delivered through thick, meconium-stained amniotic fluid should have the mouth, nose, and oropharynx cleared on the perineum before the thorax is delivered [9]. Unnecessary delays may allow aspirated material to disseminate into the peripheral regions of the lung where tracheal suctioning is ineffective. There is no evidence to suggest that pulmonary lavage with normal saline recovers additional material from the lung periphery, and it may actually increase morbidity [9].

A 5F oral or nasogastric feeding tube should be used to remove residual fluid and air from the stomach. The tube can be left in place (taped to the infant's cheek) with the open end lying at or below chest level (gravity-enhanced drainage). Nonintubated neonates with respiratory distress and tachypnea may accumulate a significant amount of air in the stomach and upper intestinal tract. During air transport, with increasing altitude, expansion of accumulated air may cause gastric or intestinal distention limiting diaphragmatic movement and further compromising the infant's respiratory status. An open gastric tube allows equilibration with changing atmospheric pressure and provides an outlet for gastrointestinal decompression. (For further discussion of the effects of changes in atmospheric pressure, see Chap. 11.)

An oral- or nasoesophageal tube is required for transporting neonates with esophageal atresia and a blind upper pouch. An 8F feeding tube should be inserted into the proximal esophageal pouch with the distal end open for continuous gravity-enhanced drainage. Frequent intermittent suctioning will help remove esophageal secretions and reduce the risk of overflow aspiration.

Airway obstruction from a mobile tongue is a particular risk in premature infants and newborns with facial malformations (e.g., Pierre Robin syndrome). Lying in the relaxed, supine position, the tongue may fall back into the posterior oropharynx, blocking the upper airway. Placing the neonate in the prone position, supporting the upper chest with a rolled towel (1–2-in. thick), and placing a large (8–10F) orogastric tube may help to prevent airway occlusion. With the face in a dependent position, gravity will pull the jaw and tongue away from the posterior oropharynx and the feeding tube will help to separate the tongue from the palate and the posterior oropharynx. If positioning alone is not effective, the use of an orotracheal tube or plastic oral airway may be necessary.

Endotracheal intubation can be an important precaution in the transport of neonates with choanal atresia. Choanal obstruction severely restricts or prevents nasal breathing. Newborn infants are predominantly nose breathers and may not adequately compensate (switch to mouth breathing) when their nares are obstructed. The additional risk of positional airway obstruction with the tongue can place these neonates in a potentially life-threatening situation if a secure airway has not been established.

OXYGENATION AND VENTILATION
Adequate oxygenation and ventilation should be achieved before the neonate leaves the referring hospital. For neonates with respiratory distress or in shock accurate assessment of pulmonary gas exchange requires a recent set of arterial blood gases. If these results are not available when the team

arrives, they should be obtained as soon as possible. Supplemental oxygen is the treatment of choice for neonates with a low arterial $PO_2$. Oxygen should be administered from a heated (body temperature) and humidified source to prevent excessive thermal and insensible water losses from the rapid movement of dry, unheated oxygen through the airway of a tachypneic neonate. The delivery of oxygen through an enclosed headbox (oxyhood) conserves oxygen supply and prevents wide swings in the fraction of inspired air as oxygen ($FIO_2$) when repeated access to the neonate or transport incubator is needed. Flow rates of 5 to 10 liters/minute ensure sufficient air turnover in the hood to prevent rebreathing of accumulated $CO_2$.

Neonates with cyanotic congenital heart disease, persistent pulmonary hypertension, or severe pulmonary hypoplasia may not respond to supplemental oxygen with an increase in $PaO_2$ or arterial saturation. When a ductus (arteriosus)-dependent cardiac malformation is suspected (e.g., transposition of the great vessels, pulmonary atresia), a continuous infusion of prostaglandin $E_1$ (0.1 $\mu$g/kg/minute) should be started to prevent spontaneous closure of the ductus. Even though a specific cardiac diagnosis may not be available, supplemental oxygen and prostaglandin infusion should be continued until the neonate reaches the center where diagnostic studies can be performed. Neither oxygen nor prostaglandin $E_1$ administered during transport is associated with serious complications if the diagnosis of cyanotic heart disease cannot be confirmed.

The concentration of administered oxygen is based on the analysis of arterial saturation and $PaO_2$. The development of portable, low-energy transcutaneous $PO_2$ ($TcPO_2$) monitors and pulse oximeters allows continuous monitoring of arterial $PaO_2$ and oxygen saturation during transport. Acceptable ranges for arterial $PO_2$ are 70 to 90 mm Hg for neonates with acute pulmonary disease and 50 to 70 mm Hg for those with chronic or stable pulmonary conditions. When pulse oximetry is used, these $PaO_2$s correspond to oxygen saturations of 90 to 95 percent for infants with acute illness and not less than 85 percent for those with chronic disease [59]. During transport it is advisable to maintain the saturation greater than or equal to 95 percent for the acute cases and greater than or equal to 90 percent for chronic cases, to allow for a greater margin of safety. The use of $TcPO_2$ monitors has been shown to increase the number of neonates with respiratory disease who arrive at the tertiary care center with $PaO_2$s in the normally oxygenated range [14,42]. With the recent addition of a combined $TcPO_2=TcPCO_2$ sensor for transcutaneous monitoring, similar control of $PCO_2$ may soon be reported.

Oxygen requirements of more than 0.60 $FIO_2$ to maintain an arterial $PO_2$ greater than or equal to 50 mm Hg indicate a need for more extensive ventilatory support. Large neonates (>2 kg) with significant volume loss (respiratory distress syndrome or atelectasis) may respond to continuous positive airway pressure (CPAP) by nasal prongs or endotracheal intubation. Although apnea is a relative contraindication to the use of CPAP, in some neonates stimulation of lower airway stretch receptors by CPAP may result in spontaneous respirations. CPAP is started at low pressures (4–5 cm $H_2O$) with subsequent adjustments based on the measurement of arterial $PO_2$ and $PCO_2$. CPAP (and positive-pressure ventilation with positive end-expiratory pressure [PEEP]) should be used cautiously in neonates with significant air trapping (e.g., aspiration) to reduce the risk of pulmonary air leak during transport. Excessive $CO_2$ retention ($PCO_2$ >60 mm Hg) and persistent hypoxia ($PO_2$ <50 mm Hg) are indications for positive pressure ventilation.

The decision to intubate a neonate may occasionally be a difficult one. However, given the limitations of most transport vehicles and the need for maximal stability, current recommendations state that intubation (and ventilation) should be started before transport whenever there is a reasonable chance that they might be required en route [25]. Absolute indications for intubation (and ventilation) include apnea (see above), respiratory failure ($PCO_2$ >60 mm Hg), or an inability to maintain an adequate $PO_2$ (see above). The endotracheal tube may be placed by either the nasal or oral route. Proper positioning of the tube should be confirmed by clinical and radiographic examination before transport (an endotracheal tube tip locator is now on the market. See Chapter Appendix I in Chapter 19.) Following placement and localization, the proximal portion of the endotracheal tube is carefully secured to prevent accidental extubation during transport. If a neonate is intubated but not mechanically ventilated, a minimal CPAP of 2 to 3 cm $H_2O$ should be maintained to prevent a loss of lung volume and increased work of breathing.

Neonates with cleft palate who require endotracheal intubation present a unique technical problem with tracheal visualization and tube insertion. The use of a wooden tongue depressor placed across the cleft with the ends extending beyond the corners of the mouth will assist with placement of the laryngoscope blade and endotracheal tube. Furthermore, in the absence of an intact palate, normal tongue thrusting behavior may force the endotracheal tube into the cleft resulting in extubation with no perceptible change in the external length of the tube [23].

ACID-BASE BALANCE
The transport team should assess the neonate's acid-base status and begin correcting any imbalance before the neonate leaves the referring hospital.

An accurate pH measurement can be obtained from an arterial blood gas or free-flowing venous sample. The most common disturbance of acid-base balance, excluding respiratory disorders, is metabolic acidosis, which may be an early sign of reduced tissue perfusion indicating a need to look closely for evidence of hypovolemia, cardiac dysfunction, or infection.

The use of sodium bicarbonate to correct metabolic acidosis is justified only after appropriate attention has been given to the underlying etiology (e.g., hypoxia, diminished tissue perfusion). Bicarbonate administration in a closed respiratory system (inadequate ventilation) may result in hypercarbia and worsening (respiratory) acidosis [46]. Correction of metabolic acidosis in hypovolemic or infected neonates without adequate volume expansion can result in severe hypotension and diminished perfusion of vital organs.

Prediluted ampules of sodium bicarbonate are available for pediatric and neonatal use. Rapid infusion of undiluted, hyperosmolar sodium bicarbonate produces significant fluid shifts between body compartments [3,55] and is associated with an increased incidence of intracranial hemorrhage [58,66]. If prediluted ampules for pediatric or neonatal use are not available, standard sodium bicarbonate (0.9 mEq/ml) should be diluted by at least half with a low osmolar diluent (sterile water). Intravenous infusion should not exceed 1 mEq/kg/minute with a total dose calculated from the following formula:

mEq (sodium bicarbonate) = 0.3 × body weight (kg) × BE

where BE represents the calculated base excess (deficit). When the base excess is not available, the total bicarbonate dose should not exceed 1 to 3 mEq/kg. The infusion may be repeated as needed for pH control; however, extensive use of bicarbonate can lead to hypernatremia. If repeated doses of bicarbonate have been given, a serum sodium should be checked immediately on arrival in the intensive care unit. Simultaneous assessment of arterial pH may be used to evaluate intratransport acid-base control.

THERMAL SUPPORT

The ideal (thermoneutral) environmental temperature for the newborn is defined as that range of ambient temperatures within which metabolic rate is at a minimum and temperature regulation is achieved by nonevaporative, vasomotor processes [4]. The temperature range that constitutes the thermoneutral environment for an individual neonate depends on the infant's basal metabolic rate. Differences in birth weight, intrauterine growth, and postnatal age affect the metabolic rate and thermoneutral requirements [30].

Table 20-3. Types of heat loss

| Type | Mechanism | Prevention |
|---|---|---|
| Conductive | Loss of heat from object to object by direct contact | Warmed bed, heating mattress, avoid cool surfaces |
| Convective | Loss of heat due to movement of surface air currents | Avoid and prevent drafts |
| Radiant | Loss of heat from one object to another by nonionizing radiation | Heat shield, double-wall incubator, radiant warmer |
| Evaporative | Loss of heat by evaporation of water from exposed surface | Dry body surface, moist wraps to exposed tissue, clear plastic body wrap, humidification |

The metabolic demands of thermal regulation and acute illness pose a significant challenge for the high-risk neonate. The importance of adequate thermal support for acutely ill neonates has been shown in controlled trials demonstrating reduced morbidity and mortality in infants managed in a warm thermal environment [18,56]. Although most neonates are capable of conserving body heat through cutaneous vasoconstriction [6], the low birth weight neonate lacks substantial subcutaneous fat and has a large surface area–body mass ratio that facilitates significant heat loss. Variations in the ambient temperature during transport may further complicate thermal regulation. Hypothermia before or during transfer has a significant effect on survival [11,12,20,31]. Management of the thermal environment for small or acutely ill neonates, or both, involves the control of excessive heat loss and maintenance of an adequate environmental temperature. Table 20-3 lists the four major avenues of heat loss and techniques to help prevent excessive losses.

The transport incubator provides a confined environment that facilitates thermal support. Environmental temperature is controlled by either manual (preset) or servocontrol (feedback) methods. With manual control, the environmental temperature is preset to correspond with the neonate's neutral thermal environment of 30 to 35° C, depending on the neonate's weight and postnatal age (see Chap. Appendix I) [30]. Smaller and younger neonates require environmental temperatures at the upper end of this range. Temperature adjustments are made by the nurse or attendant following periodic assessment of the neonate's body temperature. The consistency of the thermal environment and the variability of the patient's body temperature will be determined by the frequency with which temperature checks are made.

Servocontrol requires the use of an incubator or radiant warmer with a thermostatic sensor. A skin temperature probe from the heating unit is attached to the neonate's abdominal wall. The thermostatic sensor in the unit is set to the desired temperature and will control the output of heat in response to changes in the neonate's abdominal skin temperature. Minimal rates of oxygen consumption, metabolic activity, and normal core body temperature occur when the neonate's abdominal skin temperature is kept between 36.1 to 36.5°C [57]. Servocontrol may represent the most efficient method of thermal support during neonatal transport. Servocontrolled heat sources respond more rapidly to temperature changes, resulting in a more constant thermal environment. Interpretation of thermal responses (e.g., detection of fever) for neonates in a servocontrolled environment requires a record of the changes in incubator, skin, and axillary (core) temperatures. Consistently low incubator temperatures with a normal core or body temperature may indicate the presence of fever. Care must be taken, however, to ensure that the temperature probe remains attached to an appropriate skin site (upper, anterior abdominal wall) and remains dry. A dislodged or damp probe (blood, body fluids) may result in cooling of the temperature probe and continuous operation of the heater, subjecting the infant to potential hyperthermia.

Weather conditions and outside temperature are additional concerns for the transport team. Indyk [32] has reported unsatisfactory temperature regulation in some older-model transport incubators although performance can be improved with the use of a chemically activated warming mattress [44]. Newer transport incubators with servocontrol, high thermal inertia, double-walled construction, and built-in accessory equipment should improve heat balance and help maintain body temperature during neonatal transport [24,49]. In more severe climates, thermal wrappings (parkas) for the entire transport incubator (excluding infant viewing and control areas) and the use of plexiglass heat shields provide additional insulation.

METABOLIC SUPPORT

Hypoglycemia is a frequent complication of high-risk status during the early neonatal period. Prematurity, growth retardation and acceleration, perinatal asphyxia, and maternal diabetes (infants of diabetic mothers) are common predisposing risk factors [35,36]. Hypoglycemia is defined as a plasma glucose concentration of less than 35 dl in full-term neonates and less than 25 mg/dl in the preterm during the first 72 hours of life or less than 45 mg/dl in any neonate after 72 hours. Commercially available reagent strips provide a rapid screening method for detecting hypoglycemia from a small amount of blood. When the reagent strips provide an equivocal result, laboratory analysis of plasma or serum glucose concentrations can be used to confirm the diagnosis.

Stabilization of high-risk neonates in preparation for transport should include placement of an intravenous line and the provision of a constant glucose infusion. Early intravenous support with glucose-containing fluids has been shown to prevent hypoglycemia and to reduce morbidity and mortality in sick newborn infants [37]. A continuous infusion of glucose 4 to 6 mg/kg/minute will approximate glucose production rates from internal glycogen stores and maintain the euglycemic state [33]. Neonates with documented hypoglycemia should receive a loading dose of 2 ml/kg (200 mg/kg) of 10% D/W followed by a continuous intravenous infusion (glucose 6–8 mg/kg/minute). This will correct the hypoglycemia with a minimal risk of reactive hyperinsulinemia (hypoglycemia) [35]. If the hypoglycemia does not respond to the initial treatment, the bolus dose may be repeated and the infusion rate increased. Neonates with profound hypoglycemia or hyperinsulinemia (e.g., infant of diabetic mother) may require infusion rates as high as 9 to 12 mg/kg/minute to stabilize their blood glucose. If the fluid intake required to provide adequate glucose exceeds that which is indicated for the individual neonate, the concentration of glucose can be increased in steps up to 20 percent. Concentrations of glucose exceeding 12 percent must be given via a properly placed umbilical arterial or venous catheter [38,39]. The use of peripheral glucose infusions with concentrations in excess of 10 to 12 percent results in vasospasm, local infiltration, and cutaneous sloughs. Highly concentrated glucose infusions and bolus administrations of 25 to 50 percent glucose can produce wide swings in serum glucose concentrations and rarely have any beneficial therapeutic effect. In our experience, the use of these solutions during stabilization or transport is rarely, if ever, indicated.

The major complication of routine glucose administration is the development of hyperglycemia. Small, premature neonates weighing less than 1200 g may become severely hyperglycemic when glucose infusion rates exceed 5 to 6 mg/kg/minute [19]. Prevention of iatrogenic hyperglycemia requires careful titration of glucose infusion rates with the neonate's homeostatic abilities. Repeated glucose determinations may be required during stabilization or prolonged transport to ensure a stable blood glucose. In the very small neonate, an intravenous dextrose concentration of 5 to 7.5 percent may be necessary to maintain adequate fluid intake without risking hyperglycemia. For safety and maximum precision, the intravenous infusion apparatus should include a micro drip volume control chamber regulated by a portable infusion pump.

Glucagon, administered by either the intravenous or intramuscular route, has been used as an alternative method of treating hypoglycemia. Glucagon raises the blood sugar by stimulating glycolysis and gluconeogenesis. Neonates with deficient glycogen stores (small for gestational age neonates, prematures) or defects in gluconeogenesis are not candidates for glucagon treatment. Glucagon administration to infants of diabetic mothers may further complicate glucose control by stimulating insulin release. Since its effect is brief (15–20 minutes) and the majority of neonates with neonatal hypoglycemia have deficient glycogen stores or hyperinsulinemia and are not likely to respond to glucagon, its routine use by the transport team or referring hospital is not recommended.

FLUID AND VOLUME CONTROL

A perinatal history of placenta previa, abruptio placentae, velamentous cord insertion, third-trimester bleeding, or the presence of large fluid-losing anomalies such as gastroschisis identifies a group of patients at increased risk for hypovolemia and diminished tissue perfusion. Hypoxic-ischemic (tissue) injury occurs when perfusion and oxygen delivery are unable to meet the metabolic demands of peripheral organs. Maintenance of an adequate blood volume and hematocrit are essential to organ and tissue perfusion. Blood volume in full-term infants ranges from 79 to 98 ml/kg (depending on the time of umbilical cord clamping), whereas premature neonates have slightly higher values of 89 to 105 ml/kg. A normal hematocrit may range from 40 to 60 percent.

Early detection of hypovolemia is the result of careful attention to historical and clinical clues. Persistent, unexplained tachycardia may be the earliest clinical sign of reduced vascular volume. Delayed micturition (> 24 hours with no history of urination in the delivery room) or urine output of less than 1 ml/kg/hour is indicative of reduced renal blood flow. Severely hypovolemic neonates will present with a pale, ashen color, weak arterial pulses, and prolonged capillary filling time. Extremity blood pressures may be difficult to obtain without placement of a peripheral or umbilical arterial catheter for direct measure and may be misleading initially because many neonates are able to maintain a normal blood pressure in the face of significant hypovolemia. A low arterial pH and increasing base deficit are indicative of a metabolic acidosis as a result of diminished tissue perfusion.

The hematocrit is a poor indicator of acute volume loss even though frank hemorrhage may have occurred. A fall in hematocrit is not evident until the volume loss has been partially replaced by internal fluid shifts or exogenous volume expansion. It may be several hours before the degree of anemia accurately reflects the volume of blood lost.

A significant reduction in vascular volume can occur in neonates with peripheral edema and increased total body water. Small premature neonates with hypoalbuminemia may lose a significant portion of their blood volume to the extravascular compartment due to reduced intravascular oncotic pressure. Severely asphyxiated or septic infants can develop capillary leak syndrome as a result of extensive damage to the capillary endothelium.

The treatment of hypovolemia and anemia is directed toward the restoration of circulating blood volume and red blood cell mass before permanent hypoxic-ischemic injury occurs. In the severely hypotensive neonate, direct access to a large, central vessel is essential. At low perfusion pressures, cannulation of small peripheral vessels can be a time-consuming and frequently impossible task. In addition, small peripheral vessels will usually not accomodate the rapid infusions required to correct acute volume loss. In emergency situations, immediate intravenous access can be obtained by placement of a large (5F) catheter through the umbilical vein [39]. With restoration of blood pressure and perfusion, the umbilical vein catheter should be replaced with an umbilical (arterial) or peripheral venous catheter.

The treatment of choice for acute volume loss is replacement with fresh whole blood. Unfortunately, the treatment of hypovolemic infants frequently cannot await the availability of properly crossmatched blood (or plasma). Vascular expansion can be rapidly achieved with 5% albumin (10–20 ml/kg) or lactated Ringer's solution (10–20 ml/kg). Neonates with reduced oncotic pressure and increased total body water (edema) may respond to intravenous salt-poor albumin (25% albumin; 1 g or 4 ml/kg) by mobilizing extravascular fluid. However, a sudden increase in the intravascular oncotic pressure can be dangerous in infants with compromised cardiac function (e.g., hydrops fetalis). The use of uncrossmatched blood should be reserved only for the emergency situations. Repeated assessment of blood pressure, capillary filling, limb perfusion, and pulse pressure provides the most reliable guidelines for continued treatment. Continuous measurement of systolic, diastolic, and mean arterial blood pressure can be obtained from an arterial catheter (preferably umbilical artery) attached to the pressure port of the cardiorespiratory monitor through an inline pressure transducer.

Following the restoration of circulating blood volume, transfusion with packed red blood cells may be necessary to correct severe anemia. In acutely ill neonates, the maintenance of a normal hematocrit (40–60%) is a reasonable goal. The appropriate volume for packed red cell transfusions can be calculated from the following formula:

$$\frac{\text{Weight (kg)} \times \text{blood volume (ml/kg)} \times \text{change in Hgb desired}}{\text{Hgb (g/dl) of packed cells}}$$

Hgb represents the hemoglobin content in g/dl (Hgb is roughly equal to one-third of the hematocrit). Blood volume is an estimated value based on standards for term and preterm neonates. The transfusion should be administered with an intravenous infusion pump and inline filter over a 1- to 2-hour period. In stable neonates, the transfusion may be administered or completed during transport although severe anemia may require transfusion before leaving for the referral center.

Care should be taken not to overload the neonate with fluid. For example, the severely asphyxiated neonate may manifest signs of peripheral circulatory failure secondary to hypoxic-ischemic damage to the myocardium with "pump" failure. Not only will the administration of excess fluid increase the risk of heart failure but associated cerebral edema may also be exacerbated.

## Stabilization for Air Transport

The use of aircraft to transport critically ill neonates raises several problems peculiar to that form of transportation. Before air transport is selected the risks and advantages of air travel must be considered in relation to the neonate's condition (see Chap. 11).

Helicopters (rotary-wing aircraft) are frequently used for low-altitude, short-distance transports. Most are relatively small aircraft; once the crew, transport team, equipment, and patient are aboard, there is very little room for maneuvering. Pretransport stabilization is essential in infants who will be transferred by helicopter. A sudden change in the infant's condition requiring additional intervention (e.g., thoracostomy, intubation) may necessitate a temporary landing.

The helicopter's engine and main rotor create an extremely high noise level. Communication with the crew or other members of the transport team may require use of the aircraft's intercom system. Careful attention must be given to the patient's condition and vital signs. Monitors with audio alarms can be difficult to hear and auscultatory evaluation of the patient may be impossible. Visual alarm systems are a distinct advantage in this environment. The physiological effects of excessive noise on newborn or premature infants have not been studied. Earplugs, which are usually required for the flight crew, may also be of benefit to the neonate.

Electronic monitors have occasionally malfunctioned during helicopter transports. Rotational and vibrational forces created by the aircraft can interfere with the cardiorespiratory oscillograph. Respiratory, ECG, and pressure wave patterns may become uninterpretable. Heart rate monitors that count off the ECG R-wave may fail to record an accurate rate or may count interference patterns. Testing of electronic equipment under flight conditions, prior to their use, may suggest instrument modifications (e.g., shock absorbers, electronic shielding) that could greatly improve their accuracy and reliability.

Fixed-wing aircraft are generally used for higher-altitude, longer-distance transports. Unlike the helicopter, there is often more room for patient care, cabin noise is significantly reduced, environmental temperature is more easily controlled and, when properly modified for transport, a sufficient number of gas and electrical outlets are available to ensure proper functioning of medical equipment.

Altitude becomes an important consideration with the use of fixed-wing aircraft. Ascent to altitude is associated with a fall in atmospheric pressure and a reduction in the partial pressure of oxygen. At an altitude of 10,000 ft in an unpressurized environment, alveolar $PO_2$ falls from 103 mm Hg (at sea level) to 60 mm Hg. Commercial and many transport aircraft are pressurized to maintain a cabin altitude of 5000 to 7000 ft [26]. At this altitude, changes in the partial pressure of oxygen have minimal consequences for healthy individuals. However, neonates with marginal respiratory function may be at risk for hypoxia. In the presence of severe or progressive respiratory disease, the use of supplemental oxygen or ventilatory support, or both, should be carefully considered before traveling by aircraft. The effect of altitude is especially important when air transport is required for infants with cyanotic congenital heart disease. Although hypoxia from a fixed right-to-left shunt is generally not responsive to supplemental oxygen, the administration of additional oxygen may prevent further desaturation of arterial blood at lower partial pressures of atmospheric oxygen.

With proper pretransport stabilization, hypoxia from altitude is rarely a problem in pressurized aircraft. In the unlikely event of a failure in cabin pressurization, descent to a lower altitude will provide the most immediate relief although it will reduce air speed, prolong transport time, and increase fuel consumption.

Collections of air in closed or semiclosed body cavities follow Boyle's law on ascent to altitude [26]: the volume of air increases in proportion to the drop in atmospheric pressure. At an altitude of 10,000 ft, the gas volume of a closed container has increased by 50 percent. The stomach and intestines are considered open cavities and are usually not affected by altitude. However, placement of an open orogastric tube will help ensure minimal gas volumes in the stomach. Increased middle-ear pressure may occur in infants much as it does in many passengers on commercial aircraft. Although it may lead to slight discomfort and agitation, it does not appear to have serious medical consequences.

Expansion of air within the lungs or thoracic cavity of neonates on closed-system ventilators is a potentially more significant problem. Patients with pulmonary air leaks, trapped alveolar air, or pulmonary interstitial emphysema (PIE) can experience significant deterioration from the expansion of trapped air during air transport. The transport team must be aware of the potential for gas expansion and the risk of pulmonary air leaks. Equipment for rapid thoracostomy and drainage of extrapulmonary air should be readily available. Pneumothoraces discovered at the referring hospital must be treated before transfer. Because of the possibility for reaccumulation, pneumothoraces in neonates with pulmonary disease or on positive pressure ventilation, or both, should be treated with indwelling thoracostomy tubes attached to an underwater seal, Heimlich valve, or suction device to ensure adequate control en route.

Enclosed air leaks that cannot be easily managed (e.g., pneumatosis intestinalis) are considerably more problematic. Depending on the severity of the neonate's condition, ground transport may be more appropriate. Where expedience remains an essential criteria, low-altitude flights with pressurization to near sea level may be unavoidable. Since this may affect aircraft performance, flying time, and fuel consumption, close coordination with the pilot and flight crew is essential.

### Role of Outreach Education in Fostering Adequate Stabilization

Despite the presence of active regional perinatal programs, premature infants who require transfer to a tertiary care center are still found to have a greater incidence of potentially preventable complications than those born in perinatal centers [13]. Early diagnosis and stabilization are the major factors contributing to differences in preventable complications [20,31]. Active outreach educational programs can influence regional perinatal care and improve the condition of neonates transferred to a regional center [29,34,45].

One of the most valuable outreach opportunities occurs at the time of a neonate's transfer. The transport team has the chance to demonstrate evaluation and treatment techniques, discuss screening procedures, and review particular medical and nursing protocols in a setting where their application is immediately obvious. Retention of new information or reinforcement of previous knowledge is likely to be most effective in this setting.

The transport team must be particularly adept at teaching to render this information in a cooperative training spirit. Regardless of the patient's condition (on arrival of the team), it is best to remember that the local hospital personnel have probably performed to the best of their ability (or training) and are likely to be quite concerned for the infant's welfare. In small communities, there may be a close personal relationship between the patient's family and the local hospital personnel. A patronizing analysis of local deficiencies or management errors may squander an excellent teaching opportunity, alienate the local staff, and destroy a referral relationship, which could adversely affect the care of future patients. The transport team should review each transfer as a potential educational experience. Members of the team should become familiar with referring hospitals, their capabilities, and the people who make them function. The objective is to develop rapport and a certain espirit toward a common goal of optimal perinatal care.

The development of community-based transport systems represents a more extensive effort at regional education. In 1975, the University of Alabama-Birmingham developed a program for decentralized neonatal transfer using community-based resources [63]. Transport personnel consisted of registered nurses and emergency medical technicians (EMTs) who were specifically trained for neonatal transport. The educational program consisted of on-site seminars with a center-based didactic and practical training course. Trained personnel were located at five large community hospitals in different regions of the state. Coordination and frequent consultation with a neonatologist at the center helped the community-based systems select appropriate candidates for transport and provided an opportunity to discuss the infant's stabilization and intratransport care. Community-based transports were most frequently used for referrals from hospitals with larger delivery services at greater distances from the center and for neonates not suffering from respiratory distress. There was no correlation between the allocation of transport personnel (central versus community based) and subsequent neonatal mortality. With adequate training and support from the regional center, community-based personnel are capable of stabilizing and transporting selected neonates without adversely affecting their outcome.

### Role of Consultation in Promoting Adequate Stabilization
Early and frequent consultation between referring hospitals and the perinatal center can have a significant impact on neonatal morbidity and mortality. Chance et al. have reported the unsatisfactory aspects of neonatal transport with limited interhospital contact and unexpected referrals [12].

In the Cincinnati area, a controlled study of frequent hot-line users (and nonusers) found significant improvement in neonatal mortality in the user hospitals without a concomitant increase in referrals to the center [47]. Of the transfers that did occur, a significantly greater portion from the user hospitals were referred following early clinical assessment (<2 hours of age) and arrived at the center in more stable condition. Enhanced survival of neonates from user hospitals was associated with an increased percentage of neonates who were transferred as a result of clinical decisions arrived at more rapidly and after better stabilization. The presence of a direct communication line to the center may be presumed to have helped overcome at least some of the inertia in the process by which transfer decisions are made. More frequent communication with the center did not appear to be an inordinate burden on regional subspecialty consultants. An average of 21 calls per day were handled by the system. Each call lasted approximately 2.5 minutes, resulting in nearly 32 minutes of consultation time per patient served. A review of the telephone log revealed several instances in which the consultant provided instructional guidance to help community hospital personnel quantify their assessment of the neonate's condition and carry out required stabilization prior to the arrival of the transport team [47].

Consultation between a referring physician and the perinatal center is of critical importance with regard to planning pretransport stabilization, intratransport care, and allocating appropriate transport personnel. On the other hand, the need for consultation does not necessarily mean a need for transfer. Situations may arise that, with proper guidance, can be adequately handled in the community hospital. The approximate 3:1 call-referral ratio using a dedicated telephone system reflects the potential importance of "consultation only" calls in a regional program [63].

## References

1. *Air Ambulance Guidelines.* DOT HS 806 703. Washington, D.C.: U.S. Department of Transportation, National Highway Traffic Safety Administration, 1986.
2. Barth, J. Staff Preparation and Training for High-risk Neonatal Transport. In S. Graven (ed.), *Newborn Air Transport.* Evansville, IN: Mead Johnson, 1978.
3. Baum, J. D., and Robertson, N. R. C. Immediate effects of alkaline infusion in infants with respiratory distress syndrome. *J. Pediatr.* 87:255–260, 1975.
4. Bligh, J., and Johnson, K. G. Glossary of terms for thermal physiology. *J. Appl. Physiol.* 35:941–945, 1973.
5. Brann, A. W. In P. Sunshine (ed.), *Regionalization of Perinatal Care. Report of the 66th Ross Conference on Pediatric Research.* Columbus, OH: Ross Laboratories, 1974. P. 27.
6. Bruck, K. Temperature regulation in the newborn infant. *Biol. Neonate* 3:65–70, 1961.

7. Butterfield, L. J. Newborn country USA. *Clin. Perinatol.* 3:281–295, 1976.
8. Butterfield, L. J. Organization of regional perinatal programs. *Semin. Perinatol.* 1:217–233, 1977.
9. Carson, B. S., Losey, R. W., Bowes, W. A., et al. Combined obstetric and pediatric approach to prevent meconium aspiration syndrome. *Am. J. Obstet. Gynecol.* 126:712–718, 1976.
10. Casson, R. I., and Sennett, E. S. Prenatal risk assessment and obstetric care in a small rural hospital: Comparison with guidelines. *Can. Med. Assoc. J.* 130:1311–1315, 1984.
11. Chance, G. W., Matthew, J. D., Gash, J., et al. Neonatal transport: A controlled study of skilled assistance. *J. Pediatr.* 93:662–666, 1978.
12. Chance, G. W., O'Brien, M. J., and Swyer, P. R. Transportation of sick neonates, 1972: An unsatisfactory aspect of medical care. *Can. Med. Assoc. J.* 109:847–852, 1973.
13. Clark, C. E., Clyman, R. I., Roth, R. S., et al. Risk factor analysis of intraventricular hemorrhage in low birth-weight infants. *J. Pediatr.* 99:625–628, 1981.
14. Clarke, T. A., Zmora, E., Chen, J. H., et al. Transcutaneous oxygen monitoring during neonatal transport. *Pediatrics* 65:884–886, 1980.
15. Cordero, L., Backes, C. R., and Zuspan, F. P. Very low-birth weight infant. I. Influence of place of birth on survival. *Am. J. Obstet. Gynecol.* 143:533–537, 1982.
16. Cunningham, M. D., and Smith, F. R. Stabilization and transport of severely ill infants. *Pediatr. Clin. North Am.* 20:359–366, 1973.
17. Danzig, D. Neonatal transport teams: A survey of functions and roles. *Neonatal Network*, October 1984. Pp. 41–45.
18. Davies, P. A., and Davis, P. J. Very low birth weight and subsequent head growth. *Lancet* 2:1216–1218, 1970.
19. Dweck, H. S., and Cassaday, G. Glucose intolerance in infants of very low birth weight. *Pediatrics* 53:189–194, 1974.
20. Ferrara, A. Evaluation of efficacy of regional perinatal programs. *Semin. Perinatol.* 1:303–308, 1977.
21. Ferrara, A., and Harin, A. *Emergency transfer of the high-risk neonate*. St. Louis: C. V. Mosby, 1980.
22. Ferrara, A., and Perotta, L. Infant transport services: An overview. *Pediatr. Ann.* 5:79–85, 1976.
23. Fletcher, M. A., MacDonald, M. G., and Avery, G. B. *Atlas of Procedures in Neonatology*. Philadelphia: J. B. Lippincott, 1983. Pp. 219–220.
24. Hackel, A. A medical transport system for the neonate. *Anesthesiology* 43:258–267, 1975.
25. Hackel, A. Ventilation. In S. Graven (ed.), *Newborn Air Transport*. Evansville, IN: Mead Johnson, 1978. P. 55.
26. Harding, R. M., and Mills, F. J. *Aviation Medicine*. London: British Medical Association, 1983. Pp. 26–37.
27. Harris, T. R., Isamen, J., and Giles, H. R. Improved neonatal survival through maternal transport. *Obstet. Gynecol.* 52:294–300, 1978.
28. Hein, H. A. Regionalization of perinatal care in rural areas based on the Iowa experience. *Semin. Perinatol.* 1:241–254, 1977.
29. Hein, H. A., Christopher, C., and Ferguson, N. N. Rural perinatology. *Pediatrics* 55:769–773, 1975.
30. Hey, E. N. The relationship between environmental temperature and oxygen consumption in the newborn baby. *J. Physiol.* 200:589–595, 1969.
31. Hood, J. L., Cross, A., Hulka, B., et al. Effectiveness of the neonatal transport team. *Crit. Care Med.* 11:419–423, 1983.
32. Indyk, L. Transport Equipment. In P. Sunshine (ed.), *Regionalization of Perinatal*

*Care. Report of the 66th Ross Conference on Pediatric Research.* Columbus, OH: Ross Laboratories, 1974. P. 67.

33. King, K. C., Adams, P. A. J., Clement, G. A., et al. Infants of diabetic mothers. Attenuated glucose uptake without hyperinsulinemia during continuous glucose infusion. *Pediatrics* 44:381–386, 1969.

34. Lazzara, A., Kanto, W. P., Dykes, F. D., et al. Continuing education in the community hospital and reduction in the incidence of intracerebral hemorrhage in the transported preterm infant. *J. Pediatr.* 101:757–761, 1982.

35. Lilien, L. O., Grajwer, L. A., and Pildes, R. S. Treatment of neonatal hypoglycemia with continuous intravenous glucose infusions. *J. Pediatr.* 91:779–784, 1977.

36. Lubchenco, L. O., and Bard, H. Incidence of hypoglycemia in newborn infants classified by birth weight and gestational age. *Pediatrics* 47:831–838, 1971.

37. Lubchenco, L. O., Delivoria-Papadopoulos, M., Butterfield, L. J., et al. Long term follow-up studies of prematurely born infants. I. Relationship of handicaps to nursery routines. *J. Pediatr.* 80:501–508, 1972.

38. MacDonald, M. G. Umbilical–Artery Catheterization. In M. A. Fletcher and M. G. MacDonald (eds.), *Atlas of Procedures in Neonatology.* Philadelphia: J. B. Lippincott, 1983. Pp. 130–145.

39. MacDonald, M. G. Umbilical–Vein Catheterization. In M. A. Fletcher and M. G. MacDonald (eds.), *Atlas of Procedures in Neonatology.* Philadelphia: J. B. Lippincott, 1983. Pp. 146–153.

40. McCarthy, J. T., and Butterfield, L. J. Newborn country USA revisited. *Rocky Mountain Med. J.* 75:208–211, 1978.

41. Merenstein, G. B., Pettett, G., Woodall, J., et al. An analysis of air transport results in the sick newborn. II. Antenatal and neonatal referrals. *Am. J. Obstet. Gynecol.* 128:520–525, 1977.

42. Miller, C., Clyman, R. I., Roth, R. S., et al. Control of oxygenation during the transport of sick neonates. *Pediatrics* 66:117–119, 1980.

43. Mondanlou, H. D., Dorchester, W., Freeman, R. K., et al. Perinatal transport to a regional perinatal center in a metropolitan area: Maternal versus neonatal transport. *Am. J. Obstet. Gynecol.* 138:1157–1164, 1980.

44. Neilson, H. C., Jung, A. L., and Atherton, S. O. Evaluation of the portawarm mattress as a source of heat for neonatal transport. *Pediatrics* 58:500–504, 1976.

45. Oh, W., Cowett, R. M., Clark, S., et al. Role of an educational program in the regionalization of perinatal health care. *Semin. Perinatol.* 1:279–282, 1977.

46. Ostrea, E. M., and Odell, G. B. The influence of bicarbonate administered on blood pH in a "closed system." Clinical implications. *J. Pediatr.* 80:671–674, 1972.

47. Perlstein, P. H., Edwards, N. K., and Sutherland, J. M. Neonatal hotline telephone network. *Pediatrics* 64:419–424, 1979.

48. Pettett, G., Merenstein, G. B., Battaglia, F. C., et al. An analysis of air transport results in the sick newborn infant: Part I. The transport team. *Pediatrics* 55:774–786, 1975.

49. Pickering, D. E. One state-of-the-art design solution for continuing intensive care of distressed infants during land and air transport. In S. Graven (ed.), *Newborn Air Transport.* Evansville, IN: Mead Johnson, 1978. Pp. 27–31.

50. Raivio, K. O., and Hallman, N. Neonatal hypoglycemia. I. Occurrence of hypoglycemia in patients with various neonatal disorders. *Acta Paediatr. Scand.* 57:517–521, 1968.

51. Rudolph, A. J. In J. Lucey (ed.), *Problems of Neonatal Intensive Care Units. Report of the 59th Ross Conference on Pediatric Research.* Columbus, OH: Ross Laboratories, 1969. P. 15.

52. Ryan, G. M., Jr. Toward improving the outcome of pregnancy. Recommen-

dations for regional development of perinatal health services. *Obstet. Gynecol.* 46:375–384, 1975.

53. Sachs, B. P., Marks, J. S., McCarthy, B. J., et al. Neonatal transport in Georgia: Implication for maternal transport in high-risk pregnancies. *South. Med. J.* 76:1397–1400, 1983.

54. Schneider, J. M. In P. Sunshine (ed.), *Regionalization of Perinatal Care. Report of the 66th Ross Conference on Pediatric Research.* Columbus, OH: Ross Laboratories, 1974. P. 27.

55. Seigel, S. R., Phelps, D. L., Leake, R. D., et al. The effects of rapid infusion of hypertonic sodium bicarbonate in infants with respiratory distress syndrome. *Pediatrics* 51:651–657, 1973.

56. Silverman, W. A., Fertig, J. W., and Berger, A. P. The influence of thermal environment upon the survival of newly born premature infants. *Pediatrics* 22:876–880, 1958.

57. Silverman, W. A., Sinclair, J. C., and Agate, E. J. The oxygen cost of minor changes in heat balance of small newborn infants. *Acta Paediatr. Scand.* 55:294–299, 1966.

58. Simmons, M. A., Adcock, E. W., Bard, H., et al. Hypernatremia and intracranial hemorrhage in neonates. *N. Engl. J. Med.* 291:6–12, 1974.

59. Solimano, A. J., Smyth, J. A., Mann, T. K., et al. Pulse oximetry: Advantages in infants with bronchopulmonary dysplasia. *Pediatrics* 78:844–849, 1986.

60. Souma, M. L. Maternal transport: Behind the drama. *Am. J. Obstet. Gynecol.* 134:904–908, 1979.

61. Special Report. *The Perinatal Program: What Has Been Learned.* Princeton, NJ: The Robert Wood Johnson Foundation, 1985.

62. *Standards and guidelines for cardiopulmonary resuscitation (CPR) and emergency cardiac care (ECC). Part VI: Neonatal advanced life support. J.A.M.A.* 255:2969–2973, 1986.

63. Sumners, J., Harris, H. B., Jones, B., et al. Regional neonatal transport: Impact of an integrated community/center system. *Pediatrics* 65:910–916, 1980.

64. Swyer, P. R. The regional organization of special care for the neonate. *Pediatr. Clin. North Am.* 17:761–776, 1970.

65. Thompson, T. R. Neonatal transport nurses: An analysis of their role in the transport of newborn infants. *Pediatrics* 65:887–892, 1980.

66. Turbeville, D. F., Bowen, F. W., and Killam, A. P. Intracranial hemorrhages in kittens. Hypernatremia versus hypoxia. *J. Pediatr.* 89:294–296, 1976.

67. Usher, R. H. Changing mortality rates with perinatal intensive care and regionalization. *Semin. Perinatol.* 1:309–319, 1977.

68. Usher, R. H. The role of the neonatologist. *Pediatr. Clin. North Am.* 17:199–202, 1970.

## Chapter Appendix I. Neutral Thermal Environmental Temperatures

| Age and weight | Starting temperature (°C) | Temperature range (°C) |
|---|---|---|
| 0–6 hours | | |
| &lt; 1200 g | 35.0 | 34.0–35.4 |
| 1200–1500 g | 34.1 | 33.9–34.4 |
| 1501–2500 g | 33.4 | 32.8–33.8 |
| &gt; 2500 and &gt; 36 weeks | 32.9 | 32.0–33.8 |
| 6–12 hours | | |
| &lt; 1200 g | 35.0 | 34.0–35.4 |
| 1200–1500 g | 34.0 | 33.5–34.4 |
| 1501–2500 g | 33.1 | 32.2–33.8 |
| &gt; 2500 and &gt; 36 weeks | 32.8 | 31.4–33.8 |
| 12–24 hours | | |
| &lt; 1200 g | 34.0 | 34.0–35.4 |
| 1200–1500 g | 33.8 | 33.3–34.3 |
| 1501–2500 g | 32.8 | 31.9–33.8 |
| &gt; 2500 and &gt; 36 weeks | 32.4 | 31.0–33.7 |
| 24–36 hours | | |
| &lt; 1200 g | 34.0 | 34.0–35.0 |
| 1200–1500 g | 33.6 | 33.1–34.2 |
| 1501–2500 g | 32.6 | 31.6–33.6 |
| &gt; 2500 and &gt; 36 weeks | 32.1 | 30.7–33.5 |
| 36–48 hours | | |
| &lt; 1200 g | 34.0 | 34.0–35.0 |
| 1200–1500 g | 33.5 | 33.0–34.1 |
| 1501–2500 g | 32.5 | 31.4–33.5 |
| &gt; 2500 and &gt; 36 weeks | 31.9 | 30.5–33.3 |
| 48–72 hours | | |
| &lt; 1200 g | 34.0 | 34.0–35.0 |
| 1200–1500 g | 33.5 | 33.0–34.0 |
| 1501–2500 g | 32.3 | 31.2–33.4 |
| &gt; 2500 and &gt; 36 weeks | 31.7 | 30.1–33.2 |
| 72–96 hours | | |
| &lt; 1200 g | 34.0 | 34.0–35.0 |
| 1200–1500 g | 33.5 | 33.0–34.0 |
| 1501–2500 g | 32.2 | 31.1–33.2 |
| &gt; 2500 and &gt; 36 weeks | 31.3 | 29.8–32.8 |
| 4–12 days | | |
| &lt; 1500 g | 33.5 | 33.0–34.0 |
| 1501–2500 g | 32.1 | 31.0–33.2 |
| &gt; 2500 and &gt; 36 weeks | | |
| 4–5 days | 31.0 | 29.5–32.6 |
| 5–6 days | 30.9 | 29.4–32.3 |
| 6–8 days | 30.6 | 29.0–32.2 |
| 8–10 days | 30.3 | 29.0–31.8 |
| 10–12 days | 30.1 | 29.0–31.4 |

From Klaus, M. H., and Fanaroff, A. A. *Care of the High-Risk Neonate* (2nd ed.). Philadelphia: W. B. Saunders, 1979. P. 102. With permission.

# Appendixes

# Appendix 1

## Sample Request for Financial Assistance for the Initiation of a Regional Perinatal Dispatch Center

### Objective

The development of a regional perinatal dispatch center (RPDC) for the Washington, D.C. metropolitan area, the first phase of a regionalized transport system.

### Background

Effective, coordinated transport systems for ill newborn infants are now available in most areas of the country. The use of these transport systems has reduced neonatal mortality rates in the regions served [3,7,9]. More recently, maternal-fetal transport programs have been developed to complement existing neonatal systems as a means to further reduce perinatal and neonatal mortality and morbidity [1,4,6].

Perinatal regional planning has become central to this nation's goal to reduce perinatal and neonatal morbidity and mortality rates [3,5,8]. Specialized facilities with highly trained personnel have been developed in many hospitals to care for high-risk pregnant women and ill newborn infants. It has been observed in large urban areas that up to 10 to 11 percent of all live births have required specialized neonatal care [2]. A great many newborns at risk can be recognized before birth. Ideally, these infants should be delivered at perinatal centers, with maternal transport being the optimal form of transport. But for various reasons, they often are not recognized prenatally, or problems do not manifest until the newborn period. Since these infants will need access to special facilities, transport becomes a necessity. The efficiency of any program attempting to meet the needs of ill newborns in a particular area will depend on the *prompt* exchange of information so that proper care can be given. To achieve this goal, an organized regional plan for centralized communication regarding infant-maternal transport must be designed.

396

The integral parts of a patient transport service begin with an effective communications system, i.e., central dispatch. The development of RPDCs in other areas of the country has significantly reduced neonatal mortality in those areas [10].

### Rationale

The time between initial stabilization and transport of the infant to an institution that can effectively care for that infant is critical. In the past to determine bed availability in the Washington, D.C. metropolitan area, the referring physician has had to call at least eight different institutions. To minimize time expended on the telephone and to optimize the infant's outcome, the development of an RPDC for both maternal and neonatal transport is crucial for the Washington, D.C. area.

Presently, individual tertiary centers are arranging each transport as the call comes to the institution. An RPDC would not change that basic arrangement but would facilitate the receipt of the call, and thus allow each hospital to dispatch their transport team much faster.

Children's Hospital National Medical Center (CHNMC) maintains a current bed census of the tertiary centers who will accept infant transfers. This information is presently available only to those referring physicians or hospitals who are using CHNMC as their first point of referral. Personnel at area tertiary centers have agreed that this information must generally be available and include data on the availability of high-risk obstetrical beds. An RPDC will aid the referring physician in acquiring bed availability data and facilitate appropriate transfer of the patient. The ultimate goal will be to improve the care of and outcome for our ill newborns in the Washington, D.C. metropolitan area. This proposal is presented as a combined effort by the institutions listed on the title page, because of their concern for newborns in our area.

### Specific Aims

1. To organize an RPDC available on a 24-hour basis to *all* metropolitan hospitals, relaying neonatal and perinatal (high-risk obstetrical) bed availability in the tertiary centers in the D.C. area
2. To offer both neonatal and high-risk obstetrical consultation to the area hospitals

## Methods

The combined efforts of CHNMC, Columbia Hospital for Women, District of Columbia General Hospital, Fairfax Hospital, Georgetown University Hospital, George Washington University Hospital, Howard University Hospital, and Washington Hospital Center will be involved in the development of an RPDC. The location will be at CHNMC for the first year and at Georgetown University Hospital for the second year, with the personnel responsible for the system based at each respective institution.

1. The physical unit will consist of a dispatch phone system. All of the above hospitals will be linked via a speed-calling centrex phone system that will enable direct communications between these institutions. (Other institutions wishing a direct line may have this placed at their request.) _____ is being asked to fund the installation and maintenance of the phone system for 2 years.
2. Consultation, bed availability information, and initiation of transport services for high-risk mothers or ill newborns will be obtained by calling the RPDC number ("the gold line") and asking for the desired tertiary center. The dispatcher will transfer the referring call to the appropriate center. Each center will have a designated "gold phone" in either or both their ICN and delivery areas. Each center will have a designated neonatologist and perinatologist available on an on-call basis (24 hours/day) for neonatal/perinatal consultations.
3. Bed census will be taken twice a day (8:00 AM and 8:00 PM) and recorded on a central board or computer terminal at the RPDC site. Log books will be kept for analysis of calls. Each tertiary center will call in the bed census to the RPDC at designated time intervals so that an up-to-date census will be maintained.
4. Dispatch personnel (for year 1) will consist of the neonatal transport team members at CHNMC, with backup personnel being the neonatal nurse practitioners who are available in the nursery at CHNMC on a 24-hour basis. Georgetown hospital staff will man the system the second year. The dispatch person is only responsible for relaying calls. *Consultations will be made with the appropriate individuals at the hospital to which the patient will be transported.*

## Evaluation of the System

The RPDC system will be evaluated by reviewing response times for transport prior to the institution of the system and after the institution of the system. The infant mortality rates will also be examined prior to and after installation, but with recognition that many factors play a role in producing this rate. Questionnaires will be sent to all metropolitan hospitals to elicit their evaluation of the system, i.e., have they felt that the RPDC has aided their efforts to transfer high-risk infants or mothers? Results of these evaluations will be made available to all metropolitan area hospitals.

## Significance
Through the combined efforts of the tertiary centers of the Washington, D.C. metropolitan area, the time between stabilization and transport should be significantly reduced by initiation of an RPDC. The RPDC will play an important role in improving area morbidity and mortality rates for high-risk newborns.

## References
1. Brown, F. B. The management of high-risk obstetric transfer patients. *Obstet. Gynecol.* 57:674–676, June 1978.
2. Ferrara, A. New epidemiological evidence (survey research) to estimate 20 and 30 neonatal bed (NB) needs in urban areas, *NYC infant transport service (ITS experience).* (abstract) *Pediatr. Res.* 12:523, 1978.
3. Ferrara, A., and Harin, A. (eds.). *Emergency Transfer of the High-Risk Neonate.* St. Louis: C. V. Mosby, 1980. Pp. 3–18.
4. Giles, H. R., Isaman, J., Moore, W. J., et al. The Arizona high-risk maternal transport system: An initial view. *Am. J. Obstet. Gynecol.* 128:400–407, 1977.
5. *March of Dimes Committee on Perinatal Health. Toward Improving the Outcome of Pregnancy.* The National Foundation-March of Dimes, 1976.
6. Merenstein, G. B., Pettett, G., Woodall, J., et al. An analysis of air transport results in the sick newborn. II. Antenatal and neonatal referrals. *Am. J. Obstet. Gynecol.* 128:520–525, 1977.
7. Modanlou, H. D., et al. Antenatal versus neonatal transport to a regional perinatal center: A comparison between matched pairs. *Obstet. Gynecol.* 53:725, 1979.
8. Sunshine, P. (ed.). *Regionalization of Perinatal Care. Report of the 66th Ross Conference on Pediatric Research.* Columbus, OH: Ross Laboratories, 1974.
9. Usher, R. Changing mortality rates with perinatal intensive care and regionalization. *Semin. Perinatol.* 1:309, 1977.
10. Vogt, J. F., Chan, L. S., Wu, P. Y. K., et al. Impact of a regional infant dispatch center on neonatal mortality. *Am. J. Public Health* 71(6):577–582, 1981.

# Appendix 2

# Job Description—Neonatal Transport Team Nurse

### Department
Children's Hospital National Medical Center Department of Nursing

### Position No. _____

### Position Title
Neonatal transport team nurse

### Responsible To
Transport coordinator—neonatal transport team

### Position Description
The transport nurse is responsible for total patient care during inter-hospital transport. The transport nurse has responsibility for assessment and stabilization of patients prior to and during transport, including the performance of necessary diagnostic and therapeutic interventions. All activities are performed within the guidelines of protocols agreed on by the medical and nursing departments, and under medical supervision as defined by protocol. The transport nurse is also responsible for performing inhouse transports and for assisting nursery staff with patient care.

### Functions and Responsibilities
I. Interhospital transport
   A. Provides direct patient care to patients during interhospital transport including
      1. Complete newborn physical assessment, distinguishing between normal and abnormal findings
      2. Assessment of status of at-risk infant

3. Performance of diagnostic and therapeutic procedures as are necessary and appropriate for the care of the patient. Such procedures include endotracheal intubation, administration of emergency medications, placement of umbilical arterial and venous catheters, needle aspiration of chest, insertion of chest tubes or equivalent treatment, venipuncture, arterial puncture, interpretation of blood gases, determination of oxygen requirements, and determination of need for respiratory assistance
4. Communication with family including giving information and support

B. Maintains communication with supervising physician during transport, per protocol
C. Communicates with staff and parents at referring hospital
D. Is knowledgeable and competent in handling of all transport equipment. Ensures that all transport equipment is available at all times
E. Completes all paperwork required for transport including database, history, permits
F. Is responsible for total patient management during transport, when physician is not present
G. Performs weekly "call-backs" to referring hospitals as assigned by the transport coordinator. Prepares letters to be sent to referring physicians

II. Inhouse transport
A. Provides for transport of inpatients within the hospital, when not involved in ambulance transport. Coordinates such transports with other hospital departments

III. Assisting in nursery
A. When not involved in transport (whether outside or within the hospital) the transport nurse will assist nursery staff in the delivery of nursing care

### Qualifications

1. R.N. licensed to practice in the District of Columbia, Maryland, and Virginia, or eligible for same
2. Graduation from an accredited program of professional nursing; BSN preferred
3. Minimum 1-year neonatal intensive care experience at CHNMC, with a minimum 3.5 score on the Slater Competencies Rating Scale
4. Demonstrated expertise in neonatal nursing, in primary nursing, technical skills, and psychosocial aspects of care

5. Has in-depth knowledge and skill to assess the acutely ill neonate
6. Is flexible: able to meet varied work schedule, function independently, identify activities that will provide relief and help in the nursery
7. Has demonstrated good verbal and written communication skills
8. Has demonstrated ability to work well with staff, physicians, and patients
9. Has demonstrated reliability in work schedule
10. Satisfactory completion of CHNMC training program for neonatal transport nurses
11. Maintains current CPR certification
12. Maintains current IV start and IV push certification

# Appendix 3

# Job Description— Transport Coordinator

**Department**

Children's Hospital National Medical Center Department of Nursing

**Position No.** _____

**Position Title**

Transport coordinator—Neonatal transport team

**Responsible To**

1. Nursing: responsible to clinical unit coordinator for the nurseries
2. Medical: clinically supervised by medical director of transport. Clinically supervised during transport by attending neonatologist on-service or on-call

Annual written evaluation of performance will be completed by clinical unit coordinator and medical director of transport.

Observed clinical evaluation will be made by medical director of transport or designate.

**Position Description**

The transport coordinator is a registered nurse whose advanced training allows for practice as a transport nurse and for clinical supervision of the transport nurses. As a transport nurse, the transport coordinator is responsible for total patient care during inter- and intrahospital transport. The transport coordinator is also responsible for all aspects of supervision and practice of the transport nurses. The transport coordinator has responsibility for designated administrative aspects of the CHNMC Infant Transport System. The transport coordinator works in conjunction with the medical director of transport in the administration of the transport system.

### Functions and Responsibilities

I. Interhospital transport

    A. Provides direct patient care to patients during interhospital transport including

        1. Complete newborn physical assessment, distinguishing between normal and abnormal findings

        2. Assessment of status of at-risk infant

        3. Performance of diagnostic and therapeutic procedures as are necessary and appropriate for the care of the patient. Such procedures include endotracheal intubation, administration of emergency medications, placement of umbilical arterial and venous catheters, needle aspiration of chest, insertion of chest tubes or equivalent treatment, venipuncture, arterial puncture, interpretation of blood gases, determination of oxygen requirements, and determination of need for respiratory assistance

        4. Communication with family including giving information, support

    B. Maintains communication with supervising physician during transport, per protocol

    C. Communicates with staff at referring hospital

    D. Is knowledgeable and competent in handling of all transport equipment. Ensures that all transport equipment is functioning and available at all times

    E. Completes all paperwork required for transport including database, history, permits

    F. Responsible for total patient management on transport when physician is not present

    G. Assigns transport nurses to referring hospitals for the purpose of conducting weekly "call-backs" for patient follow-up reports, and for preparing letters to be sent to referring physicians. Performs weekly call-backs and prepares letters for those patients/hospitals assigned to the transport coordinator

II. Inhouse transports

    A. Provides for transport of inpatients within the hospital, when not involved in ambulance transport, and transport nurse is unavailable. Maintains communication and problem solves with relevant departments concerning inhouse transport of nursery patients

III. Supervises all functions of the transport nurses

IV. Evaluates clinical performance of the transport nurses (with input from medical director of transport)

    V. Prepares work and call schedule for transport nurses. Handles all leave requests of transport nurses

   VI. Attends meetings of administrative transport committee and weekly transport review meetings

  VII. Maintains statistics for CHNMC Infant Transport System and distributes to transport committee members and referring hospitals

 VIII. When not involved in above duties, assists nursery staff, including NNPs, in delivery of patient care

   IX. Staff development

     A. Participates in continuing education programs for nursery staff or transport nurses, or both

     B. Plans and participates in orientation of new transport nurses

     C. Maintains own clinical competency and keeps informed of current trends and developments in nursing practice and infant transport

     D. Ensures that transport nurses are trained in air physiology, air transport safety and survival techniques.

## Qualifications

1. R.N. licensed to practice in the District of Columbia, Maryland, and Virginia, or eligible for same
2. Graduation from an accredited program of professional nursing; BSN preferred
3. Minimum 2-years neonatal intensive care experience including 1 year of newborn transport experience
4. Satisfactory completion of an advanced training program beyond R.N. level, preferably a neonatal nurse practitioner training or other course specific to newborn transport program
5. Is a highly motivated, well-organized individual
6. Has demonstrated excellent verbal and written communication skills
7. Demonstrated expertise in neonatal nursing in primary nursing, technical skills, psychosocial aspects of care
8. Has in-depth knowledge and skills of assessment of the acutely ill neonate
9. Is flexible: able to meet varied work schedule and function independently
10. Has demonstrated reliability in work schedule
11. Maintains current CPR certification
12. Maintains current IV start and IV push certification

# Appendix 4

# Quality Assurance Report—Neonatal Transport Program

### Children's Hospital National Medical Center

## Transports during May

| | |
|---|---|
| Total number of transports | 78 |
| Primary transports | 54 |
| Return transports | 23 |
| Shunts* | 0 |
| Other | 1 |

## OUTCOME OF PRIMARY TRANSPORTED PATIENTS

| | |
|---|---|
| Discharged | 34 |
| Expired | 8 |
| Still hospitalized | 12 |

## TRANSPORT DELAYS (DELAY DEFINED AS MORE THAN 1 HOUR FROM TIME OF INITIAL CALL)

*Reasons*

| | |
|---|---|
| Ambulance/helicopter/jet | 7 |
| Personnel delay | 2 |
| Simultaneous call | 10 |
| Elective | 11 |
| Bed availability | 3 |
| Communication | 8 |
| Weather | 0 |
| Equipment | 0 |

## QUALITY ASSURANCE QUESTIONS

1. *Was equipment clean and ready for transport?*
   Yes: 78/78 transports.

2. *Was equipment functioning properly?*
   Yes: 75/78 transports. In one case, a syringe pump was nonfunctional, requiring that IV fluids be pushed intermittently. In one case, an IV pump failed to work. In both cases, the equipment was repaired by biomedical engineering.

*Transports done as a service to another referral center.

In another case, the ventilator switch on the transport module accidentally switched from IMV to CPAP mode while en route. Biomedical engineering was called on completion of the transport, and a cover plate was placed over the ventilator toggle switch; this should prevent inadvertent movement of the toggle switch during transport.

3. *Was the equipment appropriately inspected for safety according to hospital policy?*
No: 2/78 transports. In both instances, IV pumps were outdated for inspection and appropriate personnel were informed.

4. *Was there a delay in transport (i.e., more than 1 hour from initial call)?*
Yes: in most instances, delays were secondary to the elective nature of the admission, secondary to staff unavailability, or secondary to jet or helicopter unavailability. There were eight delays related to communication; in most instances, these delays involved timely notification of the transport nurse; this was discussed with the personnel involved.

5. *Did the infant survive the transport?*
Yes: 78/78 transports.

6. *Were there problems with Emergency Communications and Information Center (ECIC), security, helicopter dispatch operations?*
Yes: 2/78 transports. In one instance, the invertor on the helicopter was not working; subsequently repaired. In the second case, security was not on the helipad at the scheduled arrival time; appropriate supervisory personnel were informed.

7. *Were the actions of transport personnel appropriate?*
Yes: 78/78 transports. There were only three instances where some minor data was not recorded on admission to CHNMC. This has already been discussed with the transport staff, and recording is notably better this month.

The Pharmacy and Therapeutics Committee has yet to approve dobutamine as a stock item for transport. The next pharmacy meeting is scheduled in one month; until then, the pharmacy will provide us with a supply of dobutamine available for transport.

Negotiations with air carrier are underway. We hope that, provided an appropriate contract can be worked out, their service will provide us with more timely air transport for our patients.

# Appendix 5

## Sample Transport Statistics

| Children's Hospital National Medical Center's Transport Data | December 1987 | January–December 1987 |
|---|---|---|
| TOTAL NUMBER OF TRANSPORTS | 60 | 758 |
| Primary transports | 41 | 562 |
| Return transports | 15 | 177 |
| Shunts[a] | 2 | 3 |
| Patient expired before transport | 1 | 6 |
| Other | 1 | 10 |
| NUMBER OF TRANSPORTS BY SERVICE | | |
| Neonatology | 23 | 341 |
| Surgery | 5 | 72 |
| Cardiology | 9 | 71 |
| Neurosurgery | 1 | 27 |
| Genetics | 2 | 12 |
| ENT | 0 | 11 |
| ICU | 0 | 10 |
| Endocrine | 0 | 3 |
| Urology | 0 | 4 |
| Medical | 1 | 8 |
| Ophthalmology | 0 | 1 |
| Infectious diseases | 0 | 2 |
| ULTIMATE OUTCOME OF PRIMARY TRANSPORTS | | |
| Discharged | 25 | 475 |
| Expired | 4 | 70 |
| Still hospitalized | 12 | 17 |
| Patients not accepted due to lack of beds or staff | 16 | 119 |
| PRIMARY TRANSPORTS BY WEIGHT | | |
| <1000 g | 6 | 73 |
| 1001–1500 g | 4 | 55 |
| 1501–2000 g | 7 | 65 |
| 2001–2500 g | 6 | 87 |
| 2501–3000 g | 5 | 80 |
| 3001–3500 g | 12 | 114 |
| 3501–4000 g | 1 | 58 |
| >4000 g | 0 | 30 |

| *Children's Hospital National Medical Center's Transport Data* | *December 1987* | *January–December 1987* |
|---|---|---|
| TRANSPORT PERSONNEL | | |
| Registered nurse only | 31 | 356 |
| Registered nurse, respiratory therapist only | 23 | 277 |
| Registered nurse, physician only | 4 | 58 |
| Registered nurse, respiratory therapist, physician | 2 | 66 |
| Physician, respiratory therapist | 0 | 1 |
| TOTALS | | |
| Registered nurse | 60 (100%) | 758 (99.9%) |
| Respiratory therapist | 25 (41.6%) | 343 (45.2%) |
| Physician | 6 (10%) | 124 (16.8%) |
| TRANSPORT TYPE | | |
| Helicopter transports | 5 (8.3%) | 69 (9.1%) |
| Fixed-wing transports | 2 (3.3%) | 28 (3.7%) |
| TOTAL DELAYS[b] | 22 | 339 |
| Reasons | | |
|   Ambulance delay/helicopter/plane | 3 | 56 |
|   Personnel delay | 3 | 25 |
|   Simultaneous call | 2 | 67 |
|   Elective | 9 | 129 |
|   Bed or staff availability | 3 | 23 |
|   Communication | 2 | 37 |
|   Weather | 0 | 4 |
|   Equipment | 0 | 3 |
| TOTAL TRANSPORT TIME (LEAVE CHNMC TO RETURN TO CHNMC) | | |
| <1 hr | 8 | 67 |
| 1–1.5 hrs | 13 | 232 |
| 1.5–2 hrs | 15 | 229 |
| 2–2.5 hrs | 10 | 115 |
| 2.5–3 hrs | 9 | 58 |
| >3 hrs | 5 | 57 |

[a] Transport done as a service to another referral center.
[b] Delay time more than 1 hour from time of initial call. Some delays may be due to more than one reason.

# Appendix 6

# Infant Transport Equipment Checklist

### CHILDREN'S HOSPITAL NATIONAL MEDICAL CENTER
### Washington, D. C. 20010
### INFANT TRANSPORT/EQUIPMENT CHECK-LIST

**TOP SHELF**

| ITEM | Check |
|---|---|
| 1 Laryngoscope | |
| 1 O Miller blade with O₂ | |
| 1 1 Miller blade | |
| Extra batteries | |
| Extra bulbs | |
| O₂ tubing | |
| Benzoin | |
| 2 Swabs | |
| 2 NS for suction | |
| 2 #22 Quick caths | |
| 2 #24 Quick caths | |
| 2 #23 butterflies | |
| 2 #25 butterflies | |
| 2 #25 short butterflies | |
| 1 Arm board | |
| 2 2x2's | |
| 1 Scissors | |
| 1 1" cloth tape | |
| 1 1" paper tape | |
| 5 Rubber bands | |
| 5 Pins | |
| 5 Alcohol pads | |
| 5 Betadine ointment | |
| 2 Op site | |
| 2 Bandaids | |

**MIDDLE SHELF**

| ITEM | Check |
|---|---|
| 2 250mg Ampicillin | |
| 1 Gentamicin (40mg/ml) | |
| 1 Narcan (0.4mg/ml) | |
| 1 Dopamine (40mg/ml) | |
| 1 Priscoline (25mg/ml) | |
| 1 Lasix (10mg/ml) | |
| 1 Cagluconate (10ml) | |
| 1 D50W (50ml) | |
| 1 Phenobarbitol (65mg/ml) | |
| 1 Heparin (1000u/ml) | |
| 1 Water for injection (30ml) | |
| 1 Saline for injection (30ml) | |
| 1 NaHCO₃ (50cc) | |
| 1 Epinephrine (1:1000) | |
| 1 Atropine (1mg/ml) | |
| 1 20cc syringe | |
| 2 6cc syringes | |
| 3 3cc syringes | |
| 3 1cc syringes | |
| 5 Alcohol pads | |
| Assorted needles | |
| 1 Aerobic blood culture bottle | |
| 1 Anaerobic blood culture bottle | |
| Assorted blood tubes | |

**LOWER SHELF**

| ITEM | Check |
|---|---|
| 1 Set monitor leads | |
| 1 Package oral airways | |
| 1 Christmas tree adapter | |
| 2 #22 Medicuts | |
| 2 T-connectors | |
| 1 Flashlight | |
| 5 Lubricants | |
| 5 Betadine swabs | |

**LOWER SHELF (continued)**

| ITEM | Check |
|---|---|
| 1 60cc Betadine solution | |
| 1 Stopcock | |
| 1 Bottle dextrostix | |
| 5 Tape measures | |
| 2 Tongue blades | |
| 2 4.0 silk on needle | |

**BOTTOM OF BOX**

| ITEM | Check |
|---|---|
| 1 250cc D10W | |
| 1 250cc 5% Albumin | |
| 1 BP cuff | |
| 1 O₂ analyzer | |
| 1 Cardiobeeper | |
| 1 Calculator | |
| 4 4x4's | |
| 2 Hats | |
| 5 OP site | |
| 2 Adaptic | |
| 1 Monitor patches pack | |
| 1 I.V. tubing set | |
| 2 #8 Fr. feeding tubes | |
| 2 #5 Fr. feeding tubes | |
| 2 #10 Fr. Replogle tubes | |
| 2 #8 Fr. suction catheters | |
| 2 #6.5 Fr. suction catheters | |
| 2 Sterile stylets | |
| 2 4.0 ET tubes | |
| 2 3.5 ET tubes | |
| 2 3.0 ET tubes | |
| 2 2.5 ET tubes | |
| **1 UMBILICAL CATHETER KIT:** | |
| 1 Tray | |
| 1 Scalpel | |
| 1 Steri-drape | |
| 2 3.5 Umbilical caths | |
| 2 5.0 Umbilical caths | |
| 2 ea. 16,18,20,23 Leur stub adaptors | |
| 1 Sterile umbilical tape | |
| 1 20cc syringe | |
| 1 Stopcock | |
| 1 Heparin flush | |
| 1 Tape measure | |
| 1 4.0 silk suture on needle | |
| **1 PRESSURE LINE KIT:** | |
| 1 Dome | |
| 1 Intraflow - 30cc | |
| 1 High pressure tubing | |
| 3 Stopcocks | |
| 1 20cc syringe | |
| 1 1cc syringe | |
| **1 CHEST TUBE KIT:** | |
| 1 Steridrape | |
| 2 4.0 silk suture on needle | |
| 2 #10 argyle catheters | |
| 2 #12 argyle cathers | |
| 2 Heimlich chest drain valves | |
| 1 Connecting tube | |
| 2 OP site dressings | |
| 2 Y tubes | |
| 2 5-in-1 adaptors | |

**TRANSPORT AMBULANCE SUPPLIES**

| ITEM | Check |
|---|---|
| 1 Laerdal bag | |
| 1 O₂ hood | |
| 1 Ventilator tubing | |
| 1 Venturi | |
| 1 PEEP valve | |
| 1 Manometer | |
| 2 O₂ tubing | |
| 1 each-1, 2, 3, 4 Bennett masks | |
| 2 Suction canister liners | |
| 2 Connecting tubes | |
| 5 #8 suction catheters | |
| 5 #6.5 suction catheters | |
| 2 250cc bottles NS | |
| 5 cups | |
| 1 Box monitor patches | |
| 2 Packages monitor leads | |
| 1 Stethoscope | |
| 1 Clamp | |
| 3 1" cloth tapes | |
| 3 1" paper tapes | |
| 1 250cc D10W | |
| 1 250cc D5W | |
| 1 250cc ⅓ NS | |
| 1 250cc NS | |
| 1 250cc Ringers Lactate | |
| 1 250cc Sterile H₂O | |
| 2 I.V. tubing sets | |
| 2 Blood administration sets | |
| 2 A-line kits | |
| Assorted blood tubes | |
| 2 aerobic blood culture bottles | |
| 2 anerobic blood culture bottles | |
| 1 each film, flash for camera | |
| 1 Urine collecting system | |
| 5 Newborn 24-hour U-bags | |
| 1 box 4x4's | |
| 1 box 2x2's | |
| 5 Adaptics | |
| 3 Klings | |
| 1 box swabs | |
| 1 box Betadine swabs | |
| 1 bottle Betadine | |
| 3 Small sterile gloves | |
| 3 Large sterile gloves | |
| 2 Pillow cases | |
| 4 Blankets | |
| 2 Chux's | |
| 1 Roll plastic wrap | |
| 1 Roll 2" stockinette | |
| 1 Roll 3" stockinette | |
| 3 Transport form packs | |
| 3 OR permits | |
| 2 Replogle tubes | |
| 2 #8 NG tubes | |
| 2 Pleurevacs | |
| 1 Chest tube tray | |
| 2 250cc sterile H₂O | |
| 2 60cc catheter tip syringes | |
| 1 Screwdriver | |

CHNMC FORM 88 (Rev 1 82) Disk 1 r 1

# Appendix 7

## Treatment Protocols for Neonatal Transport

### Children's Hospital National Medical Center's General Neonatal Transport Protocol

I. *Procedures* to be followed on all transports

    A. Team members will introduce themselves to referring physicians and nursing staff.

    B. Receive report from staff about pre- and perinatal history, clinical course, laboratory results.

    C. Perform physical assessment of patient and record significant findings on appropriate form:

        1. Check vital signs—include environmental temperature, skin or axillary temperature, heart rate, respiratory rate, BP, Dextrostix.

        2. Perform rapid glucose determination.

        3. Check fraction of inspired oxygen ($FIO_2$), ventilator settings, arterial blood gases.

        4. Record appearance, hydration, color, estimated gestational age.

        5. Describe respiratory pattern, breath sounds, signs of distress (grunting, flaring, retractions).

        6. Describe heart rate, note presence of murmur, quality of pulses, perfusion, liver size, edema.

        7. Note tone, reflexes, size of fontanelle.

        8. Note any other pertinent data, e.g., bowel sounds, skin condition, anomalies, abdominal masses, urine, stool, nasogastric output.

    D. Review all x rays.

    E. Explain plans to referring staff before beginning stabilization. If there is disagreement about management, have referring physician talk with attending neonatologist before beginning treatment.

    F. Proceed with emergency stabilization (e.g., thoracentesis for treatment of tension pneumothorax).

    G. Check identity band on patient.

    H. Record a problem list pertinent to transport. List problems in order of priority.

    I. Record plans for management of each problem prior to and during transport.

    J. Call attending physician to give assessment of problems and discuss management plans. Revise plans as necessary.

K. Reassess vital signs, blood gases, other laboratory data or x rays as indicated and record on data sheet.

L. Once infant is stabilized as much as possible, talk with parents to explain plans for care, obtain remainder of information required on data sheets, give parents phone numbers, etc.

M. Move infant into transport unit, take Polaroid photo to give to parents, collect all materials to be transported with patient (sample of mother's blood, maternal cervical culture, charts, x rays, placenta if available, particularly in suspected chorioamnionitis or intrauterine infection).

N. Call receiving nursery to inform them of expected time of arrival, condition of infant, equipment needed for infant on arrival. Discuss any further changes in management with attending neonatologist.

O. Take infant in transport unit to mother's room for family to see and touch if possible.

P. Place transport unit in ambulance, check vital signs, $FiO_2$ concentration, ventilator settings, IVs.

Q. Proceed with transport, monitoring and recording vital signs every 15 minutes or more often if indicated.

R. On arrival at receiving hospital, check temperature and blood gases before removing patient from transport unit.

S. Assist with moving infant from transport unit.

T. Give report to receiving staff concerning history, all transport procedures.

U. Complete all transport forms, restock all equipment.

Each protocol has a summary that notes the critical goals for management of patients with that particular condition. Items with an asterisk (*) denote standard operating procedures that the transport nurse may initiate during stabilization prior to consulting supervising physician.

### General Management of Genetics Cases

I. *Prior to transport,* notify clinical genetics department of potential transfers of children with either malformations or suspected genetic disorders.

   A. Patient may benefit from evaluation at the referring hospital and may not necessarily require transport.

   B. Geneticist may at times prefer to accompany the transport team to the referring hospital to assess whether the transfer is truly necessary.

II. *Prior to refusal of a patient* with malformations or suspected genetic disorder, notify the clinical genetics department.

III. For malformed infants who have died following mobilization of the transport team to the referring hospital, plan to transport the infant back to CHNMC for a postmortem genetics evaluation, autopsy, and subsequent family counseling.

   A. Notify geneticist of patient's demise and of plan to transport infant back to the referral center postmortem.

   B. Obtain written permission from parents to transfer the infant postmortem.

   C. Obtain an autopsy permit with the parent(s)' signature prior to leaving the transferring hospital.

   D. Notify the local pathologist or coroner so that the body may be released for transport. Geneticist will assist with this, if necessary.

   E. If permission for transport is not given or if there are other questions or problems, call geneticist who will discuss the situation with the involved parties.

## General Premature Care

SUMMARY OF CRITICAL GOALS FOR MANAGEMENT
Avoid cold stress, fluid overload, hypoxia, or hyperoxia.

PROCEDURES FOR STABILIZATION AND MANAGEMENT OF THE SMALL PREMATURE INFANT DURING TRANSPORT

I. Assessment and initial management

   *A. Estimate gestational age using charts, obtain accurate weight.

   *B. Check vital signs and rapid blood sugar estimation, maintain normal temperature, check frequently.

   *C. Handle gently.

   *D. Avoid excess use of tape on skin. Use cardiorespiratory jacket if possible rather than chest leads.

   *E. Assess respiratory status carefully, check blood gases, avoid hyperoxia and hypoxia.

   *F. Carefully assess fluid requirements.

      1. See fluids protocol for suggested fluid administration volumes required in first days of life.

    2. Keep accurate record of all fluids administered including IV flush volumes, which should be kept at a minimum.

    3. Keep accurate record of all blood volume losses.

\*G. Assess glucose requirements and provide glucose source.

    1. Do rapid blood sugar determination.

    2. Provide IV glucose infusion 4–8 mg/kg/minute for sick prematures to avoid hypoglycemia.

II. Special procedures for transport. Concentrate on minimizing heat losses.

\*A. Use stocking cap on head to decrease body heat loss.

\*B. Cover baby with plastic wrap before transport.

\*C. Cover outside of incubator with blanket when outside in cold weather.

\*D. Prewarm all blankets.

\*E. Move baby to transport incubator quickly.

\*F. Work through portholes as much as possible.

\*G. Keep heat up in interior of ambulance.

\*H. Use warmed, humidified oxygen.

\*I.  Consider portable warming mattress, disposable heat packs, or warm water bottles.

III. Equipment needed for transport

  A. Prewarmed incubator

  B. Blankets

  C. Plastic wrap

IV. Potential complications

  A. Cold stress

  B. Retrolental fibroplasia (RLF) or retinopathy of prematurity from excessive oxygen—In premature, monitor arterial $PO_2$ frequently or use transcutaneous oxygen ($TcO_2$) monitor to help gauge hyperoxia $PO_2 > 80–90$ torr. If hyperoxia exists take immediate measures to decrease blood $PO_2 > 50 < 80$ torr.

  C. Fluid overload

  D. Hypotension, hypovolemia from inadequate replacement of blood. Volume expand with appropriate colloid, blood, or fluid as per treatment of shock protocol.

  E. Skin burns from heat sources that are too hot or too close to skin.

### Fluids
SUMMARY OF CRITICAL GOALS FOR MANAGEMENT
Avoid fluid overload and monitor for hyper- or hypoglycemia.

I. Guidelines for fluid administration during transport
  *A. Suggested rates of fluid administration in ml/kg/24 hours

|           | <1000 g   | 1000–1500 g | 1500–2500 g | >2500 g   |
|-----------|-----------|-------------|-------------|-----------|
| 1st day   | 100–120   | 80–100      | 60–80       | 60–80     |
| 2nd day   | 120–140   | 110–130     | 90–110      | 80–100    |
| 3rd day   | 140–150   | 120–140     | 110–140     | 100–120   |

  *1. Use 10% D/W for full-term or premature infants > 1000 g who are normoglycemic.
  *2. Use 5–7.5% D/W for preterm newborn < 1000 g.
  *3. Monitor capillary blood sugar, maintain > 45 < 130 mg/dl.
  *4. Monitor urine output, maintain 2–3 ml/kg/hour with specific gravity 1.005–1.010.
  *5. Run all IV fluids on IV pumps. If more than one IV is in place and extra pumps are not available, consider giving all fluid requirements through one IV and placing others on heparin lock.
  *6. Administration of electrolytes may be deferred until after transport unless the patient is severely hyponatremic, hypokalemic, or hypocalcemic and in urgent need of electrolyte correction.
  *B. Indications for peripheral IV. May be started by transport nurse when indicated for following reasons:
    1. Fluid/electrolyte administration, blood products
    2. Drug administration
    3. Glucose maintenance or correction
    4. Access to vascular space for potential emergency drug administration
  C. Indications for umbilical venous catheter (UVC). May be inserted by transport nurse after consulting with supervising physician for following reasons:
    1. Monitoring CVP with shock or congestive heart failure
    2. Exchange transfusion
    3. Access to vascular space for emergency drug administration
  D. Indications for umbilical arterial catheter (UAC). May be inserted by transport nurse after consulting with supervising physician for following reasons:
    1. Central arterial pressure monitoring
    2. Arterial blood gas monitoring
    3. Exchange transfusion
  E. Certain infants have unusual fluid requirements. Check with physician for specific orders.

1. Prematures less than 1500 g have increased insensible water loss and limitations in renal function.
2. Infants with a history of birth asphyxia may have
    a. renal injury secondary to asphyxia with subsequent oliguria and anuria
    b. cerebral edema
    c. cardiac dysfunction
3. Surgical patients have increased losses from exposed bowel, "third spacing" with dissemination of fluid into extravascular sites, and nasogastric loss.
4. Infants with congestive heart failure usually require cautious fluid restriction to approximately three-fourths of maintenance for normal infant.
5. Electrolyte supplements usually should begin on first day of life if renal function is normal, but may be delayed in first day until after transport has occurred. In very low birth weight infants hypernatremia may be a problem in the first few days of life, therefore it may be necessary to curtail sodium administration. Electrolyte supplementation may include
    a. NaCl 2–3 mEq/kg/day
    b. KCl 2 mEq/kg/day after urine output is established
    c. Elemental calcium 20–40 mg/kg/day

### Neonatal Hypoglycemia
SUMMARY OF CRITICAL GOALS FOR MANAGEMENT
Maintain rapid blood sugar determination in 45–130 mg/dl range, correct hypoglycemia promptly, and maintain glucose infusion thereafter.

I. Definition. Whole blood glucose level of <30 mg/dl (<35 mg/dl serum or plasma) in full-term infant, <20 mg/dl (<25 mg/dl serum or plasma) in prematures in first 72 hours of life. After 72 hours, whole blood glucose <40 mg/dl (<46 mg/dl serum or plasma) in any infant.
II. Recognition of causes
   A. Hyperinsulinism—infant of diabetic mother, erythroblastosis, islet cell hyperplasia or hyperfunction, Beckwith's syndrome, maternal chlorpropamide therapy
   B. Decreased stores—prematurity, intrauterine growth retardation
   C. Miscellaneous—sepsis, shock, asphyxia, exchange transfusion, glycogen storage disease, fructose intolerance, galactosemia, adrenal

insufficiency, maternal treatment with propranolol, sudden discontinuation of IV glucose supply, etc.

III. Symptoms
- A. Lethargy
- B. Limpness
- C. Tremors
- D. Apnea
- E. Cyanosis
- F. Seizures
- G. Weak or high-pitched cry
- H. Poor feeding
- I. None (always check)

IV. Differential diagnosis
- A. Adrenal insufficiency
- B. Maternal drug or alcohol use or abuse
- C. Heart disease
- D. Hypocalcemia
- E. Hypo- or hypernatremia
- F. Hypomagnesemia
- G. Pyridoxine deficiency
- H. Renal failure
- I. Liver failure
- J. Sepsis

V. Assessment and initial management
- *A. Obtain good history for predisposing causes.
- *B. Assess with physical exam.
- *C. Measure capillary blood sugar using tape test.
  - *1. If blood sugar is less than 45 mg/dl, draw blood glucose then start IV infusion for glucose administration. If arterial line is placed, the tip should be below the coeliac axis (pancreatic blood supply) and kidneys at $L_3-L_4$ level or well above the coeliac axis between $T_6$ and $T_{10}$. Begin with 6–8 mg/kg/minute glucose infusion. Glucose is given 0.36–0.48 g/kg/hour as 10% D/W. Recheck capillary blood sugar 20 minutes after starting IV. Infusion rate may be increased stepwise to achieve euglycemia, up to 15 mg/kg/minute glucose infusion.
  - *2. Rates of glucose administration greater than 15 mg/kg/minute should be given only through a central venous line.
  - *3. If blood sugar is 25 mg/dl or less *or* if infant is symptomatic, draw blood glucose, then give 2–3 ml/kg 10% D/W IV push

(0.2–0.3 g/kg of glucose). Immediately thereafter, begin 10% D/W infusion as above at 6–8 mg/kg/minute glucose infusion rate. Recheck capillary blood sugar in 20 minutes.

  *4. If blood sugar remains low, consult with neonatologist regarding further management.

VI. Equipment needed for transport. Standard transport equipment and kit to begin IV infusion; rapid glucose determination test material (Dextrostix, Chemstrip, or Accuchek).

VII. Potential complications
  A. Seizures
  B. Apnea
  C. IV infiltration and skin slough when giving hyperosmolar glucose infusion
  D. Liver damage due to infusing hyperosmolar glucose solution into misplaced UVC.

## Clinical Uses of Assisted Ventilation During Neonatal Transport

I. Relative indications for ventilatory support during transport
  A. In severe acute respiratory distress with hypercarbia, severe hypoxia, or patient exhaustion
    1. Hyaline membrane disease
    2. Aspiration syndromes, e.g., meconium aspiration, tracheoesophageal fistula (TEF) with aspiration
    3. Significant upper airway obstruction
    4. Pneumonia
    5. Persistent pulmonary hypertension (PPHN)
    6. Congestive heart failure, pulmonary edema
    7. Pulmonary hemorrhage
  B. In chronic respiratory distress, e.g., bronchopulmonary dysplasia, respirator bound
  C. In severe respiratory depression
    1. Perinatal asphyxia
    2. Seizures
    3. Severe apnea of prematurity
    4. Sepsis, meningitis
  D. With certain surgical lesions requiring airway or respiratory stabilization
    1. Diaphragmatic hernia
    2. Large gastroschisis or omphalocele
    3. Severe upper airway obstruction

E. In shock
   1. Septic shock
   2. Cardiogenic shock
   3. Hypovolemic shock
   4. Congenital lobar emphysema
   5. Cystic adenomatoic malformation of the lung
   6. Severe abdominal ascites

II. Attempt to attain satisfactory oxygenation and blood gases prior to transport
   *A. Aim for arterial $PaO_2$ 55–70 torr, $PaCO_2$ 35–50 torr, pH 7.35–7.40 generally.
   *B. Use portable transcutaneous oxygen ($TcO_2$) monitor or pulse oximeter, if available, to monitor oxygenation prior to and during transport.

III. Starting ventilator settings for various disease states
   *A. If blood gases prior to transport are normal and patient is on a respirator at the referring hospital then use similar settings on transport ventilator.
   *B. If patient has *normal lungs* (assessed by chest x ray and by pressure required to bag/ventilate the infant)

| Weight | PL (cm $H_2O$) | PEEP (cm $H_2O$) | Ti (sec) | Rate/ min |
|---|---|---|---|---|
| < 1000 g | 12–15 | 3 | 0.3–0.4 | 25–30 |
| 1000–1500 g | 15 | 3 | 0.3–0.5 | 25–30 |
| > 1500 g | 15–20 | 4 | 0.3–0.5 | 25–30 |

   *C. Hyaline membrane disease

| | PL (cm $H_2O$) | PEEP (cm $H_2O$) | Ti (sec) | Rate/ min |
|---|---|---|---|---|
| Early, mild | 18–20 | 4–5 | 0.4–0.5 | 30–40 |
| Moderate, severe | 20–25 | 5–6 | 0.6 | 30–40 |

   *D. Meconium aspiration

| PL (cm $H_2O$) | PEEP (cm $H_2O$) | Ti (sec) | Rate/ min |
|---|---|---|---|
| 25–35 | 3–4 | 0.3–0.4 | 40–60 |

   E. Persistent pulmonary hypertension of the neonate (PPHN): may require fast rates or high pressures, or both, to hyperventilate

| PL (cm $H_2O$) | PEEP (cm $H_2O$) | Ti (sec) | Rate/ min |
|---|---|---|---|
| 25–35 | 3–5 | 0.3–0.5 | 60–80 |

Note: Aim to maintain blood gases on hyperventilated patient with
PPHN pH 7.5–7.55, $PCO_2$ 25–30 torr, $PO_2$ 80–100 torr
unless premature—then $PO_2$ 75–85 torr range.

IV. Approach to treating hypoxemia, $PaO_2$ < 50 torr

*A. For nonintubated patient, increase $FIO_2$ prn up to 100%. (At $FIO_2$
> 60% use gCPAP if not a cyanotic cardiac condition.)

   1. Use portable $TcO_2$ monitor or pulse oximeter to gauge response.

   2. Aim for $PaO_2$ > 50 torr.

*B. Apply nasal constant positive airway pressure (CPAP) at 5 cm $H_2O$
up to 8 cm prn if parenchymal lung disease is present and cyanotic
congenital heart disease is not highly suspect.

*C. Intubate, ventilate. Use settings as above in III and increase $FIO_2$
prn.

*D. Listen for breath sounds and observe for symmetrical chest move-
ment (excursion).

*E. Increase Ti up to 0.7 second prn.

*F. Establish positive end expiratory pressure (PEEP) range 4–7 cm
$H_2O$.

G. If $PaO_2$ is < 50 torr despite pressure limit (PL) 30–35 cm $H_2O$, Ti
0.7 second, $FIO_2$ 100%, PEEP 5–8 cm $H_2O$ then contact physician
on call.

H. Consider differential digression

   1. PPHN

   2. Congenital heart disease

   3. Complication

      a. Atelectasis

      b. Pneumothorax

      c. Disconnected $O_2$

      d. Extubation

      e. Plugged endotracheal (ET) tube

      f. Malfunctioning respirator

V. Approach to treating *hypercarbia*, $PaCO_2$ greater than 55 torr

*A. For nonintubated patient

   *1. Gently stimulate.

   *2. Check neck position to be sure airway is not obstructed due to
positioning.

   *3. Intermittently bag ventilate for 2 minutes every 30 minutes.

*B. Intubate and ventilate for

   1. Prolonged apnea

   2. $PaCO_2$ consistently greater than 60 torr in acutely ill patient

   3. Progressively rising $PaCO_2$

\*C. Pressure cycle with short Ti (0.4–0.5 second), unless contraindicated due to coexisting hypoxemia

\*D. Favor $CO_2$ elimination by

   1. Increased rate (usually 50–60 to provide adequate expiratory time)

   2. Increased pressure limit (this effectively increases tidal volume)

   3. Decreased Ti, increased Te

   4. Decreased PEEP or decreased CPAP

   5. Increased flow rate

  E. Handbagging at rapid rates of 70–100 bpm occasionally will be needed. Be careful to watch inspiratory pressure on manometer in line

VI. Approach to treating *hyperoxia*

  \*A. Decrease $FiO_2$.

  \*B. Decrease PL by increments down to 15 cm $H_2O$.

  \*C. Decrease Ti by increments of 0.1 second down to 0.3 second.

  \*D. Decrease PEEP by increments to 3 cm $H_2O$.

  \*E. Consider weaning from respirator, but do not extubate during transport. Maintain PEEP 3 cm $H_2O$ until extubated.

Note: For PPHN, maintain $PaO_2$ 80–90 torr. Decrease $FiO_2$ only by 2–3% at a time to avoid "flip-flop" phenomenon.

VII. Approach to treating *hypocarbia*

  \*A. Some nonintubated infants spontaneously hyperventilate due to hypoxia, acidosis, CNS irritation, etc. Seek the cause.

  \*B. Decrease pressure limit by increments for intubated patient.

  \*C. Decrease IMV (rate).

  \*D. Decrease Ti.

  \*E. Do not extubate immediately prior to or during transport.

  F. Addition of dead space (5–10 cc) may be used for severe hypocarbia and alkalosis.

Note: For PPHN, hyperventilation may be therapeutic choice and $PCO_2$ 25–30 torr range may be sought. *Do not* aim to correct $PCO_2$ values immediately into the normal range since the blood $PCO_2$ level has a significant effect on intracranial blood flow.

IX. Respiratory equipment checklist.

  A. Figure A-1 is an example of the inspection checklist that should be placed in the incubator prior to transport, after equipment is cleaned and restocked.

  B. Check that items on checklist are present in working order prior to leaving on transport.

| Max. Unit. | Equipment |
|---|---|
| ☐ Incubator (inside) | Hood |
| | Laerdal bag |
| | Venturi mask |
| ☐ Drawer (inside) | $O_2$ nipple (2) |
| | Resuscitation masks 1-2-3-4 |
| | $O_2$ tubing |
| | PEEP valve |
| | Extra exhalation valve |
| ☐ Drawer or mounted | Manometer |
| ☐ Storage bin | Ventilator circuit (2) |
| | Humidifier circuit |
| | Nasal prongs, 1 each size for CPAP |
| | $O_2$ quick connectors |
| | Venturi mask |
| ☐ E cylinder | 2 at 2000 lb for ventilator |
| | 1 tank—1000 lb minimum |
| | Wrench for $O_2$ tank |

Date _____     Name _____

**PLACE THIS INSPECTION CHECKLIST IN INCUBATOR**

*Fig. A-1. Respiratory equipment checklist for transport incubator.*

## Resuscitation of the Newborn

SUMMARY OF CRITICAL GOALS FOR MANAGEMENT

Establish airway, establish ventilation, establish circulation, administer drugs, if necessary.

I. Basic neonatal resuscitation is similar to that of children and adults with regard to initial priorities
  A. Call for help.
  B. Establish airway if not already done.
  C. Ventilate to ensure adequate oxygenation and removal of $CO_2$.
  D. Establish more normal circulation.
    1. Cardiac massage
    2. Cannulation of vessels—venous, arterial
    3. Correction of hypovolemia
    4. Correction of acidosis

E. Give drugs.

F. Keep good records of timing of resuscitative measures.

Note: Remember to perform all resuscitation in a warm environment. Monitor temperature and all vital signs frequently.

II. Procedures

*A. Establish airway

* 1. Make sure airway is clear, suction as needed.

* 2. Place infant in supine position, with head moderately extended (the so-called sniffing position).

* 3. Mouth-to-mouth ventilation may be done by placing resuscitator's mouth over nose and mouth of infant. Inflation of the lungs should be done gently in the form of puffs from the mouth rather than from the lungs, until the chest wall moves.

*4. When expedient, bag and mask ventilation should be performed. The bag should be set up with a pressure manometer in line to accurately assess pressures used for ventilation. Make sure that the chest wall is moving.

* 5. Endotracheal intubation should be performed if the infant does not quickly resume spontaneous respirations.

B. Establish a heart rate and more normal circulation

* 1. If a heart rate of 80–90/min or less is found and does not increase with simple stimulation or ventilation, closed-chest cardiac massage should be started. Both thumbs are placed on the body of the sternum at the junction of the lower and middle thirds, and the back is supported with the fingers. The sternum is compressed approximately two-thirds the distance to the vertebral column 100 times/minute.

* 2. Effectiveness of massage is monitored by systolic pressure, ECG, pupil size, and return of normal heart rate.

* 3. Massage must be coordinated and simultaneous with assisted ventilation 5 compressions for each ventilation.

Note: Improperly applied compression may lead to ineffective cardiac rate, fractured ribs, or laceration of the liver.

C. Resuscitation drugs

* 1. IV access for emergency resuscitation of the newborn is most quickly obtained by passing an umbilical venous catheter just far enough to obtain blood return. This should be done as quickly and as aseptically as possible if no other IV is present. Existing UAC or peripheral IVs can be used for resuscitation.

* 2. (See Table A-1 for drugs and suggested dosages.)

*Table A-1. Resuscitation drugs most commonly used in neonatal resuscitation*

| Drug | Indication | Dosage | Route | Response | Complication |
|---|---|---|---|---|---|
| NaHCO$_3$* (1 mEq/ml) | Severe metabolic acidosis (pH < 7.25) | 1–2 mEq/kg diluted 1:1 given at rate 1 mEq/kg/min | IV | ↑pH | ↑ serum osmolality, ↑CO$_2$ if inadequate ventilation, hypernatremia, metabolic alkalosis |
| Epinephrine* 1:10,000 | Flat ECG, severe bradycardia | 0.1 ml/kg | IV or ET | Flat ECG converted to rhythmic response, ↑HR, improves myocardial tone | Hypertension, ventricular fibrillation. Not very effective with severe acidosis |
| Atropine* (0.1 mg/ml) | Bradycardia | 0.01–0.02 mg/kg (minimum dose 0.05 mg). If no response within 5 min, may increase to 0.1 mg/dose | IV or ET | ↑HR | Marked tachycardia, ↓CO |

| Isoproterenol (Isuprel) 1:5000 (0.2 mg/ml) | Bradycardia, low CO | 0.6 mg × body wt in kg added to 100 ml 5% D/W. Run at 1 ml/hour to deliver 0.1 μg/kg/min | IV | ↑HR, ↑CO | Dysrhythmias, tachycardia |
|---|---|---|---|---|---|
| Lidocaine* (2% or 4% for IV use) | Ventricular tachycardia or bradycardia | 0.5–1 mg/kg | IV or ET | Revert to normal rhythm | Seizures, myocardial and circulatory depression |
| Dopamine (40 mg/ml) | Low CO, hypotension | 5–20 μg/kg/min | IV | ↑Systemic pressure, ↑CO, ↑renal blood flow | Peripheral vasoconstriction, ↓renal flow if high dose used |
| Defibrillation | Ventricular fibrillation | 2–4 watt seconds/kg | | | |

↑ = increase; ↓ = decrease.
*First-line drugs.

## *Acid-Base Balance*

I. Definition
   A. Acceptable[†] pH 7.28–7.45, $PO_2$ 50–80 torr, $PCO_2$ 40–50 torr, BD < −8 mEq/L (in arterial blood)
   B. Acidosis—pH < 7.35
   C. Alkalosis—pH > 7.45

II. Respiratory acidosis—pH ↓, $PCO_2$ ↑, BD within normal limits
   A. Causes—hypoventilation, atelectasis, parenchymal lung disease
   *B. Management
      1. Improve ventilation
      2. Check for adequate airway
      3. ↑ Rate of ventilation
      4. ↑ PL or tidal volume

III. Respiratory alkalosis—pH ↑, $PCO_2$ ↓, BD WNL
   A. Cause—hyperventilation by mechanical ventilator or spontaneously
   *B. Management
      1. ↓ ventilator rate
      2. ↓ PL or tidal volume
      3. Shorten te
      4. Add dead space

IV. Metabolic acidosis—pH ↓, $PCO_2$ WNL, BD > −6 mEq/L
   A. Causes
      1. ↑ lactic acid, anaerobic metabolism, hypoxemia, poor perfusion, hypothermia
      2. Renal disease
      3. Late metabolic acidosis of prematurity
      4. Inborn metabolic error
   B. Management
      *1. Try to correct underlying cause, i.e., improve oxygenation (↑ $FiO_2$, ↑ PL, ↑ Ti, ↑ PEEP), improve perfusion (volume expansion), promote good thermoregulation
      *2. If persists after correction of above, may require use of $NaHCO_3$. BD × weight (kg) × 0.3. Give ½ of dose diluted 1:1 with sterile $H_2O$ slowly via IV (rate not to exceed 1 mEq/kg/minute). Recheck arterial blood gases (ABG) 15–20 minutes following dose and give additional dose if needed

V. Metabolic alkalosis—pH ↑, $PCO_2$ WNL, base excess (BE) present

---

[†]These are not normal ranges. Attempts to normalize blood gases completely during ventilation can lead to unnecessary barotrauma to the lungs.

A. Causes—excessive gastrointestinal losses, chronic diuretic therapy

B. Management—treat cause

Note: In all instances of acid-base disturbances, a compensatory mechanism takes place in either the lungs or kidneys. If the compensatory mechanism is adequate, the pH value may be normalized at the expense of an altered bicarbonate or carbonic acid concentration.

## *Shock*

SUMMARY OF CRITICAL GOALS FOR MANAGEMENT

For hypovolemia, administer volume expanders. Give pressor agents for nonhypovolemic shock.

I. Definition. Peripheral vascular collapse due to a derangement of circulatory control or loss of circulating fluid

II. Causes

A. Intrapartum asphyxia

B. Hemorrhage—perinatal or postnatal

C. Sepsis

D. Cardiogenic source

E. Adrenal crisis

F. Evaporative or "third-space" loss (e.g., as with gastroschisis or peritonitis)

III. Recognition

A. Clinical findings

1. Pallor, "clamped-down" or mottled appearance
2. Delayed capillary filling time > 3 seconds
3. Tachycardia often absent in early stages of shock
4. Tachypnea due to metabolic acidosis
5. Low central venous pressure
6. Weak pulses
7. Low blood pressure may not occur until shock is very severe because of the compensatory effect of the diving reflex
8. Hypoxia, cyanosis

B. Laboratory findings

1. Hypoxia, may have low blood $PaO_2$
2. Metabolic acidosis
3. Evidence of disseminated intravascular coagulopathy—late findings— ↑ PT, ↑ PTT, ↓ fibrinogen, fibrin degradation products (FDP) positive in urine

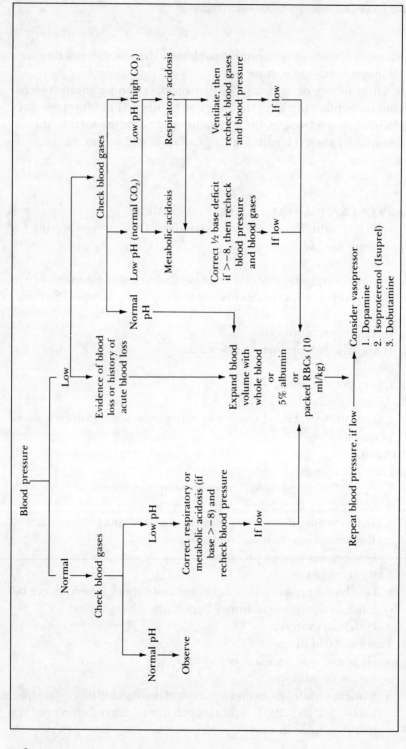

Fig. A-2. Algorithm for management of sick neonate by blood pressure monitoring.
**Note:** (1) If central venous pressure is rising with falling blood pressure, vasopressor drugs at cardiotonic dosage (e.g., dopamine 3 – 5 $\mu gm/K/min$) may be indicated as this suggests myocardial dysfunction. (2) Continued intravenous pushes of albumin can lead to cardiac failure.

428

4. Anemia in hemorrhagic shock (Hb < 14, Hct < 40 in neonate), although early in acute shock before reequilibration of blood volume, the Hb and Hct may be normal

IV. Differential diagnosis

    A. Cardiac tamponade

    B. Acute pneumothorax

V. Assessment and initial management (Fig. A-2).

    A. Physician should accompany transport of patient known to be in shock on transport.

  *B. Evaluate patient's skin perfusion and blood pressure, try to determine most likely cause for shock

      1. Check peripheral pulses and capillary filling time (normal < 3 seconds).

      2. Assess blood pressure peripherally and centrally, if possible.

      3. Consider CVP line placement. Unless a UVC can be placed quickly, with optimal localization of the tip, this is better left until arrival at the tertiary center.

    C. Consider immediate intubation and assisted ventilation.

  *D. After attempting to achieve adequate oxygenation and normal $PaCO_2$, then stabilize blood pressure by volume expansion for hypovolemic states.

    *1. Administer volume as 5 ml/kg over 5 minutes as crossmatched whole blood, 5% albumin, or normal saline. Repeat volume expander administration as necessary every 5–10 minutes until patient clinically improved and BP is in normal range.

    *2. If more than 15 ml/kg volume expander is given, consult with physician on call.

    *3. Give crossmatched packed RBCs, 10 ml/kg if anemia or hemorrhage is present and patient is shocky. O negative uncrossmatched packed red blood cells may be used in extreme emergency.

    *4. *Remember that BP may be normal in shock (especially in early stages). Do not rely on BP alone to diagnose shock.*

    *5. Notify attending physician/fellow on call of patient's shocky condition. Discuss placement of CVP line with physician on call.

    E. Consider use of pressor agents (dopamine or dobutamine) when patient is not in hypovolemic state.

      1. Consult with physician on call prior to administration.

      2. Starting doses for dopamine and dobutamine are 5–10 $\mu$g/kg/minute for renal and pressor effects.

    F. Perform rapid glucose determination and correct hypoglycemia.

G. Administer antibiotics if septic shock suspected.

H. Transport only after patient stabilized.

I. Take volume expander along on transport in case shock state recurs.

VI. Special procedures, equipment, drugs for transport

A. Dopamine or dobutamine, or both, and isoproterenol (Isuprel)

B. Type-specific whole blood or O negative packed RBCs (obtained at the referring hospital and uncrossmatched in extreme emergency)

C. Pressure transducer(s) for central pressure monitoring

D. BP cuffs and Doppler apparatus

VII. Complications

A. Cardiorespiratory arrest or arrhythmias

B. Seizures

C. Acute renal failure

D. Increased risk for necrotizing enterocolitis

E. Death

## Hyaline Membrane Disease (Respiratory Distress Syndrome)

SUMMARY OF CRITICAL GOALS FOR MANAGEMENT

Avoid hypoxia, hypothermia, acidosis. Support respiratory efforts as needed with ambient $O_2$, CPAP, or ventilator prn. Be vigilant for complications, e.g., pneumothorax.

I. Definition. This form of respiratory distress in the newborn premature infant results from a deficiency in the amount of surfactant produced in the lungs, causes alveolar collapse or atelectasis on end expiration, and leads to decreased lung compliance and inadequate surface area for gaseous exchange.

II. Recognition

A. Clinical findings—These signs can occur shortly after birth within the first 24 hours of life:

1. Tachypnea
2. Nasal flaring
3. Cyanosis
4. Retractions
5. Grunting
6. Poor air entry

B. Laboratory findings

1. ABG. Infant may be hypoxic and may show respiratory or metabolic acidosis; however, $PCO_2$ can be normal or even low during the first hours of the disease—or in large, near-term infants.

2. CBC. Hb, Hct, and differential blood count should be within normal limits providing there are no other problems.
3. Blood glucose. Hypoglycemia may occur.
   C. Radiological findings
   1. The classic x-ray finding shows a diffuse, fine, reticulogranular pattern in the lungs, with air bronchograms.
III. Differential diagnosis
Other problems that may be mistaken initially for hyaline membrane disease (HMD) are
   A. Transient tachypnea of the newborn
   B. Pneumonia—congenital or secondary to aspiration syndromes
   C. Hypothermia
   D. Hypoglycemia
   E. Metabolic acidosis
   F. Upper airway obstruction
   G. Congenital heart disease
   H. Sepsis
   I. Hypoplastic lungs
   J. Pneumothorax
   K. Tracheoesophageal fistula (TEF)
   L. Space-occupying lesions (e.g., diaphragmatic hernia)
   M. CNS pathology
   N. Acute hypovolemia
   O. Hyperviscosity
   P. Pulmonary hemorrhage
   Q. Persistent pulmonary hypertension of the neonate
IV. Assessment and initial management
   *A. View chest x ray initially to rule out surgical problems (such as TEF or diaphragmatic hernia).
   *B. Oxygenation—deliver sufficient $O_2$ to maintain $PO_2$ from 50–80 torr. If infant is requiring > 60% $FiO_2$ and has a $PO_2$ < 50 torr, CPAP or mechanical ventilation may be in indicated.
   *C. Ventilation—may require mechanical ventilation if $PCO_2$ is persistently > 60 torr or infant has severe apnea.
   D. Correct metabolic acidosis with the administration of sodium bicarbonate as warranted (see Table A-1).[†]
   *E. Watch for signs of and treat per specific protocols
   1. Hypovolemia
   2. Hypoglycemia

---

[†] Be aware that a metabolic acidosis may signal impending exhaustion in an infant using his or her accessory muscles to maintain ventilation.

3. Hypothermia
4. Sepsis

*F.  Maintain patent airway
   1. Extend neck slightly with roll under shoulders.
   2. Keep ET tube clear of secretions. Suction prn.
   3. Secure endotracheal tube well prior to transfer.

V. Special procedure for transport

*A. Check adequacy of $O_2$ supply, bag, mask, ventilator function prior to transport.

*B. Use shoulder roll to keep neck slightly extended if supine.

*C. Administer proper amount of $O_2$. Use portable transcutaneous oxygen monitor ($TcO_2$) or pulse oximeter if available to assess adequacy of oxygenation. Ventilate to maintain acceptable blood gas values (see p. 419).

*D. Suction prn.

VI. Special equipment needed for transport
   A. $O_2$ hood
   B. Oxygen analyzer
   C. Laryngoscope and ET tubes (sizes 2.5, 3.0, 3.5 Fr)
   D. Bag for ventilation and mask with proper adapters for ET tubes
   E. Ventilator
   F. Apparatus for needle thoracentesis of chest and chest tube placement and drainage should pneumothorax occur
   G. Nasal CPAP prongs

VII. Potential complications
   A. Apnea or exhaustion
   B. Air leak
      1. Pneumothorax needs to be drained by needle thoracentesis or by chest tube placement
      2. Pneumomediastinum usually not treated unless very large and under tension
      3. Pneumopericardium must be drained prior to transport because
         a. May expand during transport leading to tamponade especially if in unpressurized aircraft
         b. Very difficult to treat en route
      4. Interstitial emphysema
      5. Pneumoperitoneum may rarely require paracentesis because respiration or perfusion is compromised
   C. Infection: Do septic workup and begin antibiotics as necessary
   D. Blocked or dislodged ET tube: Suspect blocked ET tube if infant's $PCO_2$ suddenly rises or if infant appears cyanotic and is struggling

to breathe without adequate air exchange on auscultation. Suspect dislodged ET tube when a large air leak occurs when hand ventilating the infant
E. Malfunctioning ventilator or oxygen delivery bag
F. Agitation and irritability: Try pacifier, swaddle, and TLC
G. Patent ductus arteriosus
H. PPHN

## Transient Tachypnea of the Newborn
SUMMARY OF CRITICAL GOALS OF MANAGEMENT
Provide for adequate oxygenation and respiratory support if needed (rare).

I. Definition. A mild, self-limited respiratory disorder thought to be related to delayed reabsorption of fetal lung fluid
II. Recognition
  A. Clinical findings
    1. Tachypnea
    2. Cyanosis in room air may occur
    3. Retractions, usually mild
  B. Laboratory findings
    1. ABG may show mild hypoxia. Some infants may also exhibit respiratory acidosis
    2. May also be hypoglycemic
  C. X-ray findings show prominent markings with fluid present in the fissures or pleural spaces—a "wet lung"–type picture
III. Differential diagnosis
  A. HMD
  B. Pneumonia
  C. Sepsis
  D. Upper airway obstruction
  E. Congenital heart disease
  F. Persistent pulmonary hypertension of the neonate
  G. Aspiration of meconium or amniotic fluid
IV. Assessment and initial management
  *A. Oxygenation and ventilation
    1. Deliver sufficient $O_2$ by hood to maintain $PO_2$ from 50–80 torr.
    2. Consider use of CPAP or mechanical ventilation if $PO_2$ is < 50 torr in > 80% $FiO_2$.
  *B. Buffer marked metabolic acidosis with $NaHCO_3$ (BD > −8).
  *C. Watch for signs of

        1. Hypoglycemia
        2. Hypovolemia
        3. Sepsis
        4. Hypothermia
    D. Consider septic workup and antibiotics if respiratory symptoms have not improved within 24 hours after birth. (This may be done after transport by admitting physician or nurse.)
  *E. Suction prn.
 V. Special procedure for transport
  *A. Maintain patent airway—use shoulder roll to keep neck slightly extended.
  *B. Suction prn.
  *C. Deliver $O_2$ if needed and support respiratory effort.
 VI. Special equipment needed for transport
    A. $O_2$ hood
    B. Bag and mask for hand ventilation
    C. Suction equipment
VII. Potential complications
    A. PPHN
    B. Apnea due to fatigue—rarely occurs

### Pulmonary Hemorrhage
SUMMARY OF CRITICAL GOALS FOR MANAGEMENT
Prevent shock. Try to tamponade blood flow.

   I. Definition. Hemorrhage emanating from interstitial, alveolar, or both lung spaces and manifested by blood issuing from the airway
  II. Recognition
    A. Certain factors may predispose an infant to pulmonary hemorrhage
        1. Perinatal asphyxia
        2. Prematurity with respiratory distress syndrome
        3. Hypothermia
        4. Infection
        5. Oxygen therapy
        6. Breech presentation with difficult delivery
        7. Diffuse intravascular coagulopathy
        8. Hemorrhagic disease of the newborn (vitamin K deficiency)
        9. CNS hemorrhage
      10. Congenital heart disease with large left-to-right shunt

B. Clinical manifestations
1. Bleeding from upper airway occurs in about 50% of infants having pulmonary hemorrhage.
a. Bloody froth in mouth or nose is seen in nonintubated patients.
b. Bleeding from trachea suggests the diagnosis.
(1) Direct visualization by laryngoscopy may reveal a bleeding site below the vocal cords in nonintubated patient.
(2) Bloody froth welling up in endotracheal tube is very suggestive of pulmonary hemorrhage.
2. Sudden, severe respiratory distress with tachypnea, retractions, cyanosis, and rapidly deteriorating clinical picture are common findings.
C. Radiological findings are nonspecific, variable
1. Reticulogranular appearance
2. Nodular densities
3. Complete opacification of lung or portions of lung
III. Differential diagnosis
A. Trauma to trachea or bronchi due to intubation or suctioning
B. Hemorrhage from subglottic hemangioma
C. Upper airway (nasal or pharyngeal) trauma with hemorrhage
D. Gastric or esophageal bleeding with regurgitation of blood into posterior pharynx
E. Regurgitation of swallowed maternal or placental blood
IV. Assessment and initial management for transport
*A. If patient is not intubated, blood is present in posterior pharynx, and the site of hemorrhage is uncertain, perform direct laryngoscopy to ascertain whether blood is coming from below the cords.
*B. Attempt to maintain as clear an airway as possible with suctioning, but avoid prolonged suctioning.
*C. Administer oxygen. Intubate and assist ventilation.
*D. Use relatively high CPAP or PEEP (8−10 cm $H_2O$ in term infant, 6−8 cm $H_2O$ for small premature) for several hours to try to tamponade the bleeding (if patient intubated).
*E. Ensure good IV access to be ready to support intravascular blood volume.
*F. Monitor CVP or arterial pressure plus peripheral perfusion for signs of impending shock.
*G. If infant is in shock transfuse crossmatched fresh whole blood 10−20 ml/kg (or PRBCs 10 ml/kg).

*1. Obtain coagulation studies prior to transfusion.
   *a. Draw hematocrit initially, then every 3–4 hours until bleeding abates.
   *b. Obtain platelet count, PT, PTT, fibrin degradation products (fibrinogen level is optional).
   2. Repeat transfusion as required to correct shock state after consulting with supervising physician.
   H. Administer vitamin K (Aquamephyton) 1 mg IM to term infant, 0.5–1 mg IM to premature infant after coagulation studies are drawn if there is strong suspicion that the infant may have hemorrhagic disease of the newborn due to vitamin K deficiency.
 V. Equipment needed for transport. Ventilator, suction equipment, adequate PEEP valves to give up to 10 cm $H_2O$ PEEP on bag used for hand ventilation.
VI. Potential complications
   A. Obstruction of ET tube by blood clot. ET tube may require changing if suctioning fails to resolve the problem.
   B. Hypovolemic shock.

## Asphyxia
SUMMARY OF CRITICAL GOALS FOR MANAGEMENT
Recognize that all systems may be affected and anticipate renal, cardiac, respiratory, gastrointestinal, and CNS compromise. Treat seizures. Prevent hypoxia.

 I. Definition. Asphyxia occurs when adequate gas exchange fails, resulting in hypoxia and acidosis. The period of labor and delivery, as well as the first minutes following birth, carries a very high risk for asphyxia. Etiologies are diverse.
 II. Recognition
   A. Clinical findings
      1. During the delivery recognize the need for resuscitation by assessing 1 minute Apgar score.[†]
         a. If *7 or above* the infant usually will need only stimulation
         b. If *4 to 6* the infant may be moderately depressed or asphyxiated and often requires vigorous stimulation and may need ventilator with bag, mask, and oxygen
         c. If *0 to 3* the infant is severely depressed and may be severely

[†] Necessary resuscitation should be initiated concurrently.

asphyxiated. Be prepared for vigorous resuscitation that may require

(1) Positive pressure ventilation with oxygen (either bag and mask or bag to endotracheal tube)

(2) Endotracheal or nasotracheal intubation

(3) Buffer administration to help correct residual metabolic acidosis *after* establishment of adequate ventilation. Usually 1–2 mEq/kg may be given for severe asphyxia as initial dose

(4) Cardiotonic drugs (adrenaline, atropine, dopamine, Isuprel, etc.)

2. After initial resuscitation the asphyxiated infant may be

   a. Pale, shocky, or "clamped down" peripherally due to metabolic acidosis, hypoxia, cardiogenic shock, or severe intrapartum blood losses

   b. Cyanotic, if the infant has failed to make the normal transition from fetal circulatory pathways (PPHN)

   c. Hypotensive or have a normal blood pressure

   d. With seizures, usually beginning 12–24 hours after birth

   e. Hypotonic or neurologically depressed

   f. Normal, if the infant was mildly asphyxiated and received proper delivery room resuscitation

B. Laboratory findings—asphyxiated infants may manifest

   1. Hypoglycemia

   2. Metabolic acidosis, respiratory acidosis, or hypoxia on blood gas assessment

   3. Hypocalcemia with low ionized $Ca^{++}$

   4. Anemia, if prepartum or intrapartum blood loss occurred (reflected by Hb < 14 gm/dl, Hct < 40% within 6 hours posthemorrhage but not necessarily reflected acutely after the bleed)

   5. Hemoglobinuria or hematuria due to hemolysis or renal injury, or both

   6. Elevation of creatine kinase cardiac (MB) fraction will indicate significant cardiac insult.

C. X ray findings—Cardiomegaly may be noted due to hypoxic-ischemic injury with myocardiopathy or papillary muscle infarction

   Note: Diagnosis of cardiomegaly in neonate is difficult since thymus often contributes to apparently large cardiothymic silhouette.

D. Other tests that may be obtained and interpreted after transport

   1. ECG may reveal ischemic pattern, myocardial infarction pattern, or ventricular enlargement pattern.

    2. 2-D echocardiography of heart may show poor myocardial contractility, tricuspid regurgitation, papillary muscle dysfunction, right-to-left shunts foramenorale or ductus arteriosus (PPHN).

III. Differential diagnosis: Certain conditions other than perinatal asphyxia should be considered in any infant requiring a complicated resuscitation

  A. Hypoplastic lungs

  B. Diaphragmatic hernia

  C. Severe intrapartum blood loss

  D. Septic shock

  E. Severe intracranial pathology (e.g., hemorrhage, anomaly)

IV. Assessment and initial management

  *A. Determine the etiology of the asphyxia, if possible.

    1. Obtain careful perinatal history, including history of maternal illness and documentation of drugs taken or administered prior to and during labor.

    2. Review fetal monitor record, scalp, and cord blood gas analyses.

    3. Examine the placenta.

    4. Consider the differential diagnosis in *III* above.

  B. Monitor blood gases

    1. Correct severe respiratory acidosis.

    *a. Intubate if not already intubated.

    *b. If intubated, ventilate more effectively by increasing pressure limit (by $3-5$ cm $H_2O$), tidal volume, or rate on ventilator.

    *c. Alternatively, if intubated, hand ventilate at fast rates ($80-120$ per minute) with pressure manometer in line to achieve effective hyperventilation.

    *d. Use $TcO_2$ monitor or pulse oximeter if available to aid assessment of oxygenation. Use $TCO_2$ monitor to assess adequacy of ventilation.

    *2. Correct metabolic acidosis with appropriate base buffer, $NaHCO_3$, or tromethamine (THAM).

  C. Stabilize blood pressure. Correct for shock after adequate oxygenation and ventilation established. Some circulatory changes are seen with asphyxia which may mimic or mask shock. After warming, oxygenation, and correction of acidosis, anticipate that peripheral vasodilation and hypotension may occur.

  *D. Monitor and correct for hypoglycemia if present (see p. 416).

  *E. Promote normal body temperature maintenance.

  F. Anticipate development of cerebral edema with severe asphyxia.

*1. Restrict IV fluid administration. 50–60 ml/kg/day may be appropriate for severe asphyxia.
2. If considering use of steroid, consult with physician on call.
3. Mannitol or glycerol may be ordered by the physician on call. (They are unlikely to be used during transport but may be used following transport.)
4. If infant on ventilator, consult with physician on call regarding hyperventilation.
*G. Anticipate seizures in severe asphyxia.
1. Rule out metabolic causes for seizures such as hypoglycemia, hyponatremia, hypocalcemia.
2. Use anticonvulsants for therapy as per seizure protocol (see p. 444).
V. Special drugs for transport
A. Decadron
B. Mannitol
C. Phenobarbital
D. Dilantin
VI. Potential complications
A. Uncontrolled seizures compromising respirations may require intubation and ventilation (see p. 418).
B. Severe cerebral edema may result in apnea leading to respiratory arrest requiring intubation and ventilation.
C. Cardiogenic shock or heart failure may occur in severely asphyxiated infants.
D. Inappropriate antidiuretic hormone secretion. Fluid restriction will be needed.
E. Acute renal failure. Fluid restriction to insensible loss and urine output in oliguric phase is essential.
F. Fulminant hepatic necrosis.
G. Hypocalcemia.
H. PPHN
I. Necrotizing enterocolitis.

## Meconium Aspiration
SUMMARY OF CRITICAL GOALS FOR MANAGEMENT
Support respiratory needs and effort. Be alert for pneumothorax. Suspect persistent pulmonary hypertension component in severe cases.

I. Definition. The aspiration of meconium into the lungs causes obstructed airways, interferes with gas exchange, and causes respiratory distress. The passage of meconium into the amniotic fluid may result from perinatal asphyxia.

II. Recognition
  A. Clinical findings—The infant may present with the following signs or symptoms:
    1. Hyperinflation of chest wall
    2. Tachypnea
    3. Grunting
    4. Retractions
    5. Nasal flaring
    6. Cyanosis
    7. Rales
    8. CNS depression resulting from initial asphyxial insult
    9. Presence of meconium in larynx, trachea, or posterior pharynx. Meconium staining of umbilical cord or fingernails indicates meconium present a minimum of several hours.
    10. Signs of postmaturity including desquamation on distal extremities, decreased subcutaneous fat, long fingernails
  B. Laboratory findings
    1. *ABG.* Infant may be hypoxic and may show respiratory acidosis. Infant may exhibit metabolic acidosis resulting from asphyxia.
    2. *Blood glucose.* Hypoglycemia may occur, especially if infant is postmature.
  C. X-ray findings
    1. Patchy infiltrates, bilateral or unilateral
    2. "Wooly" irregular densities
    3. Hyperaeration without infiltrates
    4. Pneumothorax or pneumomediastinum may be present

III. Differential diagnosis
  A. Bacterial pneumonia
  B. PPHN
  C. Congenital heart disease
  D. Sepsis
  E. Amniotic fluid aspiration

IV. Assessment and initial management
  *A. Suction prn to remove meconium
  *B. Oxygenation
    1. Deliver sufficient $O_2$ to maintain $PO_2$ from 50–80 torr. If infant

requires $> 60\%$ $FiO_2$ and has a $PO_2 < 50$ torr, mechanical ventilation may be appropriate.

*C. Ventilation

1. May require mechanical ventilation with low PEEP (3–4 cm $H_2O$) if $PCO_2$ is persistently $> 60$ torr.
2. Usually attempt to use lowest PEEP possible to avoid air trapping, which is a particular problem for infants with meconium aspiration.

*D. Buffer severe metabolic acidosis with $NaHCO_3$ (BD $> -8$ mEq/dl).

*E. Watch for signs of

1. Hypoglycemia
2. Hypovolemia
3. Sepsis
4. Hypothermia
5. Pneumothorax, pneumomediastinum, pneumopericardium
6. Hypocalcemia

F. Administer antibiotics after sepsis evaluation when warranted.

V. Special procedure for transport

*A. Suction as needed.

*B. Administer appropriate $O_2$ therapy. Provide assisted ventilation, if necessary.

VI. Special equipment needed for transport

A. $O_2$ hood or ventilator, or both
B. Bag and mask for hand ventilation
C. Suction equipment
D. Equipment for evacuation of pneumothorax

VII. Potential complications

A. PPHN may occur if infant becomes hypoxic or hypovolemic
B. Pneumothorax and pneumomediastinum occur in at least 10% of cases
C. Blockage of ET tube due to meconium or mucus plugs
D. Dislodged ET tube

## Persistent Pulmonary Hypertension

SUMMARY OF CRITICAL GOALS FOR MANAGEMENT

Provide adequate oxygenation. Avoid acidosis. Wean slowly by small increments. Consider promoting alkalosis or using tolazoline (Priscoline) for refractory cases.

I. Definition. A syndrome characterized by persistent pulmonary hypertension (PPHN) resulting in right-to-left shunting across the patent
ductus arteriosus or foramen ovale, or both. Characteristically PPHN
is seen in infants with some form of severe in utero hypoxic ischemic
insult, and in infants with abnormal development of the lungs. Extra-
uterine insults, such as sepsis, can precipitate PPHN. The mechanisms
thought to be involved include imbalance in pulmonary vasoactive
substances and hypermuscularization of the pulmonary arteries and
arterioles.

II. Recognition

   A. Clinical findings

     The diagnosis should be considered in all cases of respiratory dis-
tress in which the oxygen requirement and progress of the disease
is not in keeping with the x-ray findings. PPHN should be suspected
with the following clinical signs and symptoms:

     1. Hypoxemia or acidosis in 100% oxygen

     2. A sustained systemic or suprasystemic pulmonary artery pres-
sure as suggested by prolongation of systolic time intervals by M-
mode echocardiography. (M-mode will be done after transport)

     3. A normal cardiac anatomy by 2-D echocardiography and normal
ECG (2-D echocardiography will be done after transport)

     4. Heart murmur may or may not be present (tricuspid regurgita-
tion blowing systolic murmur)

     5. Evidence of right-to-left shunt. A difference of 15 torr in $PaO_2$
between preductal, right radial, or temporal artery, and umbilical artery or postductal blood gases suggests a right-to-left
shunt at the patent ductus arteriosus (PDA). *Large right-to-left
foramen ovale* shunts may show no blood gas $PaO_2$ differences
between right radial and umbilical artery values.

     6. Severe respiratory distress syndrome (RDS), chronic asphyxia,
meconium aspiration, sepsis, pneumonia, or diaphragmatic hernia not responding to routine therapy.

     7. "Blue spells" or the "flip-flop" phenomenon in any infant with
respiratory distress

   B. X rays: Findings generally do not correlate with the oxygen requirement or degree of the illness. Severe meconium aspiration and
HMD may be exceptions to this

   C. Laboratory findings: Hypoxemia or acidosis at high $FiO_2$s. May
have an associated polycythemia, hypocalcemia, or hypoglycemia,
or a combination of these

III. Differential diagnosis
    A. Congenital heart disease
    B. Hypoplastic lungs
    C. Sepsis
    D. Diaphragmatic hernia
    E. Polycythemia
    F. Aspiration pneumonia
IV. Assessment and management. Acidosis and hypoxia must be treated immediately.
    *A. If respiratory acidosis is present, correct by increased ventilation. (Increase rate, tidal volume, or pressure limit, or a combination of these, depending on type of ventilator used.)
    *B. If transcutaneous oxygen monitor is available, apply monitor to right upper chest and use to help assess adequacy of preductal oxygenation. A second $TcO_2$ monitor may be applied in postductal position to help assess right-to-left shunt across ductus arteriosus.
    *C. If $FIO_2$ is not at 100%, then increase watching incrementally (the infant clinically) until $FIO_2$ 100% is reached.
    D. If infant is not intubated and step C fails, then intubate and attempt to hyperventilate with $FIO_2$ 100%, Ti of 0.3–0.5 sec, and rate 40–80 per minute. Use starting pressure limit of 20–25 cm $H_2O$ to achieve a pH 7.45–7.50 and $PCO_2$ of 25–30 torr. Watch chest-wall movement and listen for breath sounds. Increase rate, pressure limit, or both if necessary to achieve good hyperventilation. Note: Hand bagging may achieve better and quicker results than use of a ventilator for initial hyperventilation. Ventilating at fast rates may or may not achieve hyperventilation.
    *E. If metabolic acidosis is present, correct this with bicarbonate as per the acid-base protocol, p. 426. (Bicarbonate or THAM can be given as a bolus or by constant infusion.).
    *F. If anemia is present, correct this with packed RBC transfusion to improve oxygen-carrying capacity of blood.
    G. Vasodilators such as tolazoline should not be administered without a physician being present. Dose 1 mg/kg IV slowly as bolus then 1–2 mg/kg/hour as constant infusion if patient initially responsive.
    H. When weaning $FIO_2$ for infant having PPHN, decrease $FIO_2$ very gradually (at 1–2% a time) and maintain $PO_2$ in 80–90 range at least initially while weaning to avoid "flip-flop" phenomenon.
    I. Maintain normal blood pressure to prevent worsening of right-to-left shunt.

V. Special procedures for transport
  A. Take tolazoline for emergency administration.
  B. Use portable $TcO_2$ monitor if available, on right upper chest to help assess adequacy of oxygenation to the upper body including brain and retina.
  C. Have pressor agents (dopamine, dobutamine, Isuprel) available.
VI. Potential complications
  A. Pneumothorax secondary to therapy
  B. Hypotension if tolazoline is used: Applying hands to limbs as tourniquet during administration can be helpful. Have albumin (5%) or plasma substitute or FFP ready for acute volume expansion. Have dopamine or isoproterenol available. Hypotension may be fatal if the systemic pressure drops below the pulmonary artery pressure

## *Seizures*
SUMMARY OF CRITICAL GOALS FOR MANAGEMENT
Recognize that seizures may be subtle in neonates. Treat sustained seizures. Anticipate respiratory depression.

I. Definition. Seizures are caused by abnormal electrical activity in the brain frequently characterized by ocular or facial manifestations, tonic posturing, or with clonic movements of the extremities. Seizures will continue despite gentle restraint of an involved extremity. "Jitters" will stop with this maneuver.
  A. Causes of seizures
    1. Hypoxic-ischemic brain damage
    2. CNS trauma
    3. Intracranial hemorrhage
    4. Metabolic problems such as hypoglycemia, hypocalcemia, severe electrolyte imbalance, or inborn metabolic error
    5. Infections
    6. CNS malformations
    7. Drug withdrawal
    8. Kernicterus
  B. Types of seizures and their recognition
    1. Subtle seizures
      a. Eye movements
        (1) Horizontal deviation or vertical deviation of eyes
        (2) Jerking of eyes
        (3) Repetitive blinking or fluttering of eyelids

      b. Oral and buccal movements

        (1) Drooling

        (2) Sucking

        (3) Yawning

        (4) Lip smacking

      c. Tonic posturing of a limb

      d. Apnea

      e. Extremity movements with cycling or swimming movements

      f. Hyperpnea

      g. Vasomotor changes

  2. Multifocal clonic seizures present as clonic movements of limbs in a nonordered fashion, usually seen in infants over 34-weeks' gestation.

  3. Tonic seizures present as movements that are usually generalized, resembling decorticate posturing in older children; the movements are associated with eye deviation and occasionally with clonic movements or apnea.

  4. Focal clonic seizure movements involve well-localized clonic jerking.

  5. Myoclonic seizures present as synchronous single or multiple jerks of upper or lower limbs, or both.

C. Laboratory findings

  1. Hypoglycemia (see p. 416)

  2. Hypocalcemia—Ca $< 7$ mg/100 ml

  3. Hypomagnesemia—Mg $< 1.2$ mg/100 ml—is usually associated with hypocalcemia

  4. Hyponatremia—$Na^+ < 130$ mEq/liter; may result from inappropriate ADH secretion, adrenogenital syndrome, sepsis, etc.

  5. Hypernatremia—$Na^+ > 150$ mEq/liter

  6. Hyperbilirubinemia with kernicterus

  7. Urinary nontherapeutic drugs or metabolites

  8. Moderate to large ketones in urine

  9. Persistent metabolic acidosis

  10. Evidence of infection in urine, blood, CSF

  11. Anemia (e.g., intracranial hemorrhage)

D. X ray findings

  1. Skull fractures from trauma

  2. Intracranial bleed on CT scan or ultrasound (that may be done following transport). Note: Subarachnoid hemorrhage is *not* usually detected on ultrasound and may cause severe seizures. Ultrasound will not detect convexity subdural hemorrhage.

II. General approach to diagnosis of neonatal seizures
  A. Take careful prenatal and perinatal history.
  B. Examine the placenta grossly for signs of chorioamnionitis and microscopically for evidence of intrauterine infection, e.g., toxoplasmosis.
  C. Do careful physical and neurological exam including funduscopic exam and transillumination of the skull.
  D. Perform LP to rule out infection, hemorrhage.
  E. Obtain blood glucose, calcium, electrolytes, magnesium, hematocrit.
  F. When etiology is unclear, obtain serum amino acids, serum ammonia.
  G. Screen for TORCH infections as appropriate.
  H. Obtain skull films, CT scan, ultrasound, or MRI as indicated after transport is accomplished.
  I. Obtain EEG after transport is accomplished—usually not done during acute seizure period.
III. Assessment and initial management for transport
  *A. Obtain careful history including perinatal and family histories. Specifically ask for family history of metabolic disorders or of infants dying early in life, history of maternal substance abuse, family history of seizures, maternal exposure to cats (toxoplasmosis) or other infectious agents or toxins.
  *B. Obtain the placenta for gross and microscopic pathological evaluation.
  *C. Do careful physical assessment and neurological exam. Funduscopic exam and transillumination of the skull should be performed on admission to tertiary center by nurses or physicians admitting the patient.
  *D. Ensure adequate airway, and have suction, $O_2$, bag and mask for hand ventilation, laryngoscope, and ET tube available.
  *E. Describe seizure activity in detail if observed.
    1. Note parts of body involved
    2. Duration of seizure
    3. Changes in vital signs, color, blood pressure, or respiratory pattern
  *F. Position infant on side or abdomen, insert NG tube, and evacuate all stomach contents.
  *G. Ensure IV access.
  *H. Place on cardiorespiratory monitor.
  *I. Check all vital signs and make rapid glucose determination. Review all laboratory results including blood gases.

*J. Attempt to control seizures
  *1. Glucose
    *a. If Dextrostix is < 25 mg/dl, draw blood glucose then give 2–3 ml/kg 10% D/W IV push over 2–3 minutes.
    *b. Maintain glucose infusion at 6–8 mg/kg/minute (0.36–0.48 g/kg/hour) glucose infusion initially
    *c. Recheck glucose in 20 minutes.
  *2. Calcium
    *a. If hypocalcemia is present, give Ca gluconate (10%) 2 ml/kg (20 mg/kg elemental $Ca^{++}$) mixed with equal parts of water over 5–10 minutes.
    *b. Monitor heart rate during infusion since bradycardia can occur.
    *c. Do not mix calcium with $NaHCO_3$.
    *d. Do not give via UVC unless catheter is confirmed by x ray to be in vena cava. If calcium bolus is to be given peripherally, watch peripheral vein for infiltration.
  *3. Phenobarbital loading dose 15–20 mg/kg (optimum plasma level is 20–30 mg/dl).
    *a. Give as 10–15 mg/kg IV over several minutes in the presence of an active seizure.
    *b. If the seizures continue after 20 mg/kg is given, subsequent doses may be given, if necessary, if the infant is ventilated.
  K. Call attending neonatologist or fellow if seizures are not controlled by phenobarbital 20 mg/kg IV.
*IV. Special procedures for transport. Perform elective intubation for transport on any infant with repetitive seizures occurring just prior to transport. This is to ensure a patent airway if seizures occur during transport.
  V. Equipment needed for transport
    A. Standard equipment box
    B. Standard suction and initiation equipment
    C. Drugs: phenobarbital, dilantin, Valium
  VI. Potential complications
    A. Cardiorespiratory arrest or apnea
    B. Depression of respiration from seizures themselves or from drugs administered to control seizures

### Sepsis and Meningitis
SUMMARY OF CRITICAL GOALS FOR MANAGEMENT
Check CBC. Draw cultures. Treat with antibiotics. Anticipate shock.

I. Definition. Sepsis is a generalized infection with bacteria, virus, yeast-like or other agent that is spread via the blood system. Meningitis results from spread of infection into the CSF with involvement of the meninges. Sepsis or meningitis, or both, should be considered in any baby born under high-risk situations, such as PROM, complicated pregnancy and delivery, maternal fever or infectious illness, meconium aspiration, foul-smelling amniotic fluid; and in babies who are premature, or SGA. Major bacterial organisms: Group B streptococci, *Escherichia coli, Listeria monocytogenes,* enterococci.

II. Recognition
   A. Clinical findings
      1. The lung is the most commonly recognized site of infection in the newborn. These infants will therefore have clinical signs and symptoms resembling RDS of the newborn
         a. Tachypnea
         b. Apnea
         c. Grunting with retractions
         d. Nasal flaring
         e. Cyanosis
      2. Initially infected infants may be stable or may demonstrate lethargy, poor feeding, temperature instability, pallor, or cyanosis, or both, decreased skin perfusion, metabolic acidosis, low BP, petechiae, and poor urine output (i.e., septic shock)
   B. Laboratory findings—may include any or none of these:
      1. WBC low < 5000 per mm$^3$ with increased band count
            high > 30,000 per mm$^3$ with increased band count
         Note: May have an initial normal WBC that may then drop < 5000 per mm$^3$, therefore repeat WBC in 12–24 hours as indicated
      2. Hypoglycemia
      3. Hypocalcemia
      4. Decreased platelet count with increased PT, PTT, and with decreased fibrinogen and Factor VIII as DIC develops
      5. CSF: Protein—nl < 150 mg/dl (may be higher in < 1000-g infants)
         a. Glucose—$\frac{2}{3}$ peripheral blood sugar is normal
         b. WBC—nl < 30 per mm$^3$
         Note: CSF protein, glucose, and WBC may be normal in true cases of bacterial meningitis in infants. Therefore *a normal value does not rule out infection.*
   C. X ray findings

1. Group B streptococcal pneumonia may be indistinguishable from HMD (reticulogranular or ground glass pattern, hypoexpanded lungs).
2. Diffuse patchy pneumonia picture may be seen.
3. Clear lungs with only hyperinflation may be seen.
    Note: HMD and Group B streptococcal pneumonia can occur together as can meconium aspiration and Group B streptococcal pneumonia.

III. Differential diagnosis
   A. Any case of respiratory distress in the neonate
   B. Inborn errors of metabolism
   C. Drug withdrawal or intoxication
   D. Intracranial hemorrhage
   E. Bowel obstruction

IV. Assessment and initial management
   *A. Evaluate skin perfusion, capillary filling time (normal < 3 seconds), signs of pallor, or mottling. Check BP. Note: BP may be normal in the early stages of shock.
   *B. Obtain blood gases, CBC if not recently obtained.
   *C. Support perfusion with volume expansion (whole blood, 5% albumin, or NS as per shock protocol, see p. 427). If BP is decreased, then start pressor agents as per the attending physician on call (dopamine, isoproteranol, dobutamine).
   *D. Support respiratory status as per respiratory protocol (see p. 418).
   *E. Treat metabolic acidosis with $NaHCO_3$ therapy as per protocol, see p. 426.
   *F. Complete septic workup including blood culture, urine culture and latex agglutination test for Group B streptococcus antigen, and LP should be done stat. (Note: LP may be delayed in infant if too unstable until after transport.)
   *G. After cultures are obtained, give a stat dose of antibiotics. Initial antibiotics should consist of an aminoglycoside and a penicillin (example: gentamicin 2.5 mg/kg initial dose and ampicillin 100 mg/kg initial dose). If meningitis is suspected, discuss choice and dose of antibiotics with attending physician on call.
   H. Exchange transfusions may be done in severely septic infant, but this can best be done at tertiary care center.

V. Special procedures, equipment, drugs for transport
   A. Dopamine, dobutamine, and/or Isuprel
   B. Antibiotics to cover a broad spectrum of infected agents
   C. Volume expander, such as 5% albumin

VI. Potential complications
   A. Apnea
   B. Pneumothorax from ventilation efforts
   C. Persistent pulmonary hypertension
   D. Shock
   E. Disseminated intravascular coagulation
   F. Death


## Hemolytic Disease and Hydrops Fetalis

SUMMARY OF CRITICAL GOALS FOR MANAGEMENT
Determine etiology. Correct severe anemia by partial exchange transfusion. Anticipate CHF and need for respiratory support. When hydrops is severe, paracentesis (for ascites) or thoracentesis (for pleural effusion) may be indicated.

   I. Definition. Hemolytic disease in the newborn as a consequence of iso-immunization of the mother is usually caused by the passage of fetal red cells, possessing an antigen lacking in the cells of the mother, into the maternal circulation where they stimulate the production of antibody. These antibodies then return to the fetal circulation, during a subsequent pregnancy, and attach to antigenic sites on the surface of the fetal RBCs, leading to their rapid removal and destruction. The chief danger for the fetus in utero in a sensitized pregnancy is profound anemia with attendant heart failure. The most severely affected infants manifest *hydrops fetalis*. This is characterized by heart failure in utero and massive anasarca or edema with pleural effusions and ascites. Hydrops is not always associated with severe anemia, so nonimmunological causes must be considered: intrauterine arrythmias, large arteriovenous malformation, renal disease, congenital hepatitis, intrauterine infections, maternal diabetes mellitus, fetal neuroblastomatosis, umbilical or chorionic vein thrombosis, cystic adenomatoid malformation in the lung, pulmonary lymphangiectasia, chorioangioma of the placenta.
  II. Recognition
   A. Clinical findings
      1. Jaundice—not visibly present at birth even if hemolysis is severe
      2. Pallor
      3. Enlargement of spleen and liver
      4. Edema if hydropic

     5. Petechiae and purpura in severe cases

     6. May have respiratory distress and congestive heart failure

  B. Laboratory findings

     1. Anemia (Hgb < 14 g/dl but usually much lower)

     2. Increased reticulocyte count (> 6%)

     3. Increased number of nucleated RBCs on peripheral blood smear

     4. Rh disease yields a positive direct Coombs' test in the infant. If too many antibodies are present, then they may block Rh antigenic sites, and the infant's blood may type out as Rh-negative but the Coombs' test will be positive. In ABO incompatibility, the direct Coombs' test may be negative

     5. Microspherocytes are seen in ABO disease and congenital spherocytosis but not in Rh disease

  C. X ray findings

     1. May see pulmonary edema, pleural effusion, or ascites, or a combination of these in hydrops

     2. May see enlarged heart

     3. Hepatosplenomegaly may be present

III. Differential diagnosis

  A. CHD with failure in utero.

  B. Isoimmune hemolytic disorder.

  C. Ascites due to meconium peritonitis, ruptured renal papilla (posterior urethral valves)

  D. Fetal maternal hemorrhage

  E. Twin-twin transfusion

  F. Hemoglobinopathy (e.g., thalassemia)

  G. RBC defect (e.g., G6PD deficiency, pyruvate kinase deficiency)

IV. Assessment and initial management

  *A. Etiology must be considered so that proper blood studies on the mother can be drawn prior to transport and in the baby *prior to transfusion.*

  B. The severely affected infants die from progressive cardiorespiratory failure in which asphyxia and HMD play a major role. Therefore management demands a comprehensive approach including vigorous treatment of asphyxia, acidosis, hypoglycemia, and hypothermia.

  C. Assisted ventilation should be considered early in any infant with severe respiratory distress. PEEP should be used in the presence of pulmonary edema (start with 5 cm $H_2O$ and increase to 10 cm $H_2O$ as needed to improve oxygenation).

D. If significant respiratory distress is present and pleural effusions or ascites are present, these may be tapped and sufficient fluid removed to relieve the distress. Send fluid to lab for protein, cell count, and culture. Bilateral chest tubes may be inserted for drainage of pleural effusions since fluid reaccumulation after initial thoracentesis may occur.

E. In the presence of severe anemia (Hct < 35%) and respiratory distress, the fellow/attending physician should accompany the transport to evaluate the infant and decide if a partial exchange transfusion of 25–80 ml/kg of packed RBCs should be performed prior to transport.

F. Phlebotomy alone should not be performed because these infants are usually normovolemic.

G. CVP line for monitoring should be placed above the diaphragm if intravascular fluid volume is in question (normal CVP > 5 < 15 mm Hg).

H. If the infant's respiratory status can be stabilized, then it is safer to transport the infant and perform the exchange transfusion at the tertiary center.

I. Before an exchange transfusion and if the etiology is still unknown draw blood for
   1. Coombs' test—look for minor blood group incompatibilities
   2. CBC with reticulocyte count
   3. Total protein, albumin
   4. TORCH titers
   5. G6PD level
   6. Peripheral smear
   7. Alpha thalassemia—hemoglobin electrophoresis with quantitative hemoglobin levels
   8. Uncoagulated sample (hold)
   9. 1 Anticoagulated sample (hold)

J. Laboratory tests on infant
   1. CBC
   2. Reticulocyte count
   3. Peripheral blood smear
   4. Total serum protein, albumin
   5. Serum electrolytes
   6. BUN
   7. Creatinine
   8. Bilirubin (total/direct)
   9. $Ca^{++}$
   10. Coombs' test (direct)

    11. Indirect Coombs' test—look for minor blood groups
    12. Blood culture
    13. TORCH titers
  K. Placenta—look for vascular anastamoses and bring back for patho-
     logical evaluation
  L. Laboratory tests on mother (*must be drawn before transport*)
    1. Type and Rh
    2. Indirect Coombs' test
    3. Kleihauer-Betke test to detect significant fetal-maternal transfu-
       sions (anticoagulated sample)
    4. Serum TORCH titers
    5. Extra unanticoagulated sample
    6. Extra anticoagulated sample
  M. Exchange transfusion should be done at the tertiary center unless
     determined by the attending physician that the infant is not stable
     enough to move.
 V. Special procedure for transport
  A. Treat respiratory complications
  B. Fluid overload can be fatal, so monitor input and output closely and
     observe for signs of CHF. CVP monitoring may be helpful.


## Congenital Heart Disease
SUMMARY OF CRITICAL GOALS FOR MANAGEMENT
Transport promptly. If in shock, intubate for transport. Keep in telephone
contact with cardiologists for therapy guidance.

  I. Definition. Abnormal structure of or flow through the heart or great
     vessels may cause cyanosis, congestive heart failure (CHF), arrhyth-
     mias, murmurs, or absence of symptoms, depending on the lesion(s).
 II. Recognition
  A. Normal newborns may have changing heart murmurs, transient
     tachypnea, and cyanosis during vigorous crying (due to right-to-
     left shunts through PDA or PFO or both, during first hours after
     birth while transition from fetal to postnatal circulation occurs).
  B. Infants at risk for congenital heart disease (CHD) include
    1. Infants with genetic abnormalities (e.g., trisomy 21, 13–15,
       17–18, Turner's syndrome)
    2. Infants of diabetic mothers
    3. Infants with family history of or a sibling with CHD
    4. Infants infected in utero with congenital rubella or other viruses
    5. Infants born of incest or consanguinous parents

C. Clinical findings
   1. The infant may appear well for 24 hours or longer
      a. Pulmonary vascular resistance is high initially, thus protect-ing lungs temporarily from volume overload with what later may become large left-to-right shunts (e.g., ventricular sep-tal defect [VSD])
      b. Adequate flow (antegrade or retrograde) may be maintained by shunts through PDA or PFO. Once these structures close, then infant's condition quickly deteriorates with certain le-sions (e.g., hypoplastic left heart syndrome, interrupted aor-tic arch)
   2. Apgars are usually good unless there has been noncardiac-related perinatal asphyxia or heart failure in utero (e.g., as with severe Ebstein's anomaly or paroxysmal atrial tachycardia [PAT] arrhythmias in utero)
   3. Sudden weight gain or excessive weight gain
   4. Tachypnea without dyspnea; however with severe CHF and pulmonary edema, dyspnea may be present
   5. Tachycardia (> 160/minute)
   6. Cyanosis that may fail to disappear with administration of 100% $FiO_2$ over 15–20 minutes
   7. Hepatomegaly
   8. Heart murmur (often is absent even in presence of significant CHD)
   9. Abnormal pulses
      a. Weak femoral as compared to brachial pulses suggests pres-ence of coarctation of aorta, aortic stenosis, or cerebral AV fistula
      b. Bounding or jerky pulses suggest PDA, truncus with high pulmonary flow, AV fistula, or occasionally isolated VSD
      c. Generalized weakness or absence of pulses is seen with
         (1) Vascular collapse of advanced congestive heart failure (CHF)
         (2) Critically severe aortic stenosis
         (3) Malformations that are ductal dependent (e.g., aortic atresia, interrupted aortic arch, coarctation of aorta, hy-poplastic left heart syndrome)
         (4) Rarely, with myocarditis or transient myocardial ischemia
   10. Diaphoresis—sweating
   11. Edema
      a. Is a late sign of CHF in infants

      b. May be present in association with heart malformation without CHF, e.g., in patients with Turner's syndrome

12. Feeding difficulty or fatigue after initiation of feeding
13. Gallop rhythm
14. Wet lungs, rales, or wheezing on auscultation of lungs
15. Single second heart sound (heard with truncus, pulmonic atresia, transposition of the great vessels [TGV])

D. Laboratory findings

   1. Blood gases

      a. Low $PaO_2$ despite administration of high $FiO_2$ (100%) suggests cyanotic CHD or persistent pulmonary hypertension

      b. Low $PaO_2$ is seen in CHF with large left-to-right shunts and severe pulmonary congestion (since there is intrapulmonary shunting and unbalanced ventilation/perfusion)

      c. Mild respiratory acidosis may be seen with CHF

      d. In patients with severe aortic stenosis or with ductal-dependent lesions (e.g., aortic atresia, interrupted aortic arch, or coarctation of the aorta) when systemic outflow is obstructed after PDA constriction, there is initially relatively high $PaO_2$ with variable metabolic acidosis because of poor tissue perfusion

   2. ECG abnormalities using 25 mm/second paper speed

   3. X-ray findings

      a. Cardiomegaly is often difficult to assess on neonate's film

         (1) Transverse heart diameter is normally approximately 55% of thoracic width

         (2) Cardiothymic silhouette may confuse estimation of heart size

         (3) Lordotic or expiratory films may exaggerate heart size

      b. Increased pulmonary vascular markings

         (1) Seen in lesions with large left-to-right shunt

         (2) Seen in congestive heart failure

      c. Decreased pulmonary vascular markings

         (1) Seen with conditions of reduced pulmonary blood flow

         (2) Examples—pulmonary atresia, pulmonic stenosis, tricuspid atresia, tetralogy of Fallot (TET), Ebstein's anomaly

      d. Egg-shaped heart with narrow supracardiac pedicle suggests TGV

      e. Right aortic arch suggests possibility of CHD, e.g., double outlet right ventricle (DORV), tricuspid atresia, TET, truncus arteriosus

III. Differential diagnosis
   A. Pulmonary disease (e.g., HMD, TTN, pneumonia, hypoplastic lungs)
   B. PPHN
   C. Hyperviscosity syndrome
   D. Hypoglycemia
   E. Sepsis/meningitis
   F. Metabolic acidosis
IV. Assessment and initial management for transport
   A. Nonemergent cases, nonacidotic, not in shock
      *1. Review history to determine when infant developed respiratory distress, whether there has been rapid weight gain, whether there is family history for heart disease, whether mother took any substances or drugs during pregnancy that might predispose to CHD or CHF (alcohol, steroids, propranolol)
      *2. Examine infant and observe for
         a. Tachypnea
         b. Tachycardia
         c. Cyanosis
         d. Quality of heart sounds
         e. Clicks
         f. Murmurs
         g. Gallop rhythm
         h. Rales or wheezing
         i. Amplitude of pulses
         j. Edema
         k. Liver size
         l. Diaphoresis
         m. Bruits on auscultation of head and liver
      *3. View chest x ray for heart size, arch of aorta, vascularity, dextrocardia, etc.
      *4. Obtain ECG, if available
      *5. Obtain arterial blood gas, blood sugar, and hematocrit results, if available
      *6. Maintain in neutral thermal temperature range
      *7. Administer oxygen if assessed to be in CHF (30–40% $FiO_2$)
      *8. Transfer on cardiac monitor
      *9. Transfer in semi-upright (45 degree) position if in CHF
   B. Emergent cases, cyanotic with acidosis or shock
      1. Transport as speedily as possible but safely.
      2. *Physician should accompany transport.*
      3. Examine infant.

4. Administer humidified oxygen (30% $FiO_2$) when CHF suspected even in absence of cyanosis.
5. Maintain NPO. Ensure IV access for transport.
6. Buffer acidosis with $NaHCO_3$ or THAM.
7. Intubate and ventilate if severely distressed or shocky, or both.
8. Discuss with cardiologists administration of diuretics and digoxin at referring hospital, if patient in severe CHF.
9. For patient in shock with CHF, consider dopamine administration during transport (5–10 $\mu$g/kg/minute drip) to support BP and treat severe CHF. Discuss with cardiologists prior to use.
10. Be conservative with fluid administration and avoid large volume pushes.
11. Correct anemia with PRBC 5–10 ml/kg slowly (over 1 hour). If anemia severe and patient in CHF, use partial exchange transfusion.
12. Discuss with cardiologists use of $PGE_1$ to maintain ductal patency in patients thought to have ductal-dependent lesions. If decision pretransport is to use $PGE_1$, then take the medication out on transport and use only on order of cardiologist.

V. Special procedures for transport
   A. Be very prompt to transport. Do not delay.
   B. Physician should accompany transport of acidotic or shocky infant.
   C. Electively intubate if severely distressed or persistently shocky.
   D. Consider $PGE_1$ administration for suspected ductal-dependent lesion.
   E. Keep in touch with cardiologists for guidance.

VI. Equipment needed for transport
   A. Cardiorespiratory monitor
   B. Means for ventilatory support
   C. Drugs: dopamine, Lasix, digoxin ($PGE_1$, optional)
   D. Pulse oximeter or Tc $PO_2$ monitor

VII. Potential complications
   A. Cardiorespiratory arrest or apnea
   B. Arrhythmias
   C. Seizures from hypoxia (rare)
   D. Shock

## Intestinal Obstruction

SUMMARY OF CRITICAL GOALS FOR MANAGEMENT
Notify surgeons. Decompress GI tract. Keep NPO. Give IV fluids. Watch for acidosis and respiratory compromise from distension or associated sepsis or peritonitis.

I. Definition. Any condition in which transport of materials through the bowel is fully or partially blocked

II. Recognition
   A. Clinical findings—depending on where the obstruction is located. Various signs manifest:
      1. Vomiting—when bile stained, consider this a surgical emergency until proved otherwise
      2. Abdominal distension and/or discolorization
      3. Failure to pass meconium within 24–36 hours after birth
      4. Failure to develop transitional and fecal stools after passage of meconium
      5. Hematemesis or bloody stools, or both
      6. Abdominal masses
      7. Scaphoid abdomen (seen with diaphragmatic hernia)
      8. Excessive mucus and salivation (seen in tracheoesophageal fistula [TEF])
   B. Laboratory findings
      1. Electrolyte imbalance—hyperchloremic alkalosis most common
      2. CBC may show evidence of high white count and left shift
      3. Bilirubin may have prolonged elevation with bowel obstruction
   C. Radiological findings
      1. Have referring hospital obtain flat plate and cross-table lateral x-ray studies of abdomen. Upright study is difficult to obtain in newborn but may be helpful in some cases
      2. Look for distended loops of bowel, free air in peritoneal cavity, dilated stomach, and decreased or no air in intestines. Ask for left lateral decubitus abdominal film to show free air over the liver if pneumoperitoneum is suspected

III. Differential diagnosis
   A. Lower intestinal obstructions
      1. Meconium ileus
         a. Distended small bowel appears granular on x ray. Also x ray may show tiny air bubbles mixed with meconium
         b. No meconium passes through rectum even after digital stimulation
         c. May present as meconium peritonitis (calcified nodules seen on abdominal x ray)
      2. Hirschsprung's disease
         a. May present as failure to pass meconium in first 24–36 hours of life
         b. May present as enterocolitis

    c. On contrast x ray study a characteristic narrow segment with transition to dilated bowel in the area of the rectosigmoid junction may be seen

3. Imperforate anus high and low type
    a. Normal rectal opening is absent
    b. In low type a fistula may be seen on perineum, usually anterior to normal location of rectum
    c. In high type no fistula is seen on perineum but may have recto-vaginal/urethral fistula

4. Meconium or mucous plug
    a. May be relieved by digital stimulation
    b. Contrast x ray study (e.g., with gastrografin) may precipitate passage of meconium plug

B. Upper intestinal obstructions
1. Duodenal atresia
    a. Classic x ray shows double bubble of ingested air filling the stomach and blind-ending duodenum. (This lesion is commonly associated with trisonomy 21)

2. Pyloric stenosis
    a. Nonbilious vomiting (usually after first week of life)
    b. Large stomach on x ray with little or no gas found below duodenum
    c. Abdominal ultrasound may obviate need for contrast x ray study

3. Jejunal atresia
    a. X ray shows air fluid levels distributed throughout the abdomen
    b. May be seen in association with gastroschisis

4. Necrotizing enterocolitis (NEC)
    a. Infant presents with feeding problems (residuals) or vomiting, tenderness, abdominal distension, abdominal tenderness, heme-positive stools, apnea, signs of sepsis, or a combination of these
    b. On x ray, air in wall of intestines is classic sign (pneumatosis intestinalis) but is not always seen in cases diagnosed early
    c. On x ray, air in portal system is ominous sign. Look for this in right upper quadrant on PA film and anteriorly on lateral view

C. Gastric perforation—pneumoperitoneum
1. Gastric perforation
    a. Usually is seen in distressed neonates who have undergone resuscitation immediately after birth

       b. Free air in peritoneal cavity may be secondary to perforation elsewhere in gastrointestinal tract

       c. On physical exam abdominal distension is seen with elevation of the diaphragm on x ray

       d. Acute treatment by paracentesis of peritoneal cavity may diminish air and allow diaphragm to return to normal position

  D. Pneumoperitoneum due to air tracking from the thoracic cavity (will see pneumothorax or other type of air leak on chest x ray)

  E. Abnormalities of rotation

     1. Malrotation with midgut volvulus—*an emergency situation*

       a. Note bile-stained vomitus without abdominal distension

       b. Abdominal tenderness may be present

       c. X-ray findings

         (1) Show evidence of duodenal obstruction and scanty gas distributed throughout the remainder of the bowel

         (2) Airless abdomen

     2. Volvulus without malrotation

       a. See sudden onset of abdominal distension and bilious vomiting in an infant who has been having normal stools

       b. See signs of shock and sepsis

       c. X-ray findings

         (1) Dilated loops of small bowel

         (2) Possible midabdominal calcific shadow

IV. Assessment and initial management

  *A. Pass nasogastric, Levin, or Replogle tube and aspirate

     1. Empty stomach contents

     2. Keep NPO

  *B. Place IV, and start IV infusion

  C. Assess hydration, begin correction of electrolyte imbalance if possible, before transfer

  D. Do x-ray studies of abdomen, including flat plate, and cross-table lateral immediately following transport, if not already done

  *E. If signs of sepsis are present or if bowel perforation has occurred

     1. Draw cultures

     2. Treat with antibiotics

V. Procedures for transport

  *A. Place nasogastric, Levin, or Replogle tube. Aspirate frequently to evacuate contents or place to low intermittent suction. Elevate head of bed

  *B. Maintain respiratory status and vital signs as stable as possible

  *C. Maintain functional IV for fluid and medication administration

VI. Equipment needed
   A. Transport isolette
   B. IV solutions
   C. Oxygen
   D. Ventilator available
   E. NG, Levin, or Replogle tubes
   F. Antibiotics available
   G. Cardiorespiratory monitor
VII. Potential complications
   A. Vomiting and subsequent aspiration of vomitus causing respiratory distress
   B. Shock causing respiratory and cardiac distress or arrest
   C. Peritonitis due to bowel perforation
   D. Intravascular volume depletion due to "third spacing" of fluids
   E. Apnea or respiratory distress

## Abdominal Wall Defects

SUMMARY OF CRITICAL GOALS FOR MANAGEMENT
Decompress stomach. Cover bowel and minimize heat loss. If ruptured, give antibiotics. Avoid hypothermia, dehydration, and aspiration.

   I. Definitions
   A. Gastroschisis—A defect in the abdominal wall lateral to the base of the umbilical stalk through which a portion of the intestinal tract has escaped. There is no covering sac. Malrotation and intestinal atresias are frequent (20% of cases) as is prematurity (75% of cases).
   B. Omphalocele—A herniation through the umbilicus of abdominal contents. The defect is covered by a translucent membrane or sac unless ruptured.
   II. Recognition
   A. Classic clinical findings
      1. Protruding abdominal contents either covered with a sac or not
      2. May be large or small protrusion
   B. Laboratory findings not needed except to check for electrolyte imbalance
   C. Radiologic exam not necessary unless other clinical indications
   III. Differential diagnosis
   A. Umbilical cord hematoma
   B. Umbilical cord hernia

IV. Assessment and initial management
   *A. Diagnose omphalocele or gastroschisis.
   *B. If omphalocele membrane is unruptured
     *1. Limit examination and do not handle excessively.
     *2. Cover bowel immediately with sterile saline-soaked dressings (warmed saline). Cover these dressings with plastic wrap to help minimize heat loss.
     *3. Observe for discoloration or infarction caused by twisted bowel. If present notify surgeon and hasten transfer.
   *C. If omphalocele membrane covering is ruptured or for gastroschisis, follow all above steps and start antibiotics.
   *D. Prevent hypothermia, dehydration, and aspiration.
     *1. Keep infant warm.
     *2. Start IV infusion and hydrate well. Monitor capillary filling time and BP.
     *3. Pass nasogastric tube and aspirate stomach contents frequently.
V. Procedures for transport
   *A. Nasogastric tube in place.
   *B. Elevate head of bed.
   *C. Provide adequate IV access and adequately hydrate patient.
   *D. Stabilize respiratory status and vital signs. Obtain blood gases and correct severe metabolic acidosis (BD − 8 mEq/dl).
   *E. Keep the infant warm.
   *F. Position slightly to the side if possible after defect dressing is applied to avoid mass pressure on inferior vena cava that could impede venous return to the heart.
VI. Equipment needed
   A. Nasogastric tube and syringe for suction or low intermittent suction apparent
   B. Transport isolette
   C. Oxygen hood or ventilator depending on respiratory status
   D. Antibiotics needed if omphalocele sac ruptured or if gastroschisis present
VII. Potential complications
   A. Respiratory failure due to impaired abdominal movement. Plan to intubate and ventilate prn
   B. Hypothermia
   C. Electrolyte imbalance and dehydration. Give generous volumes of IV fluids and consider administering volume expander. Correct electrolyte imbalance over 12−24 hours. (Be careful. Congenital

heart anomalies can be associated with omphalocele and may pre-dispose to CHF)
D. Other associated anomalies, particularly common with omphalocele

## *Tracheoesophageal Fistula and Esophageal Atresia*
SUMMARY OF CRITICAL GOALS FOR MANAGEMENT
Suction secretions from esophageal pouch. Prevent aspiration. Keep prone with head up.

I. Definition. A condition that is an anatomical malformation of the esophagus. The esophagus usually ends (in 85% of cases) in a blind pouch extending only into the upper portion of the thorax. Usually the proximal end of the lower portion of the esophagus is connected to the trachea.
II. Recognition
   A. Perinatal history of
      1. Polyhydramnios and prematurity
      2. Inability to handle secretions in early hours after delivery. Bubbling mucus from mouth, coughing, choking
      3. Inability to pass NG tube into stomach. (NG tube may coil, however, in a large pouch and give a false sense of having passed into the stomach)
      4. Respiratory distress often from aspiration pneumonia
      5. Bowel distension (with distal TEF)
      6. Regurgitation of saliva out of infant's mouth and nose
   B. Laboratory findings—tests not needed.
   C. Radiological findings
      1. Pass NG tube prior to x ray.
      2. Isolated esophageal atresia—a blind-ending esophageal segment with gasless abdomen will be seen on x ray. Usually extends only into the upper portion of the thorax.
      3. Esophageal atresia with TEF—a portion of the distal blind-ending esophagus will be attached to the trachea and air will enter intestine.
      4. See wide air-filled pouch in the neck or upper mediastinum.
      5. May see pulmonic infiltrates due to aspiration pneumonitis. Right upper lobe (RUL) of lung is most frequently involved.

6. The NG tube, if in place, will be seen to stop at the end of the pouch at about $T_3$ or to coil in esophageal pouch.
7. Visible parts of abdomen frequently show hyperaeration of the intestines if there is a fistula.

III. Assessment and initial management

*A. Aim to evacuate secretions from esophageal pouch and prevent reflux of gastric secretions through the fistula into trachea.

    *1. Place plastic, radiopaque, sump catheter (Levin or Replogle tube) in proximal esophageal pouch connected to continuous or intermittent suction.

    *2. Pass the tube and apply suction, before x ray is done.

    *3. Maintain in prone position with head elevated (reverse Trendelenburg) to prevent gastric contents from entering distal esophagus and passing retrograde into tracheobronchial tree.

*B. Stabilize temperature.

*C. Put in IV line and hydrate the infant who must be kept NPO.

*D. Give antibiotics for aspiration pneumonitis as indicated by chest x-ray. Appropriate antibiotics, ampicillin and gentamicin, may be given.

IV. Procedures for transport

*A. Put plastic sump catheter (Levin or Replogle tube) to low suction if possible (or aspirate very frequently with syringes).

*B. Stabilize respiratory status. Maintain patent airway. Check arterial blood gases prior to leaving referring hospital. Correct severe metabolic acidosis BD > −8 mEq/dl.

*C. Maintain reverse Trendelenburg position (prone with head up).

V. Equipment needed

A. Plastic sump catheter (Replogle tube or Levin tube)
B. Transport isolette
C. Cardiorespiratory monitor
D. IV fluids
E. $NaHCO_3$
F. Oxygen or ventilator, or both, to maintain good respiratory status

VI. Potential complications

A. Poor control of secretions with regurgitation.
B. Aspiration pneumonitis
C. Abdominal distension
D. Respiratory insufficiency. Use positive pressure ventilation

## *Diaphragmatic Hernia*
SUMMARY OF CRITICAL GOALS FOR MANAGEMENT
Decompress stomach. Intubate, provide $O_2$, and ventilate as necessary. Correct acidosis. Transport quickly and notify surgeons at tertiary center.

  I. Definition. Failure of complete development of the posterolateral portion of the diaphragm results in persistence of the pleuroperitoneal canal or foramen of Bochadalek leading to presence of bowel in the chest, usually on the left side. In a right-sided diaphragmatic hernia, liver and bowel may herniate into the chest. The lung on the involved side will be hypoplastic (the lung on the contralateral side may also be hypoplastic to a lesser degree).

 II. Recognition

   A. Clinical findings

     1. History of sudden onset of respiratory distress at any time in the newborn period. These symptoms may progressively worsen.

     2. Bowel sounds in the chest (not frequently detected).

     3. Breath sounds louder on one side than the other, usually the right.

     4. Heart sounds loudest in one hemithorax, usually the right. Point of maximum impulse (PMI) may progressively shift to opposite side of chest as air enters gut.

     5. Unequal movement of chest wall.

     6. Scaphoid abdomen.

     7. Supraumbilical midline abdominal defects may be present occasionally.

   B. Laboratory findings

     1. Blood gases usually indicate hypercarbia, respiratory acidosis, or hypoxia, or all of these.

   C. Radiological findings

     1. A bowel gas pattern or mass effect is seen in one hemithorax.

     2. Mediastinal shift is seen with compression of the contralateral lung.

     3. The diaphragm may be markedly elevated or indistinct.

     4. Abdominal bowel gas is sparse or absent.

     5. Right hemithorax may opacify due to presence of liver in chest cavity.

     6. Pneumothorax may be present.

 III. Differential diagnosis

   A. Eventration of the diaphragm

   B. Congenital cystic adenomatoid malformation of the lung

  C. Multiple pulmonary cysts
  D. Diaphragmatic paralysis, phrenic nerve injury.
IV. Assessment and initial management
  *A. Empty stomach of air or gastric contents immediately by passing
     OG or NG tube (Levin tube if available) and aspirating. Leave the
     tube to gravity drainage. Apply suction on the tube frequently.
  *B. Give respiratory support and prevent distension of gut with air.
     *1. To avoid further dilation of the bowel, perform tracheal in-
        tubation. Avoid bag and mask ventilation.
     *2. After intubation, hand ventilate with $O_2$ or put on respirator.
     *3. For older stable infants, oxygen via hood may suffice in rare cir-
        cumstances.
  *C. Maintain infant in neutral thermal environment.
  *D. Obtain chest and abdominal x-ray AP (portable only).
  *E. While at the referring hospital, call back and notify pediatric sur-
     geons about the case.
  F. Put in venous and arterial lines immediately.
     1. Adequately hydrate the infant.
     2. Draw arterial blood gases. Maintain $PO_2$ of at least 50–60 torr if
        possible.
     3. Monitor arterial blood pressure at least every 10–15 minutes
        (ideally by in-line arterial pressure transducer).
  *G. Observe carefully for pneumothorax.
     *1. Listen for decreased breath sounds on unaffected side.
     *2. Listen for decreased heart sounds.
     *3. Observe for sudden change in cardiac status (hypotension, bra-
        dycardia) or respiratory status.
     *4. Transilluminate chest as baseline, if possible, and periodically
        thereafter or on suspicion of air leak.
  H. If pneumothorax occurs
     *1. Aspirate air from chest until patient's clinical condition im-
        proves, preferably using thoracentesis catheter device.
     2. Insert chest tube or use thoracentesis device as temporary in-
        dwelling catheter.
  *I. Correct base deficit if > 8–10 mEq/dl or pH < 7.25. Administer
     $NaHCO_3$.
  *J. Observe for hypoglycemia. Check by rapid glucose assessment
     technique (Dextrostix, Accu-check, Chemstrip).
V. Procedure for transport
  A. Physician should accompany team if known diaphragmatic hernia.

    \*B. Be sure to maintain NG or Levin tube to decompress stomach and bowel. Maintain NPO.
    \*C. Elevate head of bed.
    \*D. Turn infant so affected side is down.
    \*E. Maintain volume support with IV twin administration.
    \*F. Maintain normal blood gases and acid-base balance.
    \*G. Transport as promptly as possible.
    \*H. Notify surgeons of estimated time of arrival.
  VI. Equipment needed
    A. Transport isolette
    B. NG or Levin tube and syringes for suction
    C. Cardiac monitor
    D. Respiratory support equipment, including ventilator
    E. Proper IV fluids and pumps for both UAC and venous lines.
 VII. Potential complications
    A. Cardiorespiratory arrest
    B. Pneumothorax
    C. Inability to ventilate
    D. PPHN

## *Choanal Atresia*

SUMMARY OF CRITICAL GOALS FOR MANAGEMENT
Maintain stabilized patent oral airway or intubate for transport.

   I. Definition. A condition in which one or both nares are not patent.
  II. Recognition
    A. Clinical findings
      1. Restlessness, and moderate-to-severe retractions
      2. Cyanotic spells when quiet. Pink when crying.
      3. Apnea
      4. Noisy breathing (when choanal atresia is partial and unilateral) present when breathing through nose but absent when mouth breathing
    B. Laboratory findings. Not needed
    C. Radiological findings
      1. *Not* necessary at referring hospital or for transport
      2. May be helpful later to determine degree of obstruction by instilling small amount of radiopaque contrast media into nostril and obtaining several roentgenograms of nasopharynx

    III. Differential diagnosis
        A. Choanal stenosis (may present with chronic nasal discharge)
        B. Other causes of upper airway obstruction
    IV. Assessment and initial management
      *A. Diagnose by attempting to pass NG tube (5F) through nostrils.
      *B. Establish an airway with an oral airway or McGovern nipple device
           (a regular nipple with a large hole in it).
      *C. Assess if bilateral or unilateral atresia. Cover opposite nares and
           mouth and hold wisp of cotton in front of test nares to discern air
           movement in and out on inhalation and exhalation.
      *D. IV should be inserted for transport.
        E. Intubate for transport or if infant has continued respiratory dis-
           tress despite oral airway.
     V. Procedures for transport
      *A. Maintain airway—ET tube or oral airway.
      *B. Hydrate adequately
           1. IV therapy for transport
      *C. Place in prone position with face to one side with slight roll under
           upper chest.
    VI. Equipment needed
        A. Transfer isolette
        B. Oral airway or ET tube
        C. Cardiorespiratory monitor
   VII. Potential complications
        A. Acute apnea, respiratory arrest
        B. Chronic right-sided heart failure from chronic upper airway ob-
           struction and hypoventilation. This is a long-term effect and would
           not usually be seen during transport for the acute problem


## *Meningomyelocele or Meningocele*
SUMMARY OF CRITICAL GOALS FOR MANAGEMENT
Avoid placing infant on back. Cover the lesion and aim to keep sac or cover-
ing intact. If sac ruptured, administer antibiotics.

    I. Definition. Incomplete closure of the dorsal midline of the spine
       causes variable-sized deformities including supporting structures and
       at times including nervous tissue.
       A. Meningocele. A dysrhaphic disorder with a defect in soft tissues
          and bony vault with a protruding meningeal sac that does *not* con-
          tain neural tissue.

B. Meningomyelocele. A dysrhaphic disorder containing both meningeal and neural tissue components.

II. Recognition
  A. Clinical findings
    1. The lesion is apparent on visual examination of back
    2. Palpate bladder and assess anal sphincter tone. A full, paralyzed bladder may necessitate catheterization prior to transport.
  B. Laboratory findings
    1. Not necessary
  C. Radiological findings
    1. Not necessary at referring hospital

III. Differential diagnosis
  A. Lipoma
  B. Teratoma

IV. Assessment and initial management
  *A. Place infant on side or on abdomen. Avoid placing infant on back.
  *B. Cover lesion with sterile Vaseline gauze dressing.
  *C. Try to keep sac or covering intact.
  D. If sac ruptures, administer antibiotics prophylactically (to cover for *Staphylococcus epidermidis*, *Staphylococcus aureus* and gram-negative enteric organisms).
  E. Hydrate adequately.

V. Procedure for transport
  A. Place on abdomen or side.
  B. Cover lesion with sterile Vaseline gauze.

VI. Equipment needed
  A. Transport isolette
  B. Vaseline gauze dressing
  C. Equipment for bladder catheterization[†] including #8 feeding tube for infants > 1800 gm, No. 5 feeding tube for infants < 1800 gm.

VII. Potential complications
  A. Sepsis/meningitis
  B. Hydrocephalus
  C. Urinary retention

---

[†]For technique for catheterizing a prone patient with hydromeningocele see E. C. Denny, Bladder Catheterization. In M. A. Fletcher, M. G. MacDonald (Eds.), G. B. Avery (Assoc. Ed.), *Atlas of Procedures in Neonatology*. Philadelphia: Lippincott, 1983. P. 91.

# Appendix 8        *Aircraft Profiles*

It must be emphasized that weights and speeds, in most cases, do not reflect manufacturers' published data or claims but instead are based on actual aircraft being used today in hospital-based service. For instance, in most cases, speeds are average cruise speeds that these aircraft are experiencing when loaded with two medical attendants and full fuel at an average summertime temperature. Weight loading that is at or near the maximum allowable, or very high temperatures, may reduce these speeds.

Weights are from actual aircraft in service and reflect accessories and final configuration that we recommend.* Additional equipment and crew weights will of course reduce additional weight-carrying capacities. Maximum gross weight, in most cases, *does not* give a realistic comparison of performance but is a *legal limit*. For landing and taking off from difficult or very restricted locations, safety and comfortable performance margins demand that the aircraft operate at some point below these weights. At maximum gross weight, any two different models of aircraft will have different performance characteristics.

Although the comparisons shown here include a maximum fuel load, many programs do not normally operate with full fuel for weight-saving reasons. Consideration must also be given to the fact that the maximum fuel weight is usually only experienced when taking off from the home heliport without a patient on board. Depending on the aircraft, fuel will be used at a rate of between 400 and 600 lb for each hour it flies on its way to pick up a patient. Therefore most of these aircraft have comfortable patient-carrying capacities unless a flight is extremely short.

The advantages listed are opinions based on years of experience, safety considerations, and comments we hear most often from medical and flight crews *in hospital-based service* and do not necessarily reflect our opinions for other types of work. Aircraft not listed among these, we feel are not as well suited to the particular area and mission profile.

---

*Adapted with permission from *Omniflight Background Information,* January 1988. Omniflight Airways, Inc. P.O. Box 15440, Baltimore, MD 21220.

## Single-Engine Helicopters
BELL 206 L-1 LONG RANGER

| | |
|---|---|
| Empty weight (in medical configuration) | 2529 lb |
| Maximum fuel capacity | 634 lb |
| Pilot | 180 lb |
| Attendant 1 | 180 lb |
| Attendant 2 | 160 lb |
| Medical equipment and supplies (average) | 300 lb |
| Total | 3983 lb |
| Maximum allowable gross weight | 4150 lb |
| Range in hours with full fuel | 2 hrs 45 min |
| Cruise speed | 130 MPH |
| Range (distance) with 20 minutes reserve (no wind) | 314 statute miles |

*Advantages*

1. Smoothest, quietest ride of any helicopter.

2. Three-attendant seat capacity, two patient (one above the other, staggered). Excellent patient working height.

3. Good separation of pilot compartment from crew and patient area.

4. Good visibility for steep approaches. This is important in EMS especially for "scene" approaches at night. Pilot visibility forward and down is important to see wires and obstructions.

5. Reliability and reduced out-of-service time. There are more hospital-based programs currently using this aircraft than any other single helicopter model.

## Light Twin-Engine Class Helicopters
MBB BO105 CBS

| | |
|---|---|
| Empty weight (in medical configuration) | 3290 lb |
| Maximum fuel capacity | 1041 lb |
| Pilot | 180 lb |
| Attendant 1 | 180 lb |
| Attendant 2 | 160 lb |
| Medical equipment and supplies (average) | 300 lb |
| Total | 5151 lb |
| Maximum allowable gross weight | 5512 lb |
| Range in hours with full fuel | 2 hrs 20 min |
| Cruise speed | 143 MPH |
| Range (distance) with 20 minutes reserve (no wind) | 286 statute miles |

*Advantages*

  1. With high-skid option, this helicopter has the best tail rotor clearance of any of the helicopters now being used in EMS service. This gives an added measure of safety and means it is particularly well suited to land in rough terrain or high grass. Because personnel protection from the tail rotor in EMS service must receive a high priority, this is an important consideration.

  2. Excellent pilot visibility for steep approaches. EMS service, especially landings to unimproved locations, at night often demands slow, steep approaches. Visibility forward and downward is important. This is particularly important for spotting wires and other obstructions.

  3. Ease of patient loading. Because of the rear "clamshell doors" and the height of the bottom of these doors when the helicopter is on high skids, patient loading is direct and relatively easy. The high tail rotor allows patients to be loaded through the rear safely with the rotors turning with specific safety procedures and training for crew.

  4. Side-by-side patient configuration and seating for three medical attendants in most configurations. One attendant can sit at the head of the patient.

  5. The best reliability and lowest "down time" of any of the twin-engine helicopters evaluated.

### Medium-Size Twin-Engine Class Helicopters
MBB BK117

| | |
|---|---:|
| Empty weight (in medical configuration) | 4334 lb |
| Maximum fuel capacity | 1227 lb |
| Pilot | 180 lb |
| Attendant 1 | 180 lb |
| Attendant 2 | 160 lb |
| Medical equipment (average) | 300 lb |
| Total | 6381 lb |

Maximum allowable gross weight

| | |
|---|---:|
| Model A-1* | 6288 lb |
| Model A-3* | 7056 lb |
| Range in hours with full fuel | 2 hrs 20 min |
| Cruise speed | 150 MPH |
| Range (distance) with 20 minutes reserve (no wind) | 300 statute miles |

---

*The differences between the earlier model A-1 and the later model A-3 are primarily changes made to the tail rotor and stabilizer and do not reflect any changes to the engines or horsepower available or any actual increased lift.

*Advantages*

1. The best combination of cabin size and patient loading configuration. The width and height of the cabin is excellent and is often preferred by medical crews.

2. Good tail rotor height, which is important for rough terrain, high-grass areas, and personnel safety.

3. Loading of patients through rear "clamshell" doors is direct and simple.

4. Many systems incorporate a collapsible transport gurney similar to the type used in many ambulances. This further simplifies loading procedures and raises the patient to a comfortable working height.

5. Side-by-side patient configuration that includes four attendant stations in many of the aircraft now in service. Seating for at least one attendant at the head of the patient.

# Appendix 9

# Aeromedical Operator Checklist (Omniflight)

Modified from *OMNIFLIGHT Aeromedical Operator Checklist*, Baltimore, MD: Omniflight, Inc. With permission.

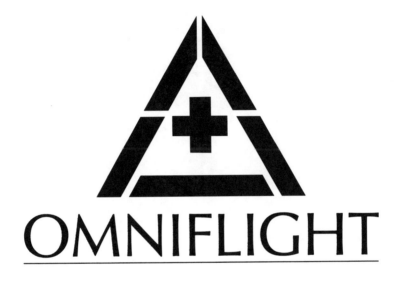

# OMNIFLIGHT

**Aeromedical
Operator
Checklist**

# INTRODUCTION

The business and technology of transporting patients by helicopter have changed rapidly in recent years. Medical procedures performed in-flight, tasks in management of the total system, the helicopters themselves, all have become more complex and demanding.

The structure of helicopter operating firms is also changing. The "classic" operator has been one who invested his future in the residual value of his aircraft. In doing so, he invested heavily in support infrastructure, such as maintenance, to protect his investment. Today's "leasee" operator is at the other end of the spectrum. He may have minimal infrastructure and little operating experience. The "leasee" operator typically owns no equipment, but has strong marketing skills and, at least initially, is well-capitalized.

The "ideal" EMS operator in the late 1980s may be found somewhere in mid-spectrum between "classic and leasee." One thing, however, is certain: successful hospital systems must demand strong aviation management if they are to be safe and mission-effective. And strong aviation management cannot exist without adequate support infrastructure. This leaves little room for the operator who "leases" its certificate to a hospital customer.

The mission of the helicopter service company should be to operate a system that is safe, efficient, and responsive to its customer's current and future needs. This is a challenging job to do profitably in the face of ever-changing economics and technology.

The questions posed in this book are tough ones for a helicopter service company. They penetrate every important element of airborne EMS capability. **Asking them of each operator you're considering will give you "apples to apples" comparisons and leave candidates with "nowhere to hide."**

Most important, they will help your organization to select the company that best delivers a complete service, that provides value, safely.

For your convenience, questions are organized in sections relating to the elements of an Airborne EMS system:

I.   ORGANIZATION
II.  SAFETY AND TRAINING
III. FLIGHT STANDARDS
IV.  PERSONNEL
V.   FINANCIAL
VI.  MAINTENANCE
VII. SUPPORT ISSUES

Copyright Omniflight, Inc. 1986

1

# I. ORGANIZATION

A customer purchasing so complex a product as a helicopter EMS system should understand the provider organization. Chances are good that if the helicopter company's organization is not clear and orderly, its performance and accountability will be even more elusive.

1. **May we have the names and phone numbers of all the EMS customers for whom your company has flown?**
   (References will quickly tell the story of almost any service company. Take the time to interview each reference in detail. If hospital contracts have been lost by the vendor, find out if it was for service, financial, bid process, or other reason.)

2. **Other than hospital clients, who are your six "oldest" current customers, name and phone numbers?**
   (Again, references will help show a company's pedigree. A long, safe, mutually profitable contract should be the goal of both parties.)

3. **How is your firm owned? When was the last change in ownership?**
   (Is it a public corporation, a partnership or privately owned? The hospital wants a company with long-term commitment; that has the financial strength and the management flexibility to serve the hospital marketplace.)

4. **Can you show me a copy of your organization chart?**
   (The chart should be clear in its organization. Both safety and maintenance quality control should receive special attention in the organization.)

5. **How long have you been in the helicopter business?**
   (Although longevity does not alone translate into quality, it does indicate experience levels and degree of business acumen.)

6. **Are you in any business other than helicopter service?**
   (Hospitals should expect the focus of senior management to be on their primary concern, helicopter operations.)

7. **What manuals can we expect to see used at our hospital?**
   (A professional operator will ensure that lessons learned are systematized by becoming part of a written document. At a minimum, the following are necessary:
   - EMS Operations Manual
   - Safety Manual
   - Training Manual(s)
   - Field Maintenance Manual)

8. **May we see your manuals?**
   (Even a cursory review will give an indication of the depth and dedication to quality of the organization. Manuals should be complete and easy to understand.)

9. **Which employees will have possession of your manuals?**
   (Manuals do not help when they are on the shelf or only at the home office.)

2

**10. Are you an active member of the Helicopter Association International and ASHBEAMS?**

(Active membership in these two organizations demonstrates a commitment to the industry and ensures a level of communication. There are other worthwhile professional organizations — these two are a minimum.)

**11. What is your position with the helicopter airframe manufacturer?**

(Hospital customers should be well informed as to the helicopter resources available to them. A vendor with a good working dialogue with the senior management of all major helicopter manufacturers may be helpful to the hospital. The best case is an operator with experience in all helicopters suitable for your EMS mission.)

**12. What is your understanding of the current and future insurance marketplace?**

(A major cost for the helicopter operator is insurance. The customer should feel confident that its vendor is "on top of" insurance topics. As these issues become more complex, the operator must have the ability to deal with them to the satisfaction of hospital requirements.)

**13. Will management visits be made to our hospital? How often?**

(A minimum number of management visits to a contract "in the field" should be policy with a helicopter service company. Four visits per year may be adequate for a smooth running system.)

3

# II. SAFETY AND TRAINING

Safety is undoubtedly your foremost concern in selecting an operator.

Safety is not automatic. Every pilot and mechanic shares your desire for safety; their careers and their lives are at stake. But they need help. The support and involvement of management, checking to ensure that safe practices are followed without exception, and assistance with facilities such as heliports and fueling are necessary. Field personnel are subject to many pressures that can compromise their best judgement, including the critical nature of the EMS mission and the operator's need for profits.

The helicopter operator's senior management must make commitments to safety — philosophical, financial, and practical — lip service will not suffice.

14. **May we see examples of the safety activities at your EMS systems?**
    (Many safety programs "stay in the home office." A working system produces results at the hospital. Look for newsletters, posters, briefing notes, incident and hazard reports. Look for evidence of participation by medical flight crew members, pilots and mechanics.)

15. **Will our system have a safety officer? What training will he or she receive? What are his job responsibilities and who does he report to on matters of safety?**
    (Answers to these questions should be included in the operator's written description of the safety system.)

16. **Can you describe your safety program?**
    (A safety program prescribes standards for 1) safety policy, 2) safety procedures, 3) training and 4) ongoing surveillance of operations.)

17. **May we see your safety manual?**
    (A clear, concise guide is necessary in order for employees to comply with safety policy.)

18. **Who has possession of your safety manual?**
    (A manual "on the shelf" will do little good — especially if the shelf is at home base.)

19. **What is your company's safety record for *all* helicopter operations over the past five years?**
    (An aviation company should approach all its flying activities with the same view of safety priorities. The entire safety history of the company should be reviewed — not just EMS activities.)

20. **If you have had an accident, what subsequent action did your company take?**
    (Accidents are often the result of problems that can be corrected. Was an analysis made and action taken or was it treated as "one of those things?")

21. **Do you pass safety information learned in one program to other programs on a regular basis? May we see an example?**
(Operators who support more than one program have the opportunity to use safety and operational lessons learned in each, to help others prevent "known" problems.)

22. **Do you have a formal system to review operational and safety information and procedures when crew shifts change and new crew members come on duty ("shift briefing")? Is this important element left to on site staff to develop? Does it sound as if this will be handled "casually"?**
(Because of the 24 hour nature of a hospital-based helicopter system and the constant personnel rotation that is necessary, aviation organizations who manage an effective safety system have taken the time to identify risks. They will give high priority to establishing formal briefings to review safety information and operating procedures at each shift change, and will supply well-conceived checklists of important items.)

23. **Will you have written procedures for the introduction of new flight and maintenance crew members to our system?**
(Experienced operators know that the introduction of any new element, especially key crew members, greatly increases the risk of accidents or serious mistakes. The operator should be able to show you systematic procedures, such as checklists, that detail formal orientation for any new or fill-in crew member, no matter how experienced he may be in another system or environment.)

24. **Do you have a documented program of fuel quality assurance, or do you trust that the quality provided by local vendors and fixed base operators is "adequate"?**
(The operator needs to establish standards of fuel quality and have a system assuring that standard for all aircraft operated. This is essential for safe operation of modern turbine engines, especially for single user fuel systems such as hospital fuel dispensing units.)

25. **Do you plan to conduct a continuing safety surveillance program?**
(A comprehensive, continuous surveillance program is necessary to assure the safety program is working, that all hazards are being identified and, that timely corrective/avoidance action is taken. Specific time between inspection schedules should exist.)

5

**26. What will your safety surveillance program cover?**
(Safety checks should cover all areas of the company's operations, including:
- Management qualifications, responsibilities and
  organization.
- Aviation safety.
- Flight operations.
- Pilot requirements/standards.
- Heliport operations and standards.
- Aircraft maintenance.
- Maintenance personnel.
- Shops and maintenance areas.
- Aircraft services.)

**27. What measurement tools will you use to evaluate the safety effectiveness of your program? May we see them?**
(The purpose of safety measurement is to evaluate performance and compliance with prescribed regulations, policies, procedures and practices. Safety measurement tools commonly used include:

| | |
|---|---|
| • Safety Meeting Records | • Inspection Reports |
| • Hazard Reports | • Incident and Accident Reports |

These tools provide a systematic method of identifying and analyzing causes of unsafe acts or conditions. They assist in responsibility assignment for timely corrective action.)

**28. Do you have written safety responsibilities for each person associated with our program?**
(Aviation safety responsibilities should integrate safety systems and procedures into all levels of operations. Specific written responsibilities should assign each person associated with your program accountability to perform his or her duty with primary concern for safety.)

**29. May we see your training manuals for our medical crew members?**
(Training nurses and others to act as crew members is *not* something to be "worked out" at a local level. Experience and a professional approach are needed to get the job done right. This is the responsibility of the operator.)

**30. In addition to FAA required pilot training, what other pilot training will your company give the pilots assigned to our contract?**
(The highest quality operators will require 6 month check rides, IFR training and a high-quality initial checkout.)

31. **Will your pilot's go/no go decision be affected by the
    medical needs of the patient?**
    (The job of the helicopter operator is to provide safe transportation in accordance
    with the hospital's mission. The hospital is paying the operator for his safety expertise
    and good judgement. The go/no go pilot decision is a safety of flight decision only,
    not a medical decision.)

32. **Do you reserve the right not to board and fly untrained
    medical flight crews?**
    (Training requirements can have a way of ''slipping'' according to other pressures. A
    responsible operator will insist on properly trained crew members, and have the
    authority to back up that standard.)

33. **What plan do you have to minimize landing site hazards?**
    (Operators should have a system of landing site hazard identification. Further, an
    ongoing landing site improvement program will be helpful in reducing hazards both at
    scenes and at referring institutions.)

## III. FLIGHT STANDARDS

The Federal Government provides a very basic framework for the regulation of commercial flight activities in FAR (Federal Aviation Regulation) Part 135. The EMS flying
business requires regulation (control) in detail and scope that far exceeds FAR 135.
Operators need a systematic approach to the operational issues surrounding EMS (such as
an EMS Operations Manual). Weather minimums and duty times are two critical items in
today's EMS industry.

34. **Who has the authority to set program weather minimums?**
    (While local knowledge will be employed, the helicopter company operations manager
    should have final authority.)

35. **What weather minimums do you assign a system?**
    (Companies should establish minimums that are more restrictive than Federal Stan-
    dards, according to local terrain and weather patterns. The published FAA minimums
    are not sufficient criteria to govern the hospital helicopter mission.)

36. **Does your operations manager have experience in
    our location?**
    (The helicopter company's operations manager is responsible for flight standards. He
    should be familiar with your area and operation.)

37. **Do your weather minimums change over time? If so, why
    and how?**
    (A new system may fine tune weather minimums as local conditions are learned
    through experience. However, the operations manager must remain the authority.)

38. **What weather minimums do you assign a new system? A new pilot?**
   (A flexible minimums system allows variations for experience or lack thereof. Normally a new system or new pilot should have more restrictive minimums than one with experience.)

39. **What are your basic requirements for IFR flying?**
   (There is little doubt that two pilots, two engines and planned IFR flights are a minimum standard. Any other answer will probably reveal inexperience or irresponsibility.)

40. **Do you recommend IFR capabilities for our hospital?**
   (Companies that understand your hospital's mission requirements and the EMS flight environment will be prepared to discuss this topic.)

41. **Will you back up our pilots for illness or vacation time?**
   (How long will our system be short a pilot before a relief pilot is sent?)

42. **What are your relief pilots' qualifications?**
   (Relief pilot is a tough job, operating at different systems with different equipment. This is the last place to train a new employee.)

43. **How will you keep our pilots and your relief pilots current in our primary and back-up helicopters?**
   (Sometimes the back-up helicopter model differs from the primary helicopter model. Yet proficiency, safety and regulations require extensive training in both. This is a high expense obligation for the vendor that cannot be short-cut.)

44. **Will you show me the pilot flight-time limitations and rest requirement regulations from the FAA and explain just what they mean?**
   (There are several interpretations currently being used. Basically, a pilot must have eight hours *uninterrupted* sleep (isolated rest) during each 24 hour period, or he must be relieved *before* the end of the 24 hours.)

45. **If our pilot comes on duty for a 24 hour shift at 12 Noon and flies at 6:00 p.m., 12 Midnight and 4:00 a.m., do you have to take any action?**
   (If the answer is anything other than "get a relief pilot," you should pursue this question. An "easy" and erroneous interpretation of the regulation is probably being made.)

46. **How many pilots will be permanently assigned exclusively to this contract and live in this area?**
   (Three pilots is the only sensible minimum. Two pilots is an unsafe standard that probably cannot comply with regulations under any interpretation. For a very busy system where a relief pilot is constantly called in, more than three permanent pilots may be appropriate.)

47. **Will our pilots be expected to perform other duties? What kind?**
    (Most operators assign pilots other duties which are flexible in time demand, such as safety supervisor or administration. However, if other assigned duties seem time consuming and/or in conflict with duty time requirements, keep asking questions. Regulations clearly prohibit such duties. Mechanic duties for a pilot is an example of questionable and suspect responsibilities.)

48. **What are the names and telephone numbers of your FAA Operations Inspector and FAA Maintenance Inspector. May we call them?**
    (Good relations with the Federal Aviation Administration will indicate a degree of professionalism on the part of the operator. Do not expect too much comment from the FAA. Public officials are often shy, especially about negative comments.)

## IV. PERSONNEL

The pilots and mechanics assigned to your program, including relief personnel, must not only deliver safe, skillful aviation services. They must also fit in well with *your* personnel in order for you to have an outstanding aeromedical team. Good hiring, training and compensation programs and practices, and effective supervision of personnel by the aviation company are necessary for the success of the program.

Personnel selection goes beyond flight hours, ratings and mechanical qualifications. The experienced operator will also select individuals suitable for the hospital mission.

The helicopter EMS market today includes many systems where the personnel assigned to the contract end up essentially working for and reporting to the hospital, not the operator. When this happens, the hospital client is being deprived of the aviation management services for which it is paying. Also, problems sometimes develop in standards and safety issues.

It is the responsibility of the helicopter operator to manage and communicate with its employees in a way that gives the hospital full value for its investment in operator and system.

49. **May we see the job descriptions for our EMS pilots, lead pilot and mechanic?**
    (Job descriptions should be sufficiently clear and detailed for a complete understanding.)

50. **How many years have the management personnel who will control our system worked for you? What are their backgrounds?**
    (You should know who will be making the decisions that affect your system. Look for dedicated, experienced managers who are likely to remain with you through years of operations.)

9

**51. What will be the approximate compensation of our pilots and mechanics?**
(Compensation must be fair in relation to the local area and prevailing national levels in order to maintain high morale and minimize turnover.)

**52. What benefits package will you extend to the people assigned to our contract?**
(A good health, dental, profit sharing and insurance package indicates the right company attitude toward employees and helps minimize turnover.)

**53. Will the pilots receive a flight hour premium in addition to their base wage?**
(Flight hour premiums may encourage pilots to act in violation of the best interests of safety. Pilots should earn a sufficient wage to obviate the need for motivational pay that might adversely affect their decisions.)

**54. What work schedule will our pilots and mechanics have?**
(Common sense can prevail in this area. Personnel need time off to allow enough rest to function safely and effectively on the job. There are many variations in work schedules, but some being operated today raise obvious safety questions.)

**55. What is your policy if we find a particular pilot or mechanic unsuitable for our system?**
(Some people, although competent professionals in every way, do not "fit" with particular hospital teams. In that case, the operator should cooperate in changing or replacing the employee.)

**56. What is your retention history for pilots? For mechanics?**
(The operator should provide this information. The question should also be discussed with references.)

**57. What experience in hours, type of aircraft, and type of operation must a pilot have to be hired for our program?**
(Extensive prior experience is essential, especially for personnel stationed away from their main base and company management.)

**58. What prior experience must a mechanic have to be hired for our program? What training will the mechanic receive?**
(Extensive prior experience is essential for mechanics as well as pilots, especially for a mechanic "on his own" in the field. Factory or equivalent training on the aircraft model to be operated should be provided as a minimum.)

**59. What standard requirements and procedures do you have for hiring personnel?**
(Complete, detailed checks with prior employers and personal references, plus interviews conducted by operator top management may disclose personality or behavior problems not detected in interviews and flight checks.)

### 60. How do you evaluate, promote and compensate your personnel?
(A formal performance appraisal system, with promotion based on performance and not longevity or other factors, helps assure personnel know where they stand, and are given opportunities to voice their concerns.)

## V. FINANCIAL

The financial strength of your operator is of paramount importance in assuring his ability to perform for you. Operators without substantial earnings, equity and cash flow can have problems getting parts when needed, meeting payrolls on time, and funding equipment and backup aircraft essential to the safety and continued support of your service.

The helicopter industry and most operators have faced severe financial challenges during the past five years, beginning with the oil slump in 1982. During this period, many operators have failed, and major markets have declined or disappeared, particularly in the West. Aircraft values have dropped and financing has become increasingly difficult to obtain.

Virtually all operators are in worse financial condition today than they were in 1981, unless they have obtained significant new equity funding. Some have survived only because manufacturers have agreed to long term workouts of debt and elected not to foreclose on equipment that is not being paid for.

Because new aircraft cannot be operated profitably in many markets, helicopter fleets are aging, with higher and higher maintenance requirements and costs. Many of these fleets have been refinanced, resulting in debt burdens that exceed the earning capability and current value of older equipment.

Manufacturers now arrange and underwrite lease and debt financing that operators might not be able to obtain otherwise. This makes it relatively easy for weak operators to acquire complex, expensive equipment that they may not be able to afford or properly maintain.

At the same time, high revenues can be obtained by operating new equipment, particularly in EMS service. Outlays for maintaining new equipment are usually very low in the first two years, although large outlays may be required thereafter, as the aircraft reach their first scheduled major inspections and overhauls.

High revenues and initial cash flows in EMS can attract operators who may be unable to set aside or generate enough funds to pay the costs of major maintenance usually due in the third year of operation. This is likely to happen when revenues from new work must be used to pay for idle aircraft or debt and lease service that exceeds the earning ability of older equipment. In some cases, operators may underprice new work to obtain high revenues and initial cash flows, almost certainly leading to financial problems in later years.

Much new equipment is now obtained through operating leases, many as long as 10 years. This equipment and the related lease liabilities do not appear on the operator's balance sheets. This may result in financial statements indicating a strong financial position and relatively little debt when, in fact, enormous future lease obligations exist.

11

Most lessors retain all of the equity in leased aircraft, leaving the operator with no saleable asset at any time during or at the end of the lease. Many leases have no reasonable provision for early termination or disposition of the equipment, "locking in" substantial liabilities from which the operator has no escape.

**61. Do you owe substantial amounts on debt secured by older equipment, whose value may be equal to or less than the amount of the debt?**

(If so, the operator may have to use part of your revenues to pay debt service on equipment not used in your service and may not be able to generate funds through sale of equipment.)

**62. How much equipment do you have on lease?**

(Adding this equipment and related lease liabilities to the liabilities shown on the operator's financial statements may be a better indicator of "real" equity and financial resources than the amounts shown in the financial statements.)

**63. What are your future obligations for payments on leased equipment not shown on your financial statements?**

(This reveals the magnitude of lease obligations and should also show how far into the future the operator is obligated.)

**64. May we have a copy of your audited financial statements for at least the last two years?**

(Audited financial statements provide greater assurance that all information relevant to the financial position, cash flow and operations of the operator is available to you.)

**65. Who are your auditors?**

(Large auditing firms normally provide advice and recommendations on business and financial matters that smaller firms do not provide. This is an important resource to the operator that helps with good operating information and controls and effective resolution of financial issues.)

**66. What interest rates do you pay on your debt?**

(Low interest rates suggest that lenders are comfortable and confident with the operator's financial position and ability to pay, and that the operator meets its commitments to lenders and others.)

**67. How much working capital (current assets minus current liabilities) do you have?**

(Working capital and cash indicate ability to meet short term commitments, such as payrolls and payment of vendor invoices, and ability to withstand short term problems such as increases in operating costs or temporarily idle aircraft and equipment.)

**68. What is the market or sales value of aircraft and other major equipment shown on your balance sheet?**
(It is not uncommon for aircraft and equipment to be carried at values in excess of current market values, resulting in possible losses and additional cash requirements if the equipment has to be sold. The Helicopter Blue Book or McGowan's Aircraft Digest are the best places to establish current helicopter values.)

**69. What percentage of your aircraft fleet and equipment is not working or working at a loss?**
(Many operators have excess or idle equipment that must be paid for, in part, with revenues from your work. While some idle or underemployed equipment is normal, idle equipment in excess of 10% of the operator's total fleet may result in financial problems.)

**70. May we see your recent interim financial statements?**
(Significant changes in financial position, earnings and cash flow may have occurred since the date of the latest audited statements. A strong operator's statements should show improvements from the latest audited statements.)

**71. What arrangements have you made for additional borrowing or investment by your owners?**
(Availability of lines of credit and similar facilities indicate confidence in the operator by its primary banks. Access to funds for borrowing or investment shows capability to withstand financial problems.)

**72. Do you have the aircraft for our service, or confirmed lending or leasing arrangements for its acquisition?**
(Operators may have difficulty obtaining financing for additional aircraft, particularly if they are weak. This could result in delays in starting your service, and cash or profit problems for the operator, if acquiring the aircraft is more expensive than expected.)

**73. How will our aircraft be acquired?**
(It is easier to dispose of aircraft that are owned or leased short-term than aircraft leased long-term, making it easier for you to change aircraft, should you wish to do so.)

**74. How will you fund major maintenance of the aircraft to be operated for us?**
(Guaranteed cost programs, such as power by hour and regular payments to escrow accounts for leased aircraft, assure the availability of funds when major outlays for maintenance are needed. If the operator does not have in-house major maintenance capability, he will pay more to an outside provider, and the hospital will probably suffer time delays.)

**75. How many aircraft of the type we want do you operate for others?**

(Operating a number of the same aircraft usually results in lower costs of inventory, tools and training, and makes it easier to find other work for the aircraft, should you decide to change the type you operate. It also improves knowledge and experience with the aircraft, increasing safety and reducing maintenance and down time.)

**76. How much hull and liability insurance do you normally carry on your aircraft?**

(If insurance is not fully adequate to cover loss of an aircraft and possible resulting liability, the operator may have severe financial problems in the event of a loss.)

**77. What portion of any aircraft loss do you have to pay because of deductible or coinsurance?**

(High deductible and coinsurance can result in severe cash and profit problems, especially in the event of partial losses and inadvertent damage to aircraft, which occur quite often.)

**78. Have you ever missed a payroll or paid your employees later than scheduled because of inadequate cash?**

(Some operators have had this problem which, if not permanently solved, can make it impossible to effectively support your service.)

## VI. MAINTENANCE

The heart of a helicopter service company is its maintenance department. It is here that serious helicopter operators make long term investments in physical facilities, parts, and most of all, experienced manpower.

Perhaps the easiest way to separate the professional helicopter operator from the "lessor" or "pass-through" type operator is to take a close look at their maintenance departments.

79. **How close is your main support facility?**
    (Helicopters occasionally and periodically require direct support from the home base shop, where the concentration of expertise and equipment exists. The hospital can expect less delay during major maintenance interruptions if a main support base is nearby.)

80. **How often will the helicopter go back to the main base?**
    (Major maintenance should be done at a main base where technicians, tools, manuals and inspectors are located. A major shop visit once a year is a minimum.)

81. **How often will a second qualified mechanic and the Chief Inspector inspect my aircraft?**
    (A second set of eyes is important. There should be procedures to ensure this takes place on a regular basis and, for certain work, always takes place.)

82. **How is the quality of maintenance monitored? Is there a manual we can review?**
    (A good quality control system is necessary for safety and effective operation in the "field." Quality control systems are definitive and should be clearly documented.)

83. **How do you monitor component times to assure changes are made when due?**
    (To maintain a fleet of helicopters today, a computer-based aircraft status system is a must. Ask for a copy. Can you understand what it says? It should be clear to you.)

84. **How are airworthiness directives and service bulletins tracked and put into effect?**
    (The computer and an aircraft status system, under the supervision of the Chief Inspector, should be used to handle important items.)

85. **What major support capability and authorization do you have?**
    (An absolute minimum is a FAA-certified repair station. The operator should also be a factory authorized service station for the helicopter you plan to operate.)

86. **How long have you been a repair station and a factory authorized service station?**
    (Factory service station authorization can "come with" a new purchase, in which case experience, training and parts may not be all they should be. Experience counts especially high when dealing with complex aircraft.)

15

**87. What other support capabilities do you have?**
(In-house engine, avionics, overhaul and completion capabilities will help you. If the helicopter service company has to rely on subcontractors, confusion, delays and more down time may result. The best case exists when the operator has full maintenance capabilities, including completions.)

**88. How much inventory is included with the aircraft?**
(Each hospital system requires a basic stock of parts and supplies, depending on model and hours flown. Experience will dictate what is an adequate "basic stock" of parts.)

**89. Do you have in-house avionics capability for rapid response?**
(Modern helicopters, especially in EMS work, contain sophisticated avionics that require considerable support. Without having and understanding wiring diagrams, troubleshooting may be a problem.)

**90. Where are the special tools required to maintain the helicopter? Do you have to "rent" them or do you own them?**
(All helicopters require expensive special tools that differ for each model. If the operator has to rent the tools from the manufacturer, there may be service delays if the tools are "out" when needed.)

**91. How do you assure the mechanics have the latest information?**
(A good notification procedure for verbal and written notices is important. There must be no chance of a missed service bulletin, manual revision, or other communication.)

**92. To whom does the mechanic report? How does he communicate with maintenance managers?**
(Hospital mechanics should report to a *maintenance* manager, not a general manager or flight manager. Checks and balances are important. The mechanic should talk with his maintenance manager on a scheduled basis.)

**93. What is your support response procedure in case our aircraft is grounded?**
(Operators should have plans in place in advance of a service interruption. A priority shipping protocol should be part of these plans, which should be in writing.)

**94. Who in your maintenance organization is an FAA Authorized Inspector?**
(Although not required by regulation, the helicopter company's Director of Maintenance or Chief Inspector should be an FAA Authorized Inspector.)

**95. Does your company have an FAA-Approved Minimum
Equipment List for our helicopter?**
(Without an MEL, the aircraft must be grounded even for the malfunction of items
not necessary for safe flight. Down time may be increased if the operator has not done
his homework by designing and having approved MELs.)

**96. Does your company have an FAA-Approved Aircraft
Inspection Program for our type of helicopter?**
(Manufacturer inspection programs are rarely ideal for the EMS situation. An
operator with experience and understanding of mission demands should design and
have approved a system to maintain safety and dispatch availability.)

# VII. SUPPORT ISSUES

The helicopter service operator has knowledge to share with the hospital client, concerning all those items which support the helicopter and flight team. Aircraft selection, interior design, back up systems, marketing, heliport design and installation, public relations, fuel systems and financial planning are a few areas where the experienced operator can help the hospital avoid "reinventing the wheel."

97. **Do you plan to provide a back-up aircraft if ours is out of service for maintenance? How?**
(Helicopters will require out of service time for maintenance, especially the larger, more complex aircraft. Pitfalls to watch for include: dependence on sources for aircraft outside the operator's control, such as equipment supplied by the manufacturer; one back-up ship to cover too many systems; or back-up helicopter locations too far away. The best answer is a full time back-up ship on location, although that is rarely financially possible. Anything else is a compromise from "ideal back-up." The least compromise from the ideal will separate the serious, professional operator from the others.)

98. **What are the serial numbers, condition, and equipment (configuration) of your back-up helicopters? May we see photographs?**
(Hospital systems will need back-up helicopters. Make sure their equipment is compatible with your operation. Check the ownership of a serial number to be sure the operator has total control of the aircraft.)

99. **What assistance can you provide us with regard to physical facilities planning, especially heliports?**
(Heliports, both at your hospital and the referring hospitals, require an experienced operator's knowledge. Communication centers, pathways, lighting and fuel systems are areas of operator responsibility. Ask to see manuals, designs, plans of past projects.)

100. **What will you do to help get us started? Whom do we go to with questions?**
(The lead pilot of a new system will be a very busy man. He cannot cover all the planning and activities necessary to get the program going. The best case for the hospital is a "start-up manager," whose sole function is to get the system operating on a safe and successful basis, as soon as possible.)

101. **How many hospitals have you started? May we have their names and contact phone numbers?**
(Checking with all references may be the best way to gauge future support.)

**102. How will we equip the helicopter to be used at
our hospital?**
(If the operator has completion capabilities, he and the hospital can sit down and
design the interior most suitable for the particular mission. Then, if changes need to
be made during the contract, the helicopter operator can do so with a minimum of
disruption. Also, the completion center is the best place to engineer "fixes" to
mechanical service interruptions. The operator who must rely on outside completion
services often has to rely on the same outside services for repairs and alterations.)

**103. What analysis have you performed concerning the type
of helicopter our hospital wishes to operate?**
(The professional operator will do a great deal of "homework" prior to bringing a
new model helicopter into his fleet. Without an analysis beforehand, how can an
operator expect to deal with the complexities that come with a new machine?
Mechanical design, flight characteristics, inspection schedules, and parts support are
just four areas of concern. The hospital should ask for documentation of the
analysis. This is not an area for casual approach.)

## POSTSCRIPT

No operator is perfect for all hospital EMS requirements. Each healthcare institution contemplating a helicopter system must look to the aviation industry with regard to its own unique needs. Hopefully, the preceding questions will assist *your* hospital in its selection of an aviation partner.

Just as the technical aspects are important in a helicopter transportation system, so too is the total commitment of management. Without the operator's dedication to safety and service to the hospital customer, it would be difficult for a new helicopter transportation service to succeed.

## Corporate Offices

105 Wappoo Creek Drive
Suite 1-A
Charleston, South Carolina 29412
(803) 762-1620

## Regional Offices

*Eastern Region*
P.O. Box 15440
Baltimore, Maryland 21220
(301) 391-7722

*Southern Region*
105 Wappoo Creek Drive
Suite 1-A
Charleston, South Carolina 29412
(803) 762-1620

*Central and Western Region*
5300 West 63rd Street
Midway Airport
Chicago, Illinois 60638
(312) 585-9800

# OMNIFLIGHT

# Appendix 10

## Safety Guidelines for Pilots, Aircraft, and Operations—National EMS Pilots Association

Modified from *National EMS Pilots Association, Safety Guidelines for Pilots, Aircraft & Operations—EMS Helicopters*. Pearland, TX. National EMS Pilots Association. With permission.

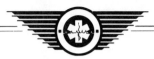

# NATIONAL EMS PILOTS ASSOCIATION

SAFETY GUIDELINES

FOR

PILOTS, AIRCRAFT & OPERATIONS

EMS HELICOPTERS

## THE NATIONAL EMS PILOTS ASSOCIATION

The National EMS Pilots Association is dedicated to improving the professionalism of EMS pilots and to increasing safety in EMS operations. The organization provides a central focus for professionals within the industry to:

- Exchange ideas and information and to monitor trends pertaining to equipment, operations and safety;
- Provide positive, professional input concerning proposed policy or operations;
- Function as a clearinghouse for statistics and other information concerning various phases of EMS operations;
- Recognize exemplary performance by those involved with EMS operations; and
- Cooperate with, and provide support for, other associations with compatible goals.

## PURPOSE OF ASSOCIATION

NEMSPA's primary concern, and force behind its creation, is safety in the EMS industry. Although a relatively new industry, emergency medical services flight programs are experiencing phenomenal growth and expansion. NEMPSA was formed to provide a forum for all interested parties in this rapidly growing industry to address safety issues in a positive, constructive manner. NEMSPA'S work will help assure the industry's continued growth.

## PILOTS - MINIMUM EXPERIENCE AND QUALIFICATIONS

**GUIDELINE - (In additions to FAA requirements)**

   I. Pilot—in—Command (P.I.C.)

      A. Flight experience

         1. 3000 hours helicopter total time
         2. 1000 hours turbine experience, helicopter
         3. 300 hours night, helicopter

      B. Ratings

         1. Commercial Helicopter
         2. Instrument Helicopter

**or**

   II. Pilot in Command Grandfather Clause

      A. Flight experience of 2000 hours total helicopter time, plus one of the following:

         1. One year EMS pilot experience, or
         2. 300 hours as an EMS pilot, or
         3. 200 EMS missions

      B. Ratings

         1. Commercial Helicopter
         2. Instrument Helicopter

1

III. Co—Pilot

    A. Flight experience

        1. 1500 hours helicopter total time
        2. 500 hours turbine experience

    B. Ratings

        1. Commercial Helicopter
        2. Instrument Helicopter

    C. May upgrade to P.I.C. by meeting requirements of
        Grandfather Clause

## PURPOSE:

A minimum experience level requirement for EMS pilots is necessary because of the type of missions being performed. More than aircraft handling proficiency is demanded in EMS flying; a well developed judgment in operational decision-making, based upon long and varied experience, is necessary as well. An EMS pilot must be prepared to operate (in most cases) single pilot, both day and night; there is often no time for flight planning; and takeoff and landing at unprepared sites requires an experience level greater than that in most other operations.

Because of individual differences, it does not naturally follow that everyone meeting these guidelines will be competent to perform EMS missions. However, we feel that this is the minimum experience necessary before being assigned as an EMS pilot.

2

## MINIMUM INITIAL PILOT TRAINING

### GUIDELINE - (In addition to FAA requirements)

I. Less than 100 hours in aircraft type

    A. Factory school or equivalent (ground and flight)

    B. 25 hours as P.I.C. in aircraft type prior to EMS missions

II. Over 100 hours in aircraft type

    A. Part 135 check ride

    B. 5 hours local area orientation

III. Less than one year EMS experience

    A. 12 duty days at hospital participating in a structured training program in an EMS aviation environment

IV. Over one year EMS experience

    A. 6 duty days at hospital participating in a structured training program in an EMS aviation environment

### NEW PROGRAMS:

Strongly recommend that in addition to P.I.C. requirement the lead pilot should have minimum of two years EMS experience.

### PURPOSE:

Surveys indicate that a pilot needs 4-6 months to feel comfortable in a new aircraft and new environment. In some instances it is necessary to eliminate one of these learning experiences so the pilot can concentrate on the other. This guideline is designed to protect the pilot from information overload and prepare the pilot with the most information prior to attempting an EMS mission where all aspects must come into play at the same time.

3

## MINIMUM RECURRENT PILOT TRAINING

### GUIDELINE—(In addition to FAA requirements)

I. All Programs

    A. Semi-annual training flight oriented toward realistic EMS operations including: day and night operations; IMC procedures; scene work; unimproved area operations; instrument training; egress and survival training; emergency procedures and limitations.

    B. Recommend instrument currency and proficiency for all pilots.

### PURPOSE:

A pilot operating in marginal weather conditions must have suitable equipment and be prepared for instrument flight. Due to the large number of EMS accidents relating to spatial disorientation brought on by inadvertent IMC meteorological conditions, pilots must be trained (and maintain their proficiency) in operations without visual reference to the ground. Even if the program conducts only VFR flights, the number of inadvertent IMC occurrences is great enough to necessitate this type of training.

IMC = instrument meteorological conditions; VFR = visual flight rules.

4

## AIRCRAFT TYPE AND EQUIPMENT

### GUIDELINE - (In addition to FAA requirements)

I. Aircraft type

A. Recommend IFR certified helicopters for all programs flying other than day, VFR only. Recommend programs presently flying VFR aircraft convert to IFR certified equipment when they upgrade or change vendors.

II. Equipment

A. Recommend IFR certified aircraft, and/or stability augmentation, and/or two-pilot operations.

### PURPOSE:

For EMS pilots to operate in marginal weather conditions it is necessary to have equipment suitable for flight in instrument conditions. Even if the program conducts only VFR flights, the possibility of going IMC is too great to be unprepared for this eventuality. A large number of fatal EMS accidents are the result of inadvertently flying into clouds or fog. Proper equipment to recover from this type of situation is a must.

IFR = instrument flight rule.

5

## MINIMUM STAFFING REQUIREMENTS

### GUIDELINE - (In addition to FAA requirements)

    I. Single helicopter contracts

        A. Four crews

        B. In addition to A above, one relief crew available to cover holidays, sick days, vacation, training, etc.

    II. Multi-helicopter contracts

        A. One additional crew above the minimum for each additional helicopter. (i.e., 2 helicopters=9 crews)

## PURPOSE:

The number one problem identified by pilots across the country is understaffing. Pilot error has been identified as a factor in well over 90 percent of the EMS accidents. Every piece of evidence collected to date has pointed to the number of hours a pilot spends on duty as being the most treacherous hazard to flight safety. The stress and emotion associated with EMS flying in conjunction with fatigue produces an unsafe operating condition. It is estimated that more than 90 percent of EMS accidents could have been prevented by the addition of a second pilot in the aircraft. Second to that, the single most beneficial step to promote safety at hospital programs is to adhere to these minimum staffing guidelines.

6

## DUTY TIME LIMITATIONS

### GUIDELINE - (In addition to FAA requirements)

I. 12 hour shift maximum (recommend no more than four shifts in a row) or average 42 duty hours in a seven day period.

II. Limited rotation between days and nights

### DUTY TIME:

Time spent on training, public relations, maintenance, etc. is considered duty time. Duty time begins upon arrival at the hospital and ends upon leaving the hospital. For hospitals other than your home base hospital, duty time begins when you depart your home and ends when you return home.

### PURPOSE:

Due to the response time mandated by the EMS mission, it is not possible for a pilot to be at his peak of performance for more than the times indicated in this guideline. Twenty-four hour shifts will inevitably catch pilots, at some time, when they are in an unsafe condition. As fatigue cannot always be self-determined, and in most cases it may not be apparent until serious errors are made, it is necessary to avoid the environment that would promote these conditions.

7

## VFR WEATHER MINIMUMS

### GUIDELINE - (in addition to FAA requirements)

I. Day

   A. Local

      1. 500 ft ceiling/1 mile visibility

   B. Cross Country/Not Local

      1. 800 ft ceiling/2 miles visibility

II. Night

   A. Local

      1. 500 ft ceiling/2 miles visibility

   B. Cross Country/Not Local

      1. 1000 ft ceiling/3 miles visibility

**LOCAL** - is defined as locale of urban area with enough ground lighting at night for suitable ground reference. This generally should not extend beyond 30 nautical miles

### PURPOSE:

The guidelines depart from the traditional method of establishing weather minimums and call for a realistic appraisal of each program with emphasis on mission requirements.

Actual weather minimums must include careful consideration of terrain, over-water operations, obstacles, local weather patterns and phenomena, local area flight activity, aircraft performance and equipment, instrument recovery procedures (in the event of IMC), and pilot familiarity and may vary accordingly. These guidelines are for ideal conditions and should be increased as flying area demands.

8

## MEDICAL ATTENDANTS ON BOARD THE AIRCRAFT

### GUIDELINE - (In addition to FAA requirements)

I. All attendants

A. All attendants who routinely fly must receive an aircraft and operations orientation that is designed to introduce attendants to EMS missions and should include safety awareness training, operating standards, and communications. This shall include ground and flight orientation

II. Other than regular attendants

A. Must be briefed prior to each flight

### PURPOSE:

Although no one else can assume responsibility for any aspect of aviation-safety related matters, in the interest of safety it is necessary to make all who fly aware of as much as possible. Without proper understanding of safety measures and practices it would be possible for medical attendants to inadvertently create or contribute to an unsafe condition. This type of training must be ongoing and recurrent.

9

## SAFETY PROGRAM

### GUIDELINE — (In addition to FAA requirements)

I. Each program will implement an active safety program

II. Each program should be subject to an annual evaluation by an independent party.

### PURPOSE:

An active safety program promotes safety awareness and commits an organization to the concept of good safety practices. A formal safety program allows pilots and others to address safety concerns without fear of reprisals. Not only can all safety matters be brought to the appropriate person's attention, but some kind of action is then required. Problems will not tend to be swept under the carpet.

An outside safety evaluation allows an unbiased observer to address issues that may have gone unnoticed and reinforce the safety attitude of everyone with the flight program.

10

# HELICOPTER AND EMERGENCY MEDICAL SERVICES

## *HELICOPTERS SAVE LIVES*

1. Over one million lives saved in the past forty years.

2. That is more than 25 lives saved for each of the nearly 40,000 civil and military helicopters operating in the world today.

3. Helicopters, because of their unique characteristics, can save lives that can be saved in no other way.

## *HOW DO HELICOPTERS SAVE LIVES?*

1. Helicopters can get the seriously injured to shock trauma centers within the hour.

2. Survival rates for those receiving the appropriate treatment within the "Golden Hour" is 90%.

3. Helicopters can get to and from places that other vehicles can't.

4. How many ambulances can pick up an injured hiker at 20,000 feet in the Himalayas?

5. How many ambulances can pick up an injured soldier in a steamy jungle?

6. Helicopters were instrumental in saving one of the few survivors of the tragic Air Florida crash in Washington, D.C. in 1982.

7. Helicopters conducted the initial, and for a long time, the only rescue activity at Mount St. Helens and the volcano in Columbia, South America, where helicopters alone were credited with saving 4000 lives!

**(Reprinted from an article by John Zugschwert, NEMSPA Member and Executive Director of the American Helicopter Society.)**

### Philosophy

In the ever expanding helicopter EMS Industry, our role as pilot is unique among our aviation peers. With the hostilities of our flying environment ever challenging and the pressure of knowing that our decision may at times determine the outcome of the life and death struggle for another human being, ours is a special position.

In consideration of this uniqueness we, the National EMS Pilots Association, intend to offer the leadership necessary to establish operations and safety standards, a forum for the exchange of new ideas, the framework for the dissemination of knowledge and the sensible guidance to formulate positive change in our profession.

Finally, it is not our intent to set ourselves apart from our aviation peers but rather to set an example as responsible professionals. It is our intention however, that with a broad constituency represented, we may offer the expertise required to help our industry prosper safely and to enhance the delivery of health care in our respective regions.

*Author: Michael Burke*

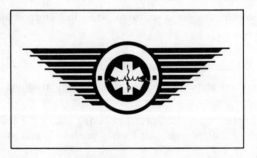

**National EMS Pilots Association**
**P.O. Box 2354**
**Pearland, Texas 77588**
**713/997-2563**

# Appendix 11

## Preparing a Landing Zone—National EMS Pilots Association

Reprinted with permission of National EMS Pilots Association.

## Selecting An On-Scene LZ

First, determine if the area is large enough to land a helicopter safely. The landing surface should be flat and firm, free of debris that would blow up into the rotor system.

Touchdown Area. Small helicopter: the touchdown area should be a square with 60-foot sides, 100 x 100 ft. at night. Medium-size helicopter: the touchdown

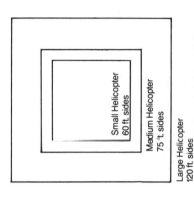

Small Helicopter
60 ft. sides

Medium Helicopter
75 ft. sides

Large Helicopter
120 ft. sides

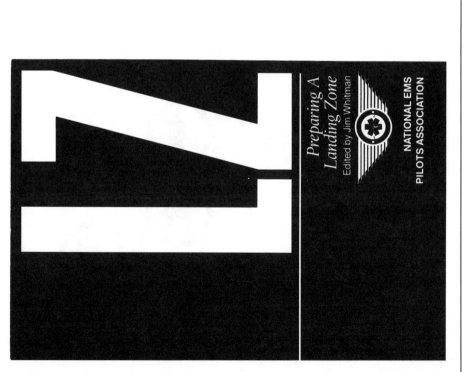

*Preparing A Landing Zone*
Edited by Jim Whitman

NATIONAL EMS
PILOTS ASSOCIATION

## Wind Direction & Touchdown Area

Consider the wind direction. Helicopters land and take off into the wind.

Is the approach and departure path free of obstructions (wires, poles, antennas, trees, etc.)? If there are obstructions, please tell helicopter crew on initial radio call.

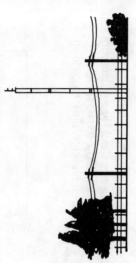

area should be a square with 75-foot sides, 125 ft. at night. Large helicopter: the touchdown area should be a square with 120-foot sides, 200 ft. at night.

The landing site should be clear of people, vehicles, obstructions such as trees, poles and wires. Keep in mind that wires cannot be seen from the air. The landing site must be free of stumps, brush, posts and large rocks.

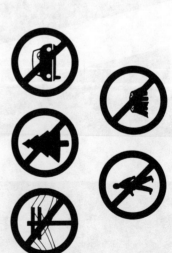

## Personnel Safety & Night Landing

Keep spectators at least 200 feet from the touchdown area. Keep emergency service personnel at least 100 feet away. Have fire equipment (if available) standing by. Assure that everyone who will be working near the helicopter wears eye protection. If helmets are worn, chin straps must be securely fastened (no loose hats blowing up through rotors). Have firefighters wet down the touchdown area if it is extremely dusty. When the helicopter has landed, do not allow anyone to approach the aircraft.

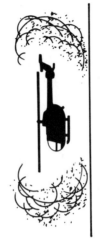

Mark the touchdown area with five lights/road flares (one in each corner and one indicating wind direction).

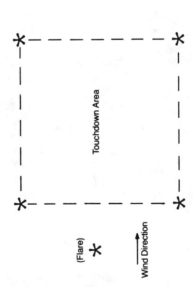

Touchdown Area

(Flare)

Wind Direction

## Ground Guide

When you see the helicopter, one person should help guide the helicopter in to a safe landing. That person must wear eye protection. He should stand with his back to the wind and with his arms raised over his head to indicate the landing direction.

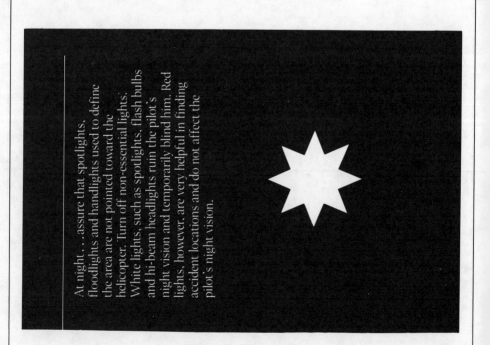

At night . . . assure that spotlights, floodlights and handlights used to define the area are not pointed toward the helicopter. Turn off non-essential lights. White lights, such as spotlights, flash bulbs and hi-beam headlights ruin the pilot's night vision and temporarily blind him. Red lights, however, are very helpful in finding accident locations and do not affect the pilot's night vision.

## Assisting The Crew

Once the helicopter has landed, do not approach the helicopter. The crew will approach you when it is safe to do so.

Please be prepared to assist the crew by providing security for the helicopter. If asked to provide security, do not allow anyone but the crew to approach the helicopter.

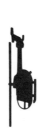

As the helicopter turns into the wind and begins a descent, the ground guide should begin directing the approach using approved hand signals. The ground guide should be far enough from the touchdown area that he can maintain eye to eye contact with the pilot.

## General Helicopter Safety Rules

When working around helicopters, never approach from the rear. Always approach and depart the aircraft towards the front so you can see the pilot, and he can see you. When approaching the helicopter, remember to keep low to avoid main rotor, because winds can cause the rotor to flex down.

If the helicopter is landed on a slope, approach and depart from the down-slope side only.

Once the patient is packaged and ready to load, allow the crew to select two or three personnel to assist loading. When approaching or departing the helicopter, always be aware of the tail rotor and always follow the crews directions for your safety.

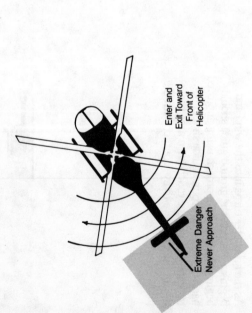

Extreme
Danger
Never
Approach

Enter and
Exit Toward
Front of
Helicopter

Extreme Danger
Never Approach

## Hazardous Materials

Accidents involving hazardous materials require special handling by Fire/Rescue units on the ground. Just as important are the preparations and considerations for helicopter operations in these areas.

Those hazardous materials of concern are those which are toxic, poisonous, flammable, explosive, irritating or radioactive in nature. Helicopter ambulance crews normally don't carry protective suits or breathing apparatus to protect them from hazardous materials.

The helicopter ambulance crew must be told of hazardous materials on the scene, in order to avoid the contamination of the crew. Patients/victims contaminated by hazardous materials may require special precautions in packaging before loading on the aircraft for the medical crew's protection.

When the helicopter is loaded and ready for take off, keep the departure path free of vehicles and spectators.

If an emergency were to occur, we would need this area to execute our landing.

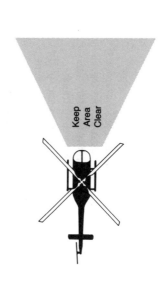

Keep
Area
Clear

## Hazardous Chemicals/Gases

Hazardous chemicals and gases are extremely dangerous to the unprotected person and may be fatal if inhaled or absorbed through the skin.

Upon initial radio contact, the helicopter crew must be made aware of any hazardous gases in the area. Never assume that the crew has already been informed. If the aircraft were to fly through the hazardous gases, the crew could be poisoned and/or the engines could develop mechanical problems.

Poisonous or irritating gases may cling to a victim's clothing and go unnoticed until the patient is loaded and the doors of the helicopter are closed; the crew is then compromised.

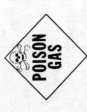

## Radioactive Materials

Some radioactive materials are more dangerous than others, depending upon the type and amounts of those materials. In general, radioactive materials are difficult to ignite, but will burn and the smoke is toxic to humans.

Helicopter crews should be advised if victims may be contaminated by radioactivity.

## Hazardous Material LZ's

Helicopter landing zones must be selected to avoid *all* possibility of compromising the safety of the helicopter and its crew.

When explosives, poisonous gases/vapors, or chemicals in danger of exploding and burning are on site, helicopter landing zones must be prepared *upwind*, at least *one mile* from the hazardous material accident site and never in low-lying areas. The toxic gases or vapors may be heavier than air and gather in these low-lying areas.

For hazardous material accidents involving radioactive materials, the helicopter landing zone must be prepared *upwind*, at least *one-quarter mile* from the accident, unless there are *radioactive gases* (steam or smoke), and in that case, the landing zone must be at least *one mile upwind* of the accident site.

## A Final Note

This helicopter ambulance can serve you only if we arrive safely. Our safety and the safety of the people on the ground depends on you, the professionals on the scene.

### NOTICE

**The National EMS Pilots Association assumes no responsibility or liability for incidents or damages in connection with the use of this product. This material is intended for informational use only and does not purport to address all safety considerations involved with aircraft operations.**

**1st Revised Edition: June 1987**

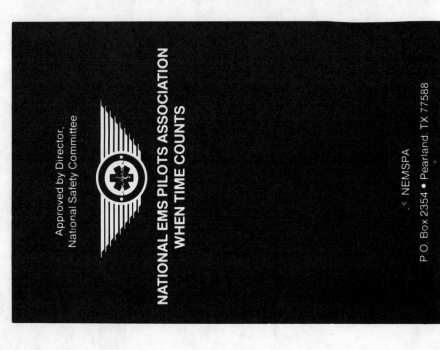

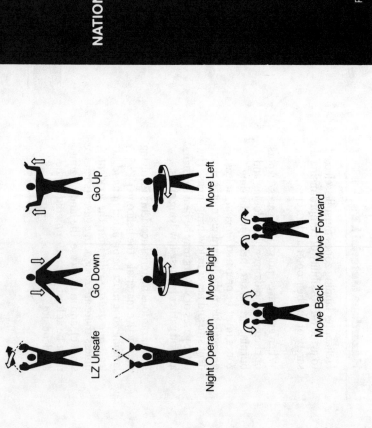

# *Index*

# Index

Note: Page numbers followed by *f* designate figures, by *t* tables, and by *a* appendixes.

*Darling v. Charleston Community Memo-*
    *rial Hospital,* 160
*Davis v. Wyeth,* 166
Death(s)
  neonatal
    See also *Neonatal mortality.*
    after neonatal vs. in utero trans-
        port, 261–263, 262t, 263t
    imminent, 172, 174
  notifying referral hospital of, 60
  perinatal, as outcome variable, 131
Deceleration injuries, 249
Decompression
  gastric, 464a
  gastrointestinal, 376, 386, 456a, 460a
  rapid, in aircraft, 248
Defendant, transport service as, 161
Defensive medicine, 166
    See also *Legal issues in transport.*
  in maternal transport, 181
Defibrillation, neonatal, 425a
DeLee, Joseph, 17
Delivery of pregnant patient
  en route, 52, 208, 308, 336
  mode of, and survival, 139
  tocolysis to delay, 265, 266, 285,
      324–326, 326t
Dhooley, 92f
Diabetes, maternal
  and neonatal hyperinsulinism, 416a
  and neonatal hypoglycemia, 381–
      383
  transport in, 266
Diabetic ketoacidosis, maternal, 266,
    318–320, 319t
Diagnosis-related groups, 77, 89
Diaphragmatic hernia, 463a–465a
Digitalization, maternal, 321
Director of neonatal transport, 359,
    360
  See also *Medical director.*
Dispatch, ambulance, 93
Dispatch center, 96, 101f
Dispatch procedure, in neonatal trans-
    port, 343, 344, 349
Dispatcher, 49, 51, 93, 94, 96, 101f
  liability of, 154
Diuresis
  in pregnant patient, 317, 318t, 321,
      327
Donor, organ, neonate as, 173
Dopamine
  in neonatal resuscitation, 425a

in neonatal shock, 428a, 429a
in pregnant patient, 317
Doppler monitoring, fetal, 292
Down's syndrome, 171
Dressings, 296a
DRGs, 77, 89
Drive, Nelson, 13
Driver, ambulance, 51, 160
Drugs. See *Medications.*
Ductus arteriosus, patent, 377, 441a,
    452a
Dunant, Henri, 9
Duty to care, 154, 158
Dwarfism, 172
Dying infant, 172, 174
Dysraphism, 467a

E cylinders, 221, 222t, 222f
E-911, 93, 94
Ear pressure, 387
Ear protection, 197, 246
  for neonate, 385
Ebstein's anomaly, 453a, 454a
Eclampsia, 272, 326–328, 327t
Economic variables affecting parental
    response, 186
Educational conferences
  in maternal-fetal transport, 315
Educational objectives
  for neonatal transport nurse, 372t
Educational programs
  See also *Outreach educational programs.*
  in neonatal transport, 340
Educator, perinatal nurse, 282, 282t
Electric ambulance, 10
Electrical power supply in neonatal
    transport, 213, 222–224, 227,
    231
Electrocardiographic monitor, 217
Electrode, Clark, 221
Electrolyte disorders, 318, 319, 378,
    379, 423a, 426a, 444a
Electrolyte supplements, for neonate,
    416a
Electromagnetic interference of bat-
    teries, 239
Electronic monitoring equipment, 198,
    200, 201, 209
  malfunction of, 385
Emergency aeromedical transport. See
    *Aeromedical transport service.*
Emergency medical communications,
    93–96

flow pattern in, 303, 304f
follow-up communication after, 308, 312a
geographic considerations in, 277, 287
gestational age in, 261, 262t, 264–266
helicopters for, 44, 52–54
indications for, 129, 130, 261–273, 265t, 315
  and choice of conveyance, 267–269, 272
  fetal age and, 261, 262t, 264–266
  obstetric problems, 264–267, 265t
  prenatal risk and, 267, 268t–272t
initial phone call, 303, 303t
legal issues in. See *Legal issues in transport.*
levels of care in, 286
managing maternal illness, 315–329
  See also *Pregnant patient.*
mechanism of, 303–309, 304f
one-way vs. two-way, 43, 44
outcome assessment in, 262, 263
patient records in, 306, 307t, 310a
patient selection in, 38
principles of care in, 195, 208–211
psychological effects of, 38, 130, 178–191, 264
  See also *Psychological effects of transport.*
  minimizing, 187, 187t
receiving staff in, 308
referral forms for, 107a, 109a
sample cases of, 288–291
selection bias in, 262, 263
specialty teams for, 45, 49
stabilization of patient in, 209–211, 315–329
  See also *Pregnant patient.*
stage of labor and, 323
transfer criteria in, 39
transport team in, 277–295
  See also *Obstetric transport team.*
vehicles in, 209, 291, 291t
weather conditions in, 288
Maturation, fetal, 265
Mechanical ventilation
  See also *Ventilatory support.*
  of pregnant patient, 318
Mechanics
  helicopter, 485a–487a, 492a
  role of, 254

Meconium aspiration
  transport protocol in, 439a–441a
  ventilatory support in, 418a, 419a, 440a
Meconium ileus, 457a
Meconium plug, 458a
Med-Evac units, 16
Medical conditions of mother, 317–328
  See also *Pregnant patient.*
Medical control officer, 50
Medical crew, 509a
  safety training for, 245, 248–254
Medical director, 146, 147
  in neonatal transport, 359, 360
  obstetric, 279, 280, 280t
  of perinatal transport program, 45f, 46
  role in communications, 98, 100
Medical equipment, for air transport, 238, 240
  See also *Equipment.*
Medical gas systems, 220f, 221, 231
Medical instruments, in neonatal transport
  maintenance of, 229–232
  mounting of, 231, 232f
Medical records, 150, 306, 307t, 310a
Medical supply panniers, 342f
Medical technician, emergency. See *Emergency medical technicians.*
Medical torts, 163
Medical transport. See *Aeromedical transport system; Maternal-fetal transport; Neonatal transport; Perinatal transport.*
Medications
  for advanced life support, 298a
  for obstetrical care, 299a
  in neonatal resuscitation, 423a, 424a
  in neonatal transport, 346, 347, 363a
Medicine, defensive, 166
  See also *Legal issues in transport.*
Membrane rupture. See *Premature rupture of membranes.*
Meningitis, neonatal, 173, 447a–449a
Meningocele, 467a
Meningomyelocele, 467a
Mental illness, parental, 185, 186, 191
Metabolic acidosis
  maternal, 318, 319
  neonatal, 379, 423a, 426a
Metabolic alkalosis, neonatal, 426a